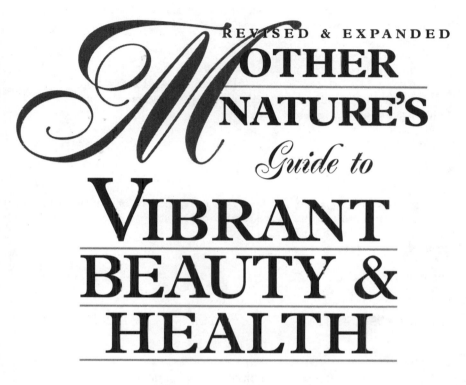

REVISED & EXPANDED

MOTHER NATURE'S

Guide to

VIBRANT BEAUTY & HEALTH

MYRA CAMERON
THERESA FOY DIGERONIMO

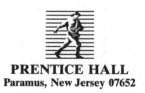

PRENTICE HALL
Paramus, New Jersey 07652

Library of Congress Cataloging in Publication Data

Cameron, Myra.
    Mother Nature's guide to vibrant beauty and health / Myra Cameron
with Theresa DiGeronimo.
        p.   cm.
    "Revised and expanded"—T.p. verso.
    Includes bibliographical references and index.
    ISBN 0-13-845314-4 (cloth). — ISBN 0-13-845018-8 (pbk.)
        1. Skin—Care and hygiene.   2. Cosmetics.   3. Beauty, Personal
4. Health.   I. DiGeronimo, Theresa Foy.   II. Title.
RL87.C36   1997
646.7'2—dc21   96-52951
                                                                                    CIP

Printed in the United States of America

10 9 8 7 6 5 4 3 2 1   *10 9 8 7 6 5 4 3 2 1*

ISBN 0-13-845314-4 (c)   ISBN 0-13-845018-8 (p)

ATTENTION: CORPORATIONS AND SCHOOLS

Prentice Hall books are available at quantity discounts with bulk purchase for educational, business, or sales promotional use. For information, please write to: Prentice Hall Career & Personal Development Special Sales, 240 Frisch Court, Paramus, NJ 07652. Please supply: title of book, ISBN, quantity, how the book will be used, date needed.

PRENTICE HALL
Career & Personal Development
Paramus, NJ 07652
A Simon & Schuster Company

On the World Wide Web at http://www.phdirect.com

Prentice Hall International (UK) Limited, *London*
Prentice Hall of Australia Pty. Limited, *Sydney*
Prentice Hall Canada, Inc., *Toronto*
Prentice Hall Hispanoamericana, S.A., *Mexico*
Prentice Hall of India Private Limited, *New Delhi*
Prentice Hall of Japan, Inc., *Tokyo*
Simon & Schuster Asia Pte. Ltd., *Singapore*
Editora Prentice Hall do Brasil, Ltda., *Rio de Janeiro*

OTHER BOOKS BY MYRA CAMERON:

Home-style Microwave Cooking
The G.N.C. Gourmet Vitamin Cookbook
Treasury of Home Remedies
Lifetime Encyclopedia of Natural Remedies

How This Book Will Help You Look and Feel More Vibrant and Naturally Beautiful

Suppose there was a miracle product that could help clear up your skin problems, put a sparkle in your eyes, leave your hair looking thick and shining, and your body muscles lean and limber. Chances are you'd buy that product! In fact, Americans spend millions of dollars each year on fast-fix health cure-alls and commercial cosmetics that promise the world, but seldom deliver.

Yet, with a bit of help from you, and at practically no expense, radiant health and beauty can be yours. *Mother Nature's Guide to Vibrant Beauty and Health* offers a complete guide to genuine, do-it-yourself beauty care for women *and* men—without harsh, irritating chemicals or additives. In a world deluged by synthetics, reverting to nature's plan gives you safe and easy options for each of the many phases of beauty.

By combining centuries-old beauty secrets with up-to-date advice from modern dermatologists, nutritionists, physicians, and fitness experts, this *Guide* offers up-to-the-minute, time-tested secrets, and all-natural remedies for tackling many of the beauty problems you thought were unsolvable.

Here are some of the many benefits you'll discover in this book:

- Tips on protecting your skin from seasonal changes
- Four everyday products from nature that safely remove makeup and clean skin
- An all-natural, updated recipe for making your own soap
- How to prepare your own skin-care products
- Do-it-yourself moisturizers for dewy-fresh skin
- How to give yourself an at-home facial with professional, salon-like results
- Natural masques from nature that rejuvenate and nourish your skin

- The safe way to eliminate blackheads and whiteheads
- All-natural treatments for clearing up skin discolorations
- Tips on nourishing maturing skin
- Herbs that enhance your bath
- How to play it safe in the sun—with natural remedies for relieving sunburn pain
- Natural remedies for correcting seven common foot problems
- 25 herbs that make effective mouth rinses
- Time-tested secrets for beautiful hands
- Nine soothing compresses and poultices for refreshing tired, irritated eyes
- Natural colorants to perk up your hair and shampoos you can make yourself
- How to snack nutritiously all day long
- Six-minute shape-up guide for toning and limbering
- Nine natural aids for combating stress

You'll find *Mother Nature's Guide to Vibrant Beauty and Health* to be an invaluable resource for healthful products and remedies. Radiant health and beauty *can* be yours—with the help of Mother Nature!

PREFACE

You can employ beauticians to glamorize your face with cosmetics, temporarily minimize wrinkles or bulges, and coif you with a wig. Playing Cinderella for an evening might be exciting; having genuine, do-it-yourself beauty is more rewarding. It reflects in your mirror at dawn, in the way you move, and in the eyes of your beholders. Clear skin, sparkling eyes, shining hair, and lithe muscles do not disappear when the clock strikes twelve. Beauty is the total you; it comes as a package deal. Nutrients you ingest, muscles you move, the way you cope with stress; all play a role in your beautiful image.

Along with her gift of a body, complete with a permanent covering of skin, Mother Nature has provided the wherewithall for its care. In a world deluged by synthetics, reverting to nature's plan may be wise because foods affect your exterior as well as your interior. The body's outer surface absorbs or reacts to substances with which it comes in contact, so why not feed your face (and your hands, feet, nails, and hair) with low-cost, healthful products instead of endangering them with expensive, chemically contrived beauty aids?

By correlating centuries-old beauty secrets with up-to-date advice from modern dermatologists, nutritionists, physicians, and fitness experts, *Mother Nature's Guide to Vibrant Beauty and Health* offers safe and easy options for each of the many phases of beauty. With its explicit step-by-step directions you can concoct your own facial masques, toners, and lotions. From the dietary guidelines you can create your individualized regimen of eating for beauty and energy. You can customize your personal muscle-toning and life-extending fitness program by selecting your choices from the exercises described. For your inner self there are mood-changing techniques to relieve tension or entice sleep; and, for your Prince Charming, there are "handsome" treatments and tips—men, too, have skin, nails, and hair.

Nurturing Mother Nature's gifts to make the most of your visible assets is not vanity. When you look and feel your best, you radiate an aura that attracts others and makes them receptive. Neglecting appearance and health isn't noble; it diminishes self-assurance, "turns off" those around you, and accelerates the aging process. The axiom "Pretty is as pretty does" still applies; it takes conscious effort to be beautiful. With this book as a guide, and a bit of your help, Mother Nature can be your fairy godmother—transforming you into a vibrantly lovely, full-time Cinderella. No matter what your age may be at this moment, *now* is the time to begin your transformation.

Contents

Section 2
HEAD-TO-TOE BEAUTY   123

Section 3
LIFETIME BEAUTY AND HEALTH: DIET, EXERCISE, AND STRESS MANAGEMENT   193

Section 4
TAPPING INTO NATURE'S OWN REMEDIES 263

༄ *Section One* ༄

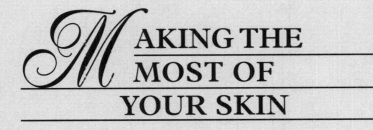

MAKING THE MOST OF YOUR SKIN

1

HOW TO HAVE BEAUTIFULLY HEALTHY SKIN

You can hide your hair beneath a wig and wear a mu-mu to conceal figure faults, but until veiled hats come back in style, your face is up front for everyone to see—and even professional makeup can only temporarily mask skin that has been ignored or mistreated. The men in your life can also reap the benefits of skin pampering. Fifteen years ago, the few men who entered prestigious Madison Avenue skin-care salons sidled through rear entrances. Today, conscious of the importance of outward appearance in business and social life, over half the salon clients are men.

SKIN: THE VITAL STATISTICS

MIRACLE COVERING SUBSTANCE

Lightweight & Flexible—conforms to any shape
Elastic—will expand up to 40 times its original size
Waterproof—forms a two-way barrier between fluids
Self-mending—reseals itself if burned, cut, or punctured
Washable & Durable—one coating lasts a lifetime

The response to the above advertisement would be a line of prospective purchasers encircling the globe. Most of life's best sensations pass through the outer covering, yet skin is not for sale, it is a miraculous gift from Mother Nature. Even its vital statistics are fascinating: skin varies in thickness from $1/50$ of an inch over the eardrums

3

to $^1/_4$ of an inch on the soles of the feet. The 15 to 20 square feet of skin required to encase an adult weighs approximately 20 pounds. It protects us from environmental pollutants, contains an early-warning device to inform us of impending danger from extreme heat or cold, and is an automatic thermostat that helps regulate body temperature.

There is more to skin than meets the eye. The epidermis, the surface we see, is composed primarily of dead skin and melanocytes (pigment cells) performing their protective duties while waiting to be sloughed off. Beneath the epidermis lies the dermis, a veritable beehive of activity. Within it flourish collagen and elastin (the fibrous supportive system), hair follicles, tiny blood vessels, and the sebaceous glands which supply fluids to fuel and lubricate the skin. A resilient subcutaneous layer below the dermis further supports the skin and cushions internal bones and organs from shock. The amount of sebum (a waxy-oily substance) exuded by the sebaceous glands is largely responsible for the type of skin we have.

Dry, *oily*, or *normal* are the stereotyped labels for skin. *Combination* or *mosaic* is how most facial skin really is, and it usually has a "T-zone" of oiliness across the forehead and down the nose, with dryness on the cheeks. Whatever your skin type may be at the moment, it is subject to change with very little notice.

TIPS ON PROTECTING YOUR SKIN FROM SEASONAL CHANGES

Like the exterior walls of your home, your skin is your body's shelter. Exposed to the elements and to your physical environment, it has an outer as well as an inner life. It copes with summer heat and wintry chill; industrial fumes, smoke, fog, smog, dust, and soot; plus sudden fluctuations in temperature caused by air conditioning and forced-air heating.

HOW TO WINTERIZE YOUR SKIN

Winter is beauty's enemy. Outdoor cold and wind attack your skin, indoor heat robs it of moisture. Dry skin suffers more than oily skin, but every type of skin benefits from these defensive measures:

❧ Tone and moisture (see Chapters 3 and 4) after each cleansing to preserve and replenish the moisture in your skin. Use a moisturizing night nourisher every evening. Apply a daytime moisturizer around your eyes and on dry-skin areas each morning.

❧ Add skin-pampering ingredients to your bath (see Chapter 8) to prevent allover dryness.

❧ Wait 30 minutes after bathing, or washing your face, before going out into frigid air. Splash your face with cool water when you come back inside. Extreme temperature changes can burst capillaries near the skin's surface.

❧ Moisturize indoor air by plugging in a humidifier, by placing a damp towel or a pan of water near the heat source, or by surrounding yourself with growing plants.

HOW TO SUMMERIZE YOUR SKIN

Although summer is kinder than winter to dry skin, it accentuates oily-skin problems and necessitates a different skin-protective campaign.

❧ Give your face an extra cleansing each day and always clean your face after strenuous activity. Warm weather means more active oil glands. Perspiration makes dirt cling to your skin.

❧ Use a "light" night cream and daytime moisturizer. Smooth on only a few drops to compensate for the extra washing and perspiring that remove the skin's invisible shield. Use additional moisturizer when you travel by plane; pressurized air is excessively dry.

❧ Watch out for the sun; too much of it makes skin lined, leathery, and old before its time.

SEVEN WAYS TO PROMOTE— AND PROLONG— A MORE YOUTHFUL APPEARANCE

Skin is more than just a covering; it is a barometer that registers the state of our health and reveals the story of our lives. The decline and fall of our epidermis does not become apparent until we pass the 30-year milestone, but it actually begins at birth. Our "perfect" baby skin alters with puberty; undergoes more variations from hormonal fluctuations during menstrual cycles, pregnancy, and menopause; then gradually becomes thinner, drier, and less supple as cell functions slow with age. Chronologically, we all grow old at the same rate. Visibly, we age at an individual pace—and it's never too early or late to start improving your skin.

Life expectancy is now double what it was a few centuries ago, more than triple the original design which anticipated death shortly after the conclusion of a short span of reproductive ability. Evolutionary alterations to delay the biological processes of approaching old age are a future probability. Meanwhile, if we are to save our twentieth-century faces, it's up to us to assist Mother Nature. Prolonging a youthful appearance by keeping up with changes as they occur is easier than rejuvenating the ravages wrought by Father Time.

Acne (see Chapter 6) attacks more boys than girls during the teenage years, but besets more women than men because oral contraceptives, menstruation, and menopause cause hormone levels to surge and wane.

Pregnancy profoundly affects the skin. For the first five months, increased estrogen production suppresses the natural skin-lubricating oils to make skin drier than normal. Use a mild, nondetergent cleanser, a nourishing moisturizer during the day, and apply a rich night cream before retiring. During the latter half of pregnancy, an upswing of progesterone hormones may make skin oilier and more subject to blemishes. Cleanse your skin thoroughly, use an astringent toner, cut back on your moisturizing routine, and guard against the brown splotches of a pregnancy mask by applying a potent sunscreen before venturing forth in daylight.

While waiting for the fountain of perpetual youth to be discovered, you can prolong a youthful appearance if you:

1. Incorporate more moisturizing in your daily-care routine to compensate for the reduced activity of sweat and sebaceous glands, which causes gradual drying and thinning of the skin.

2. Forestall photoaging by applying a sunscreen and sunning safely (see Chapter 9).

3. Exercise regularly to maintain the blood circulation essential for bringing nourishment to the dermal vessels and for carrying off

wastes from the skin. Reclining on a slantboard also improves circulation, and the "downhill" position negates some of the sags, wrinkles, and droops attributable to gravity.

4. Deliberately relax away tension (see Chapter 17) to help prevent "expression lines" in your face and other stress-related skin problems.

5. Get sufficient sleep so your skin can receive its fresh supplies of oxygen and nutrients.

6. Keep your weight fairly constant to avoid the saggy wrinkles that can develop when yo-yo dieting leaves stretched skin without underlying support.

7. Eat a well-balanced diet to help maintain and rebuild the supportive tissues, and to preserve the visible surface.

INSIDE-OUT CARE FOR A FLAWLESS COMPLEXION

HOW TO CARE FOR YOUR SKIN FROM THE INSIDE

What you eat, or don't eat, is revealed by your skin: nutrients absorbed into the bloodstream nourish it through loops of capillaries close to the surface. Radiantly healthy skin is one of the dividends of eating a nutritionally balanced diet (see Chapter 15), taking supplements when needed, and drinking six to eight glasses of water each day. Fruit and vegetable juices or herbal teas may be substituted for some of the water. Alcoholic drinks and caffeine-containing beverages, (regular coffee, tea, some herbal teas, many soft drinks) act as mild diuretics to dehydrate your system, so they shouldn't be counted on for filling the quota. Drinking two glasses of barley juice each day is credited with maintaining the flawless complexions of British royalty.[110]

Here's how to prepare your own *Royal Barley Juice*: Simmer $1/4$ cup pearl barley in 5 cups of water in a covered saucepan for 1 hour. Squeeze 1 lemon and 3 oranges, reserve the juice, add the rinds to the saucepan, and let stand until cool. Strain the liquid into a pitcher, stir in the reserved juice plus honey to taste, then store in the refrigerator.

Protein: Skin is predominantly protein, requires a daily supply from the foods you eat because protein molecules are not absorbed through the epidermis into underlying tissues,[47] and registers a deficiency by becoming slack and loose. Collagen-containing protein foods (avocados, brewer's yeast, dried legumes, nuts, sesame and sunflower seeds, whole grain cereals) help prevent and smooth out wrinkles. Other protein foods (fish, meats, poultry, eggs, dairy products, vegetable proteins) help your body equalize the balance between new and dying cells.

Fats and Oils: The unsaturated fats in vegetable oils assist assimilation of fat-soluble vitamins A, D, and E; contribute to your own natural oils to give your skin a sheen, plump out fine lines, and create the fresh-faced look of youth. One or two tablespoons a day can be used as salad dressing or whizzed in the blender with milk, fruit, or vegetable drinks.

Fruits, Vegetables, and Fiber: In addition to varying amounts of protein and the complex carbohydrates needed for energy, fruits and vegetables provide the fiber (grandmother called it roughage) to keep you vibrantly beautiful and healthy by flushing toxins out of your body and avoiding constipation. If you run short, a tablespoon of miller's bran each day should help. Fresh, raw foods also contain enzymes that act as the body's housekeepers to keep the bloodstream clear, and, cooked or uncooked, fruits and vegetables offer an appetizing supply of vitamins and minerals necessary for skin health.

Vitamins and Minerals: Overindulging in anything, particularly fat-soluble vitamins A, D, and E, can be dangerous. Some of the following supplements may be in order, however, because individual requirements may be higher than the official RDA (recommended dietary allowance), and because eating sufficient quantities of their natural food sources (see the Vitamin and Mineral Chart) is either impractical (6 oranges equal 500 milligrams of vitamin C) or would lead to unwanted weight gain.

- Vitamin A is used to preserve a smooth skin texture, prevent dryness, and avoid blemishes or hasten their healing.

- B vitamins are vital for clear, luminous skin. Only about 1 percent of the water-soluble, must-be-replenished-daily B complex ingested is routed to the skin, and, because they function interactively, a deficiency of any of the B's can cause skin problems. Insufficiencies may make themselves apparent by inflamed fissures at the angles of the nose and mouth, scaly lips, premature wrinkles, or by other skin disturbances.[58] Studies show that 40 percent of dermatitis sufferers lack B vitamins.[33]

꿈 Vitamin C, in conjunction with protein, is necessary for the production of collagen—the glue that holds us and our skin together and circumvents sags or wrinkles. Combined with bioflavinoids, vitamin C helps prevent the pigment clumping that the sun turns into "age spots," and strengthens capillaries to avoid easy bruising or the tiny hemorrhages that become spider veins. Vitamin C also helps the oil-secreting glands function properly to keep the skin from drying out. If you're a cigarette smoker, supplemental C is advisable. Cigarettes devour at least 500 milligrams per pack, or up to 5,000 milligrams, according to Irwin Stone, author of *Vitamin C Against Disease* (Grosset & Dunlap, 1972).

꿈 Vitamin E, necessary for healthy, moist skin, is an antioxidant present in vegetable oils; yet additional amounts of E are required to prevent the E in the oils from oxidation within the body. Biochemical research has demonstrated that large doses of vitamin E double healthy cell reproduction to slow the aging process and forestall premature wrinkling.[20] *Caution*: If you have diabetes, high blood pressure, or an overactive thyroid, check with your physician before taking supplemental E.

꿈 Minerals all contribute to our beauty and well-being. Two of the most essential for skin care are

> Copper—important for the production of skin pigment and for the prevention of blotches under the skin from ruptured blood vessels. It also cooperates with other nutrients to preserve the integrity of the elastic-like fibers supporting the skin.

> Zinc—aids in the formation of collagen, helps prevent dry skin and stretch marks, and promotes blemish healing. Without enough zinc a deficiency of Vitamin A can occur even though the intake of that vitamin appears adequate.

How to Care for Your Skin from the Outside

If you treat your skin with tenderness, it will respond with finely textured dewy freshness. If you neglect your skin, overexpose it to the sun, abuse it with harsh soaps and abrasive cleansers, irritate it with stinging astringents, or suffocate it with leftover makeup and heavy creams, it will retaliate by flaking away, erupting in bumps, developing splotches, bursting its capillaries, and wrinkling prematurely. Caring for your skin gently and consistently is the key to extending its youthful appearance.

The once-held belief that skin is an impenetrable barrier turns out to be a myth. Laboratory studies reported in *Health* (May, 1986) indicate that many substances are absorbed through the skin, reach the bloodstream, and are transported throughout the body. Iodine, for instance, can be detected in the urine shortly after it is applied to unbroken skin. Dermatologists now agree that *everything* permeates to some extent. According to Dr. Peter M. Elias of the University of California at San Francisco, the degree of absorption varies with the substance and the body area. The face is ten times more permeable than any other part of the body, with water and alcohol solutions (colognes and astringents) penetrating most easily; water and oil-based emulsions (moisturizers) next; and little absorption from sunscreens or the brief contact of cleansers. "Feeding your face" is more than just a witticism. Tests conducted at Purdue University show that natural foods benefit the skin when used cosmetically (see Chapter 3); they are not only harmless, they are often more effective than chemical-containing commercial cosmetics.[141]

Skin's response to a program of systematic care is almost instantaneous, and, as young cells migrate up through the dermis to replace dead cells sloughed off the surface in a constant process of self-renewal, we have a "new" face every 28 days. "Regimen" sounds intimidating. A daily routine of skin care requires no more than ten minutes and requires only three simple steps—cleanse, tone, and moisturize—each evening and morning.

Night care

1. Cleanse. Remove any makeup with cleansing cream or a natural makeup remover. Wash with mild soap or other cleanser, rinse, and pat dry.

2. Tone. Apply an acid-containing solution to restore the pH balance and protective shield. For dry skin, use a mild freshener-toner. For oily skin, use an astringent preparation.

3. Moisturize. Splash on cool water or mist with a spray bottle. Blot, but do not dry completely—moisturizer magic relies

more on retaining moisture than in providing it—then
smooth on a few drops of your moisturizer.

Day care

1. Cleanse lightly to remove nighttime accumulations, refresh
   your face with a few splashes of water, and pat dry.

2. Tone by applying a freshener or astringent.

3. Moisturize around your eyes. If your face is excessively dry,
   mist or splash with water, blot, then lightly cover with moisturizer.

2

TIPS ON SAFELY AND GENTLY CLEANSING YOUR FACE AND THROAT

Clean skin is essential for both beauty and health; we breathe through skin pores as well as through nose and mouth. Horror tales of circus performers perishing after being coated with gilt paint do not create a precedent for sudden death following one night of sleeping with the day's accumulation of perspiration and pollutants. However, habitually retiring uncleansed may damage more than your pillow case: dry skin areas can become more sensitive; normal or oily skin can develop enlarged pores, blackheads, blemishes, or similar unpleasantries; and your skin may lose its luminosity.

BEYOND THE KITCHEN: FOUR EVERYDAY PRODUCTS FROM NATURE THAT SAFELY REMOVE MAKEUP AND CLEANSE SKIN

If you wear makeup, getting all of it off your face is the first stage of cleansing. Commercial creams or lotions are not the only options; Mother Nature offers a full line you can share with your favorite male if he makes "on camera" appearances. (Stage makeup is harsher than the department store products; he should allow several hours between shaving and its application.)

1. Mayonnaise. Bottled or homemade (see Glossary for recipe), mayonnaise is surprisingly effective. Smooth on, tissue off, or remove with a damp washcloth.

2. Milk. Shake 2 tablespoons of warm, whole milk with $1/4$ teaspoon oil. Apply with a cotton ball, then tissue off.

3. Vegetable oil. Dip a cotton ball into your favorite salad oil, swish over eyes and lips, and gently wipe off. Saturate another cotton ball to coat your face, wait a few seconds for it to permeate, then remove it with a tissue or damp cloth.

4. White vegetable shortening. This can be smoothed on like a cleansing cream, allowed to remain for a minute, then removed with gentle, upward sweeps of a tissue or damp washcloth.

An ALL-NATURAL, UPDATED APPROACH TO MAKING YOUR OWN SOAP

Even if you don't wear makeup, the day's conglomeration of contaminants should be removed. What should you use to cleanse your face? Soap (which emulsifies the particulates and skin oils lurking on the surface) and water (which can't go it alone but is essential for rinsing) are the most popular and most efficient of many choices. The soap-making art has advanced considerably in the 2,000 years since the Romans boiled goat tallow with wood ashes to duplicate the foamy suds that billowed up when rain fell on the charred remains of sacrificed animals. Today's detergent-deodorant soaps and those containing abrasive granules are too harsh for facial use, but there are superfatted and cold-cream beauty bars scented with perfume, liquid soaps in pump dispensers, transparent soaps filled with glycerin, floating soaps filled with air, pure castile cakes that smell like soap, and do-it-yourself options.

❧ Homemade Natural Glycerin Beauty Bars ❦

This homemade soap contains a natural glycerin (formed by the chemical reaction of fat and caustic but removed from commercial products for separate sale), so much skin-softening oil it is low-sudsing, and you can manufacture 10 pounds of it without butchering a beast or building an outdoor fire. The equipment required is minimal: an 8-quart enamel or nonmetal cooking pot; an immersible thermometer that registers as low as 90 degrees Farenheit; a long-handled wooden spoon; cheesecloth, muslin, or plastic wrap; and three 9-by-14-inch glass baking pans or cardboard boxes, or an array of custard cups. The ingredients can be obtained from your grocery or drugstore.

5 pounds pure lard

2 cups hot water (chlorine free)

2 cups olive oil

6 cups cold water (chlorine free)

1 twelve-ounce can 100% lye

³/₄ cup almond or coconut oil

1 tablespoon tincture of benzoin

optional perfume: 2 tablespoons oil of lavender, lemon, lemon grass, musk, or other fragrance

Place the lard and hot water in the cooking container and heat until the fat is melted. Remove from heat, stir in the olive oil, and let stand until the temperature drops to 100 degrees. Pour the cold water into a 4-quart glass bowl, slowly stir in the lye with the wooden spoon. Let cool to 90 degrees. Gradually stir the lye-water into the melted fat, stirring until it is thick and creamy, then beat in the almond or coconut oil, benzoin, and perfume (if used).

Line the pans, boxes, or dishes with plastic wrap or wet cloth. Ladle in your "soap" to a depth of about 1-1/8 inch. Let stand for 8 to 16 hours (until firm), remove from the containers and cut into bars. "Cure" for at least two weeks by layering the bars in a carton on sheets of cardboard.

❧ Oatmeal Beauty Bars ❧

Grind 2 cups of oatmeal in an electric blender or food processor. After half the creamy soap has been transferred to its mold, beat the oatmeal into the remainder and proceed as with the natural glycerin bars.

"Bonus Bar" is Richard's name for this oatmeal variation. He had been skeptical about Sally's "kettleful of grease" ever turning into soap, had even questioned the project's necessity. "Why don't you just buy some? Stores do sell soap," he said, "ready-made, cut into bars and everything." However, Sally's skin felt so soft after a few days of using her homemade beauty bar that Richard agreed to experiment—just in case it might smooth up his flaky forehead. It did—so successfully that he volunteered to assist with cooking up the next batch of soap!

THREE NO-FUSS WAYS TO IMPROVE STORE-BOUGHT SOAP

For "no curing required" soaps, try one of these mixtures. The bars have a base of two 4-ounce cakes of white castile soap, grated by hand or in a food processor.

Scented Soap for Softening and Whitening: Melt the grated soap in the top of the double boiler with $1/4$ cup alcohol *or* strained, fresh lemon juice. Stir in $1/4$ cup of your favorite cologne and 1 tablespoon glycerin before transferring to a foil-lined loaf pan to harden.

Skin-Softening Oatmeal Soap: Combine the grated soap with $1/4$ cup almond oil in the top of a double boiler. Heat until the soap melts, then stir in $1^1/3$ cups uncooked oatmeal (pulverized in an electric blender, if desired). Transfer to a foil-lined loaf pan to harden.

Almond-Meal Softsoap: This mild, liquid soap was a favored complexion cleanser during the 1800s. For easy preparation with modern equipment, blend 2 tablespoons almond meal with $1/2$ cup rose water and one-fourth of a 4-ounce bar of unscented castile soap grated into a food processor. Process with a cutting blade while gradually adding more rose water until the mixture looks like milk. (A hand grater, mixing bowl, and rotary egg beater may be used for nonelectric preparation.) Strain, then funnel into a pump-dispenser container.

NINE EASY-TO-FIND SOAP SUBSTITUTES FROM MOTHER NATURE

Makeup-remover pads (homemade or purchased at a cosmetic counter) premoistened with a freshener or astringent can be used in an emergency or for midday oily-skin cleansing. Cold cream or cleansing cream (originating from a second-century Greek formula of olive oil, beeswax, and water which produces a cooling effect as the water evaporates) is fine for makeup removal but leaves a residue. In addition to the commercial foaming-liquid facial cleansers that appear to have resulted from a mating between cleansing cream and shampoo,

Mother Nature offers soap equivalents. Indians in Colombia and in the Southwest of North America created an acceptable cleanser from chopped yucca roots. Botanicals such as soapbark, soapberry, soapwort, and the flowers of the sweet pepper bush were used by Native Americans and early pioneers. The following cleansers are more convenient:

- **Alcohol**, mixed with water, was the cleansing solution recommended to travelers in the nineteenth century. (They were also advised to wash as infrequently as possible.)

- **Ammonia**, in the proportions of $1/4$ teaspoon ammonia to 1 quart of water, is said to clean out the pores and take the place of soap. (Warning: Don't use near your eyes.)

- **Glycerin**, smoothed on and wiped off, is believed to thoroughly cleanse your face.

- **Kelp granules**, blended with white vegetable shortening in the proportions of 1 teaspoon kelp to 2 tablespoons shortening, have healing as well as cleansing properties. Work the mixture into your face with a soft, moist sponge; remove with a damp washcloth.

- **Milk** is amazingly versatile. Plain whole milk, applied with a cotton ball and tissued off, replaces soap and water for a dry-skin cleanser. For normal or oily skin: make a paste with instant, nonfat dry milk and water, gently massage your face with the mixture, then rinse off with lukewarm water.

  Sour cream is an enriching cleanser for dry skin. To increase its benefits, squeeze the contents of a 5,000-IU vitamin A capsule into $1/2$ cup of sour cream. Blend thoroughly and store in the refrigerator.

  Yogurt, with or without the addition of a capsuleful of vitamin A in each half cup, can replace soap for normal or combination skin.

- **Oatmeal** can be ground to a powder or used as is. Dry oatmeal mixed to a paste with milk or cream, then smoothed on and rinsed off, is an exemplary soap substitute.

- **Oil** was the cleanser for the glamour-conscious Golden-Age Greeks, who did not use soap. They oiled their faces and bodies, scraped off the excess, and left a thin film to conserve their skin's moisture. You can follow their precept by smoothing on any vegetable or nut oil and wiping it off with a tissue.

- **Potato** (raw), grated and massaged into your face, then removed with a wet washcloth, is an effective cleanser with blemish-healing properties.

- **Wheat flour**, mixed to a paste with a little water, cleanses and smoothes skin when massaged in and rinsed off.

TEN DEEP-CLEANING EXFOLIANTS THAT CLEAN AND PROTECT YOUR SKIN WITHOUT HARSH CHEMICALS OR IRRITANTS

The dead cells clinging to your skin are oldies, not goodies. If they aren't sloughed off occasionally, they can enlarge your pores, muddy your complexion, and prevent their replacements from emerging. Shaving deposes most of this debris for men. Barbers recommend that electric-shaver users lather up and shave with a blade razor once a week. Dermatologists suggest occasional deep cleaning of facial areas that aren't de-whiskered.

The sloughing process (exfoliating or epidermabrading) should not be irritating. "Scrub" is a misnomer in that you don't "scrub"; you smooth, pat, or gently massage the exfoliant onto your clean, moist face, then rinse it off, pat dry, and apply your toner and moisturizer. How frequently you need to deep clean depends on your skin: from every day (if it looks dull, is very oily, or feels rough), to once a month if it is clear, dry, and sensitive. "Combination skin" may rate a weekly epidermabrasion on only the forehead, nose, and chin. Summer's upbeat schedule of increased cell production and shedding may call for more frequent sloughing. A complexion brush, moistened and stroked with feathery, rotary motions from throat to forehead over your usual cleanser may suffice; any of the following deep-cleaning exfoliants will also speed the departure of unwanted dead skin cells.

ALMOND MEAL

- **Almond meal** smoothes skin while it cleanses. Make a thin paste with a tablespoon of almond meal and water, milk, and/or honey.

Almond-citrus oatmeal sounds like a breakfast cereal but is intended for external feeding: Mix $1/4$ cup of leftover, cooked oatmeal with $1/4$ cup almond meal and 1 teaspoon *each* dried lemon and orange peel. Store in a wide-mouth jar. To use: scoop a spoonful of the mixture into the palm of your hand, drizzle in a bit of hot water, then massage your face with gentle, circular motions. Rinse off with tepid water.

Almond-lanolin-egg is excellent for dry skin. You can make enough for several scrubs by combining the following ingredients in an electric blender and refrigerating the mixture.

> *$1/3$ cup almond meal*
> *$1/4$ cup lanolin*
> *1 raw egg yolk*
> *1 teaspoon each almond extract and honey*
> *$1/2$ teaspoon tincture of benzoin*

Almond-papaya oil is another gently effective exfoliant that will keep for a week or two in the refrigerator.

> *$1/3$ cup mashed papaya (fresh or canned)*
> *$1/4$ cup almond oil*
> *2 tablespoons water-dispersible lecithin powder*
> *2 teaspoons almond meal*
> *1 teaspoon lemon extract*

Whir in an electric blender until very smooth. Massage into the skin, gently remove with tissues; reapply and tissue off again, then rinse with tepid water.

Almond shortening is recommended for dry skin. Mix $1/4$ cup *each* almond meal and white vegetable shortening with 2 teaspoons of honey. Store in a wide-mouth jar.

Almond yogurt, $1/4$ cup yogurt blended with 1 tablespoon almond meal, is great for blemished skin.

BAKING SODA

  🍂 **Baking soda**, mixed to a thin paste with water and smoothed over the face, is an anti-inflammatory agent as well as an exfoliant. Do not scrub with the soda; simply rinse it off with splashes of water.

CORNMEAL

- **Cornmeal** deep cleans and softens. Wet your face with warm water, moisten a tablespoon of yellow cornmeal with water or milk, then rub it gently into your skin with fingers or a complexion brush. Remove with a washcloth, rinse with cool water. (Note: Preparing the cornmeal paste in advance reduces its coarseness.)

   Cornmeal-verbena cleanser can be made by softening $1/2$ teaspoon of dried lemon verbena in 1 tablespoon warm water for 2 minutes, then stirring in 2 tablespoons cornmeal, plus additional water if needed, to make a thick paste.

LEMON OR LIME

- **Lemon face peel** is good for normal or oily skin. Combine the grated rind and juice from one lemon. Cover and let stand for 8 hours. Pat the mixture over your face, let dry, then remove by gently rubbing with a damp washcloth. Rinse with cool water and apply a moisturizer.

- **Lemon scrubber.** Juice a lemon half (reserve the juice for other use), scoop out the lemon pulp and mix it with 2 tablespoons yogurt plus enough almond meal, cornmeal, or oatmeal to make a thick paste. Press the mixture into the lemon shell and wrap it in moistened cheesecloth. Rub the open end of the scrubber over your face for several minutes. Remove its traces, along with expired skin cells, with a damp cloth.

- **Lime juice**, diluted in the proportions of $1/2$ lime to 1 cup warm water, can be used to dissolve the flaky top layer of skin. Dip a washcloth in the liquid, squeeze out the excess and cover your face for several minutes, then gently rub with the washcloth before rinsing off.

MILK

- **Milk** can be used for a before-bed exfoliant-soother. Mix 2 tablespoons powdered whole milk with enough water to make a thick paste. Spread over your face and throat, rub in with fingers or a complexion brush, rinse off with tepid water. Apply a second coating of the milk paste and let it dry for a minute or so until it is sufficiently rubbery to roll off with your fingers. After rolling off this puttylike film, do not rinse and do not put anything else on your skin; the milk residue will continue conditioning your skin overnight.

OATMEAL

☙ **Oatmeal** is a superb cleaner-softener. You can tie a handful of dry oatmeal in a square of gauze, swish it around in warm water, rub it over your freshly cleansed face, then let the oatmeal liquid dry for about 5 minutes before rinsing off.

Or, you can make a paste from oatmeal and water, milk, cream, or yogurt; smooth it over your face and throat, and let it dry before rinsing off. Caution: Oatmeal paste can be messy to apply, and hazardous to your skin if you live with a cat. One feline fancier spread a beach towel on the floor to protect it from oatmeal droplets, then lay down on the towel while the mixture dried on her face. She smiled as her affectionate tabby licked off some of the oatmeal paste. She was shocked upright when the cat took a bite that included part of her chin!

PAPAYA TEA

☙ **Papaya tea** contains an enzyme that dissolves surface cell debris. Squeeze a washcloth in strong, hot, papaya (or papaya-mint) tea. Cover your face with the cloth for a total of 15 minutes, redipping and rewringing every 2 or 3 minutes. Or, immerse a papaya tea bag in enough boiling water to cover it, let cool until comfortably warm, then smooth the tea bag over your face. Allow the liquid to dry before rinsing off.

PINEAPPLE

☙ The bromelain enzyme in fresh pineapple is another dead-cell dissolver. Press the juice out of a slice of fresh pineapple or puree fresh pineapple chunks in a blender. Smooth over your face and let dry. Rub gently with a dry washcloth before removing with a wet washcloth. To intensify the exfoliating benefits, saturate strips of gauze or cotton cloth with the pineapple juice and apply as a 5-minute compress over your original coating.

Pineapple-carrot juice is advised for blemished skin. Mix equal amounts of fresh pineapple juice and carrot juice and use as directed above.

SALT: EPSOM, SEA, AND TABLE

Blend $1/_2$ teaspoon *each* epsom salt and table salt (or 1 teaspoon sea salt) with 1 tablespoon white vegetable shortening. Massage into your skin with your fingertips for 3 minutes. Leave on your face if you are going to "steam" as part of a facial (see Chapter 5), or remove with warm water and a washcloth.

Instead of epidermabrasion, you can indulge in a "salabrasion" every week or two by dissolving 1 teaspoon *each* epsom salt and table salt (or 2 teaspoons sea salt) in $1/_4$ cup hot water, sponging on the saline solution, and allowing it to dry before rinsing off with warm water.

Buttermilk salt is recommended for oily skin. Mix a spoonful of buttermilk with enough table salt to make a grainy scrub. Massage into your face, then rinse off.

SUNFLOWER SCRUB

&. Sunflower scrub, made by mixing ground sunflower seeds with milk, can be massaged in and rinsed off; or the ground seeds may be substituted for almond meal in any exfoliant.

BACK TO BASICS: THE *RIGHT* WAY TO WASH YOUR FACE

Step-by-step directions for this fundamental process seem as ridiculous as instruction for tying shoe laces, but every skin care expert has a long list of adamant rules. Water—hot versus warm, cold versus cool—is a prime bone of contention. Rinsing with a washcloth or splashing with water a certain number of times is another point of debate. "Wash with hot, rinse with cold" proponents contend this method cleanses more efficiently, opens and closes pores, and stimulates circulation. Other dermatologists declare that hot rinsing arouses the *lipids* (oil glands) into reestablishing the skin's pH balance. The "warm/cool" and the "keep it tepid" brigade believe that skin should never be shocked with either hot or cold and agree with the

American Medical Association's statement that pores neither open nor close.[159] Among these extremes are some facts: skin around the pores does contract and expand to have the effect of opening and closing pores; warm-to-hot water is comfortable for washing; and a splash of cold water is refreshing as a final rinse. Here's the basic process for properly washing your face:

1. Moisten your face with water. Work up a lather by rubbing the soap between wet palms. Using your fingertips (not the bar of soap), massage the lather into your face and throat.

2. Rinse thoroughly with a washcloth or with splashes of water. A three-to-one ratio of rinsing time to lathering time is considered adequate; the important thing is that you remove all of the soap so any caustic it contains won't burn your face, and so your face won't be left with the film equivalent of a bathtub ring.

3. Blot dry with a soft towel; vigorous rubbing with coarse material aggravates and tugs at your skin.

3

TONING: FRESHENERS AND ASTRINGENTS TAILOR-MADE TO FIT YOUR FACE

Thorough cleansing removes more than makeup, grime, and cellular debris: it strips your skin of its protective shield. Toners, fresheners, and astringents restore the pH balance of the acid mantle; remove any lingering vestiges of makeup, oily cleanser, or soap film; make pores seem smaller and fine wrinkles less noticeable. They should not be harsh enough to irritate your skin. If your face is sensitive and powdery-dry, rose water or other botanical water may be all you need; if it is extremely oily, a stronger astringent will dispense with the excess sebum as it tones.

HOW TO MAKE YOUR OWN SKIN-CARE PRODUCTS

According to Federal Regulations Code #21, cosmetics are "articles to be applied to the body for cleaning, beautifying, promoting attractiveness or altering the appearance," and are not subject to the same standards as foods and drugs. We may feel condescendingly superior to the sixteenth-century courtesans who wasted away as a result of powdering their faces with white lead, but label-scrutinizing can reveal some surprises about the cosmetics now on the market. The same chemicals used in insecticides are often incorporated in beauty products to prolong shelf life,[171] formaldehyde may be included in lotions as well as in nail hardeners,[13] while other potentially hazardous ingredients contribute color and scent to beautify the product, not the skin to which they are applied. It's no longer "un-macho" for men to care for their skin; industry analysts reveal that sales of masculine cosmetic preparations rose from 20 million in 1985 to 40 million in 1987. Skin bracers and after-shave lotions—consisting primarily of alcohol, water, and scent—provide little more than sting.

Concocting your own natural cosmetics is amazingly easy and rewarding. You can tailor the formulas to fit your face. If your skin is a normal combination, you can bottle two-thirds of your prepared toner-astringent to use on your oily T-zone; then dilute the remainder for toning your cheeks and throat. By pouring a little of the full-strength mixture over pressed-cotton puffs in an airtight container, you can manufacture your own makeup-remover/skin-freshener pads.

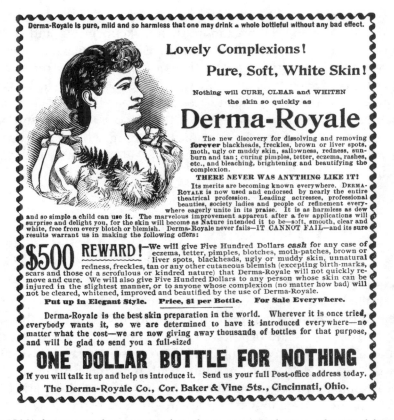

This 1890's beauty product may not have been as miraculous so advertised, but it was safe to drink.

Equipment and Ingredients: Your "cosmetics lab" requires only standard measuring spoons and cups, an enamel or glass pan, a fine sieve, and a funnel. A medicine cup or jigger with graduated markings is a convenient time saver (one fluid ounce equals two tablespoons): if your tap water contains chlorine or fluoride, you may have more satisfactory results if you use bottled water. For aesthetic appeal, you can add a few drops of vegetable food coloring, or exotic scents from the essential oils, fragrant oils, or extracts available in beauty supply houses, health food stores, or supermarkets. Alcohol, benzoin, vinegar, and witch hazel are natural preservatives for your lotions and potions. Fruits and vegetables are perishable, however, so it is wise to prepare small quantities and refrigerate any surplus.

HOW TO CODDLE YOUR COMPLEXION— AND BUDGET—WITH EIGHT SKIN-FIRMING MIXTURES

AROMATIC, BOTANICAL WATERS

These waters may be used alone for a mild toner or added to astringents as a "strength reducer." For increased astringency, stir in one or two teaspoons of lemon juice. For skin texturizing and product preserving, add a tablespoon of tincture of benzoin. As a bonus, you can mix a bit of lemon juice with the strained botanical remains and utilize them as a facial pack.

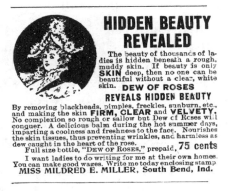

• **Rose water**, the most versatile beauty liquid, can be purchased in pharmacies. If you would rather do it yourself, you can acquire *rose otto* (attar of roses, rose oil) by having a lackey collect the oil floating on your moatful of drifting rose petals—as did a sixteenth-century Persian princess—follow the example set by Napolean's Josephine who considered rose water a love potion and cultivated over 250 different types of roses, or opt for one of these methods:

Attar of roses: Fill a large jar with unsprayed, freshly picked, rose petals. Add distilled water to cover, then top with a fine screen. Place the jar in the sunshine each day, bring it indoors at night. As the rose oil rises to the surface, lift it off with cotton balls and squeeze it into a small glass vial with a tight lid. Continue the process for a week or until no more oil appears.

Rose water from attar of roses: Dissolve $1/4$ teaspoon of the rose oil in $1/2$ cup rubbing alcohol. Add 5 cups distilled water, mix thoroughly, then decant into small bottles for storage.

Rose water astringent: Mix $3/4$ cup rose water with $1/4$ cup rubbing alcohol—adjust to the desired degree of tingle by adding more of either liquid.

Quicker, easier and milder *rose water* can be produced by following the directions given with floral waters, below.

Floral waters. Acacia flowers, clover blooms, elderflowers, orange or lemon blossoms and leaves, rose petals or buds, or violets can be simmered in just enough water to cover, allowed to cool, then strained, and the liquid bottled.

Herbal waters have long been used by men as well as women to firm skin tissue and retain its youthfulness. To make camomile, chervil, comfrey or sage water: Place $3/4$ cup of the fresh herb in a glass jar with 1 cup of water. Cover tightly and shake each morning and evening for 2 weeks. Strain and bottle.

A quick mint tonic can be made by liquefying a handful of fresh mint leaves with an ice cube in an electric blender.

Vegetable waters. Stir $1/2$ cup grated cucumber, or $1/2$ cup finely minced celery and leaves, with 1 cup of water. Let stand for 1 hour, then strain through doubled cheesecloth and squeeze out all the liquid. Bottle and refrigerate.

Cucumber or celery astringent can be made to order by mixing $1/4$ cup of the vegetable water with a tablespoon or so of rubbing alcohol, vodka, or witch hazel.

REFRESHING TEA TONERS

Herbal teas, made double-strength and steeped for several hours, are not only facial toners with mildly astringent properties; they provide a facial treatment if allowed to dry on your skin for 30 minutes. Comfrey or camomile tea offers the same skin firming benefits as a "water" made from the fresh herb. Chervil tea is ideal for fair skin. Mint or sage tea is a gentle astringent for normal, combination, or oily skin.

- **Camomile-rosemary refresher,** made from 2 camomile tea bags plus 1 tablespoon dried rosemary steeped in $1^1/_2$ cups water and strained, is especially recommended as a postexercise unisex skin refresher.

- **Strawberry-mint tea,** prepared by steeping 1 tea bag of each in 1 cup of boiling water, is a delightfully scented skin freshener-toner.

COSMETIC VINEGARS

Apple cider vinegar, white vinegar, or wine vinegar can be splashed on as an acid-mantle restorer when mixed with water in the proportions of one teaspoon to one tablespoon of vinegar to each half-cup of water, depending on personal preference and the dryness of your skin. Cosmetic vinegars, first concocted by medieval alchemists and still sold in European herb shops, have olfactory appeal as well as additional benefits, and are used as after-shave lotions by German barbers. When you make your own, dilute with a little rose water or other botanical water for use as a toner on oily skin and dilute with a lot of the water for dry-skin toning.

- **Floral vinegars.** Pour 2 cups slightly warmed white vinegar over 2 cups fresh, unsprayed petals from carnations, honeysuckle, lavender, roses, violets, or other scented flowers. Mix well. Steep in a lidded glass container for 2 weeks, shaking daily, then strain the liquid into a smaller glass bottle.

- **Herbal vinegars.** Prepare from camomile, dill, lemon grass, rosemary, sweet basil, thyme, or other pungent herb by pouring

2 cups of warm white vinegar over 1 cup of fresh snippets (or $1/4$ cup of the dried herb), and following the directions for floral vinegars.

Instant mint vinegar. Mix 1 cup cider vinegar, 1 cup boiling water, and $1/4$ teaspoon oil of peppermint. For scent, add $1/4$ teaspoon oil of rose geranium.

Minute mint vinegar. Mix 1 cup double-strength peppermint tea with 1 cup cider vinegar.

Rose-camomile vinegar. Steep 1 cup fresh rose petals and $1/2$ cup fresh (or 2 tablespoons dried) camomile flowers in 2 cups white wine vinegar for 1 week. Strain, then add 1 cup rose water to the liquid.

Scented vinegar. Steep 1 tablespoon *each* dried lavender, mint, rosemary, and thyme in 1 quart white vinegar for 2 weeks, shaking the bottle daily. Strain and bottle.

Variegated vinegar. Pour 1 pint of boiling white vinegar over $1/4$ cup *each* fresh camomile, orange flowers, orange leaves, orange peel, rosebuds, rose hips, rose leaves, and white willow bark. (The willow bark may be omitted, and 2 teaspoons dried camomile substituted for fresh, if desired.) Let the mixture steep in a tightly closed container, shaking the bottle once each day, until the botanicals lose their color. Strain, add 1 cup rose water, let settle for a few days, then decant the clear liquid into a smaller bottle.

- **Lemon vinegar.** For a mild astringent that requires no advance preparation or refrigerated storage: Blend $1/2$ cup water with $1/4$ cup apple cider vinegar and 1 teaspoon lemon extract. Shake well before using.

- **Strawberry vinegar.** Stir $1/4$ cup mashed ripe strawberries into $1/2$ cup white vinegar. Cover and let stand for several hours, then strain out the seeds and blend the liquid with $1/4$ cup rose water.

PEROXIDE

Hydrogen peroxide, in the 3 percent solution available from drug stores, is a gentle toner and an antiseptic that helps eradicate existing blemishes and prevent new ones from appearing. (When used daily, it also bleaches facial hair—be cautious around your eyebrows and hairline.) Peroxide gradually loses strength and eventually turns into just plain water—discard it after the expiration date printed on the bottle.

WITCH HAZEL

The commercial product is a freshening-toning-antiseptic liquid extracted with alcohol from the leaves or bark of the witch hazel shrub, then reduced with water. For a quick-mix freshener or after-shave with sparkle: combine $1/4$ cup witch hazel with 1 teaspoon lemon or peppermint extract from the kitchen shelf.

If your skin is especially dry dilute the witch hazel with rose water, or make your own alcohol-free witch hazel water by boiling 3 tablespoons witch hazel leaves or bark in 2 cups of water for 5 minutes. Let cool, then strain and bottle.

COSMETIC COCKTAILS

Your face needn't be a teetotaler, even if you are. Vodka has less odor than rubbing alcohol and is a smoother mixer for toners and astringents.

> ❧ **Russian rose refresher.** Pour $1/2$ cup rose water into a glass or plastic bottle with a screw cap. Add $1/4$ cup 80-proof vodka and $1/4$ teaspoon glycerin. Shake to blend. Test on your skin, then adjust for the precise amount of tingle you want by adding either vodka or rose water.

Paul and Jennifer had a shelf cluttered with skin bracers and fresheners, each of which was either too harsh or too mild. Weary of playing Goldilocks sampling the bears' porridge, Jennifer concocted her own "just right" Russian refresher and was so delighted with the results she decided to create a lotion for Paul.

❧ HOLIDAY AFTER-SHAVE ❧

$1/4$ cup white rum
2 tablespoons double-strength camomile tea
$1/4$ teaspoon rum extract
2 drops maple flavoring

Paul says it smells like a Christmas party and reminds him of their vacation breakfasts in Vermont. He is so happy to have his "just

right, just for him" lotion that Jennifer hasn't admitted she was thinking of the aroma of her father's pipe tobacco when she added the
rum and maple flavorings!

- **Whiskey toner.** Blend $1/3$ cup whiskey with 1 teaspoon tincture of benzoin. Add 1 cup water, stopper tightly, then shake.
This was a favorite, "perfectly harmless," complexion reviver during the 1800s. The instructions called for diluting the mixture
with more water, if desired, sponging it over the face and throat,
and letting it dry.

FRUITFUL FRESHENERS

- **Apple juice** gives your face a refreshing lift.

- **Grape.** Split a grape, remove any seeds, then run the cut halves
over your face and throat for toning and refreshing.

- **Grapefruit juice.** Squeeze a teaspoonful of fresh grapefruit juice
into the palm of your hand. Smooth over your face and throat.

- **Lemon,** because of its astringent properties, is especially recommended for oily skins.

    Cooked lemon astringent: Cook 1 chopped lemon with $1/2$
    cup water in a small, covered pan until tender. Whir in an elec-
    tric blender, strain to remove any fragments of peel, then
    dilute with water to the desired strength.

    Lemon frost: To duplicate a famous salon's skin refresher used
    as an after-shave or after-masque toner: Blender whir $1/4$ cup
    each distilled water and lemon juice with 2 ice cubes and 1
    teaspoon olive oil.

    Lemon milk: Stir 1 tablespoon lemon juice into $1/4$ cup milk.
    Apply generously, then blot off the excess. For a stronger solu-
    tion, substitute water for milk.

    Lemon-lime freshener: In an 8-ounce bottle, combine $1/3$ cup
    water, 1 tablespoon *each* lemon juice and lime juice, and $1/2$
    teaspoon tincture of benzoin. Stopper tightly, shake to blend,
    then refrigerate until ready to use.

- **Orange or tangerine** slices or segments may be smoothed
over the face and throat for freshening and toning.

VEGETABLE TONICS

* **Celery astringent.** Finely chop 1 large rib of celery with leaves. Simmer, covered, in 1 cup water for 20 minutes. Strain, stir in $1/4$ cup rubbing alcohol and 2 teaspoons tincture of benzoin.

* **Cucumber** is a centuries-old complexion aid still used in exclusive beauty salons and included in some of the more expensive commercial cosmetics. You can acquire cucumber's mildly astringent benefits by rubbing the meaty side of a strip of its peeling, or a slice of raw cucumber, over your face.

  Cucumber-citrus astringent: Pour the juice from half a lemon and half an orange into the container of an electric blender. Add half a cucumber, cut in chunks, and whir on high speed for a few seconds. Strain, then stir in a tablespoon of rubbing alcohol, vodka, or witch hazel.

  Cucumber-lettuce lotion is a no-alcohol astringent with masculine as well as feminine appeal. Boil the dark, outer leaves of a head of leaf lettuce in 1 cup water. Let stand until cool. Strain, then combine the liquid with the strained juice from a cucumber liquefied in an electric blender.

  Cucumber milk is a mild toner for after cleansing (or after shaving) or for mutual midday skin refreshing. Liquefy enough chopped cucumber to produce $1/4$ cup strained juice, then add 2 tablespoons milk.

  Cucumber-witch hazel is recommended for normal or oily skin. Liquefy half a cucumber (chopped) with 2 tablespoons water and 1 teaspoon honey in an electric blender. Strain, discard the pulp, then add enough witch hazel to make 1 cup. Chill before using. For very oily skin: Mix $1/4$ cup of liquefied, strained cucumber juice with an equal amount of commercial witch hazel.

  Cooked cucumber freshener: Cut half a cucumber in chunks and whir in a blender with $1/2$ cup water. (Or, mince the cucumber and stir into $1/2$ cup water.) Simmer in a covered saucepan for 20 minutes and let stand to cool. Strain through doubled cheesecloth, squeeze the liquid into a small bowl, then stir in tincture of benzoin, a few drops at a time, until the cucumber takes on a milky appearance.

❧ **Potato.** For an instant freshener-toner, rub a slice of raw potato over your face and throat.

❧ **Tomato,** sliced and rubbed over your skin (or mashed, smeared on and wiped off), is a mildly astringent toner.

FIVE CUSTOM-MADE COMPLEXION TONERS, TONICS, AND ASTRINGENTS

Here are five complexion refreshers you can make at home:

1. *Almond flower milk.* For a tissue-building skin refresher, whir $1/4$ cup almond meal in an electric blender with enough rose water to form a loosely flowing lotion. Strain, stir in $1/4$ teaspoon tincture of benzoin, then decant into an attractive container.

2. *Benzoin water.* The May 1895 issue of *The Delineator* states that the most efficacious spring tonic for enervated skin is a drop of benzoin beaten into $1/4$ cup water. It is to be sponged over a thoroughly clean face and throat, then allowed to dry without rinsing. For a skin-firming toner: Mix $1/4$ teaspoon tincture of benzoin with $1/4$ cup rose water and apply with a cotton ball. Do not rinse off.

3. *Glycerin,* mixed with rose water or other aromatic water, is an old-fashioned toner for dry to normal complexions. Test with the proportions of $1/4$ teaspoon glycerin to $1/2$ cup of the water, then add more glycerin if desired.

4. *Herbal astringent* for oily skin: Steep 1 tea bag *each* camomile and peppermint in 1 cup boiling water until cool. Remove the tea bags (pressing out all the liquid) and stir in 3 tablespoons witch hazel, 1 teaspoon vinegar, and 1 teaspoon tincture of benzoin. If your skin is encumbered by blemishes, you can add the antiseptic qualities of boric acid by stirring in $1/4$ teaspoon of crystalline powder.

5. *Honey* can be shaken with mineral water or any botanical water to make a nonsticky, skin-smoothing toner. One tablespoon honey to $1/2$ cup of the water is the usual ratio.

How Ice and Snow can Tighten Pores and Refine Your Skin

Modern dermatologists warn against shocking the skin with temperature extremes, and cite laboratory tests showing that tiny capillaries near the surface can become so traumatized that they will mar your appearance with spidery red veins. Nevertheless, beauty conscious women have been employing ice or snow for skin-refining and pore-tightening for hundreds of years. As one 93-year-old charmer replied when asked for the secret of her clear, fine-textured complexion, "I don't have any secret. All I've ever done is what my mother did: smooth on a touch of olive oil at night, and wash with soap and water—rinse thoroughly, then rub an ice cube over my face. Of course," she admitted with a smile, "when I was young, we went out and scooped up a handful of snow in the wintertime, or chipped a piece off a block of ice in the summer—we didn't have ice cubes." Our refrigerator-freezers offer more interesting alternatives.

- **Ice diving:** Fill the bathroom sink with cold water and two trays of ice cubes. Pin your hair back, or don a shower cap. Dip your face in the icy water for as long as you can hold your breath. Blot almost dry, then apply your moisturizer. A famous actor credits his daily ice dive (without the shower cap) for his non-receding hairline as well as his youthful-appearing skin.

- **Lemon freeze:** Combine strained fresh lemon juice and water to the degree of astringency you prefer. Partially fill an ice cube tray (your frozen cubes need not be more than one-half an inch thick), freeze, pop out, and store in a plastic bag in the freezer. To use: Lightly rub one of the icy rectangles over your face. Tissue off the excess lemon liquid, along with any surplus skin oil.

- **Super ice:** This duplicates the effects of "cold iron" salon treatments to increase circulation, wake up a weary face, and leave your complexion firm and dewy fresh.

Mix $1/2$ cup bottled mineral water with $1/2$ cup of your favorite freshener and $1/4$ teaspoon alum. Pour into an ice cube tray, freeze, pop out, and store in an airtight container in the freezer. When you rub a cube over your face, pause a few seconds over any noticeable lines or wrinkles before blotting off the excess liquid.

4

MOISTURIZERS AND NIGHT NOURISHERS FOR SOFTER, MORE SUPPLE SKIN

Who needs to moisturize? Almost everyone. *Cleansing* strips away the protective acid mantle and surface oil; *toning* restores the pH balance so the sebaceous glands (which commence their withering-away decline when we reach the age of 25) can proceed with their skin-lubricating chores; *moisturizing* helps retain the radiantly unwrinkled bloom of youth by sealing in water and replenishing some of the precious oils reduced by aging or removed during cleansing and toning. Race, gender, and inherited tendencies are largely responsible for all-over dry or always-oily skin; normal skin is a mosaic combination of slightly dry and slightly oily. Caucasian women have drier skin than women of African-American, Latin, or Asian origin. Men of all nationalities have more productive sebaceous glands than their female counterparts and may be able to wait until they are in their forties before moisturizing dry areas. We can't alter our ancestry or our genes, but we can make the most of the skin we have by moisturizing when and where required.

WATER: NATURE'S SECRET FOR DEWY-FRESH SKIN

Water (comprising 70 to 90 percent of skin, other body tissues, and blood) is Mother Nature's secret for dewy-fresh skin. As skin physiologist Dr. Peter T. Puglise explains in the January 1988 issue of *Health*, water moves through the body to the surface in a process called "transepidermal water loss," leaving skin pleasingly plump and firm. If your system is deficient in water, the skin's upper layers become dry and brittle. Drinking at least six glasses of water daily and eating fluid-rich fruits and vegetables help normalize dry or oily conditions, and is essential for preventing your body from hoarding its necessary moisture at the expense of your skin. In addition to internal liquid refreshment, skin requires external water replenishing. Supplying this water from the outside is something of a paradox: extended immersion first bloats and puffs your skin, then leaves it looking like a shriveled prune; water applied and allowed to evaporate untended carries away some of the skin's own moisture. Moderation in watery contacts, plus *humectants, emollients*, and *occlusives* (see Glossary) smoothed over slightly damp skin, resolve the dilemma.

TIPS ON MOISTURIZING YOUR SKIN

DRY SKIN

Facial skin reveals crinkly-wrinkly signs sooner than body skin because of exposure to the elements and more frequent cleansings. Sales of masculine moisturizers are mounting as men, too, strive to prevent the telltale evidence of aging, and wrinkle-prone dry skin is the most common problem besetting over-30 women. Including two tablespoons of unsaturated oil in your diet and taking a vitamin A supplement may lessen dry-skin discomfort and flakiness. Contrary to advertisements generated by cosmetic promoters, however, slathering on globs of elegantly packaged skin rejuvenators won't slow Father Time. Neither collagen nor elastin can be assimilated from topical application, and, according to Dr. Erno Lazlo and other skin care experts,[47,89] smothering your skin with heavy creams may enlarge pores, cause facial blemishes, and weaken its elasticity to such an extent that it will droop and sag with nature's gravitational pull. Moistening with water, then applying a thin film of air-excluding moisturizer, restores its suppleness.[159]

Night Moisturizing: Complete your cleansing-toning routine with a splash of water or a water-misting. Pat almost dry with a soft towel, then smooth moisturizer from bosom to hairline. For the ultimate benefit, allow five minutes for immediate absorption (cover your face and throat with warm washcloths to hasten penetration), then blot off any excess moisturizer with a tissue. Men may elect to skip the toner but should moisturize the delicate skin around the eye area which contains few oil glands.

Day Moisturizing: Even if you use a makeup foundation that includes a moisturizer, caressing a touch of your natural moisturizer over the freshly cleansed, toned, and dampened skin on your throat, cheeks, and around your eyes can pay beautiful dividends. Men are advised to follow a "double-dose" routine of applying moisturizer immediately after shaving, waiting ten minutes, then moisturizing again.

OILY SKIN

Oiliness, like dryness, varies with time, temperature, your endocrine system, and your emotions (stress may be responsible for a sudden outburst of oily-skin problems[173]). Cutting back on fried foods, pastries, and other saturated food fats may reduce the amount of excess oil accumulating on your epidermis. If your skin is extremely oily, three or four daily cleansings may be in order and little or no moisturizing necessary before you reach the 30-year milepost. After that point, the skin around your eyes and mouth and on your throat may benefit from a nightly moisturizing, plus a mere touch of moisturizer in the morning. If your oily skin is scaly, using a deep-cleaning exfoliant on alternate nights, and following the treatment with a light coating of moisturizer often corrects the problem.

COMBINATION SKIN

For most of us, oily areas are concentrated in the T-zone of forehead, nose, chin, with drier, moisture-thirsty skin covering the rest of the face and throat. If twice-daily all-over moisturizing accentuates the oiliness, experiment with "spot moisturizing" on alternate nights and for daytime care.

WHEN TO REMOISTURIZE

Here are three general guidelines on when to remoisturize your skin:

1. Before and after your face is exposed to wind or extremely hot or cold outdoor temperatures, or when it has had an encounter with ocean spray, swimming-pool water, or falling snow or rain.

2. When you're sitting near an open fire, when your culinary endeavors require a lot of oven-door opening and closing, or when you use hot rollers, a curling iron, or a hair dryer on its high setting.

3. When the relative humidity is low, as in pressurized airplanes, overheated rooms, and desert climates. Under these conditions your body contains a higher percentage of fluid than the air around it and loses water rapidly.

Do-IT-YOURSELF MOISTURIZERS THAT COST LITTLE AND REPLENISH MUCH

Ancient Greeks anointed themselves with sweet oil, Native Americans and hardy pioneers smeared on bear grease or skunk oil; we have many other options. To increase the benefits from your moisturizer you can incorporate vitamins A and E by snipping capsules and squeezing the contents into your homemade cosmetic. Comfrey is another beneficial additive; *allantoin*, comfrey's major component, promotes tissue building, cell restoring, and healing. Some cosmetic manufacturers blend comfrey into their night creams; you can mix a spoonful of comfrey tea with your own moisturizer, or reap even more of allantoin's skin-strengthening rewards by applying cooled comfrey tea instead of water before smoothing on your night nourisher.

Cocoa Butter, Oils, and Petroleum Jelly

These ready-to-use moisturizers double as a base for makeup and are ideal for both men and women.

- **For dry skin:** cocoa butter; almond, castor, olive, peanut, and wheat germ oils.

- **For oily skin:** corn, cottonseed, poppyseed, safflower, sesame, and sunflower seed oils.

- **For normal skin:** any of the above (warmed peanut oil is said to work wonders when massaged into a "scrawny" neck[79]) or avocado, coconut, mink, or soy oils.

Lanolin and mineral oil are effective occlusives but lanolin may instigate skin problems for those allergic to wool; mineral oil sometimes leaves an irritating residue and is suspected of robbing the body of fat-soluble vitamins. If you can wear wool comfortably, you can make a nurturing moisturizer by warming $1/4$ cup lanolin in the top of a double boiler, stirring in $1/4$ cup safflower oil, then adding 5,000 IU vitamin A and 100 IU vitamin E from pierced capsules.

This femme fatale formula is a wonder-working oil mixture similar to the one Cleopatra's handmaidens lavishly applied and then scooped off with a spatula-like "strygil."

> *3 tablespoons* each *safflower oil and sesame oil*
> *2 tablespoons* each *avocado oil and pean ut oil*
> *1 tablespoon* each *olive oil and wheat germ oil*
> *5 drops of perfume oil (optional)—musk, rose,*
> *geranium, or other favorite*

Petroleum jelly does not provide the nourishment of natural oils, yet is effective, innocuous, and versatile. Cathy discovered it to be an indispensable traveling companion when car trouble turned an afternoon drive into a weekend adventure. The mountain lodge offered comfortable accommodations and a magnificent dining room. Behind racks of candy and potato chips in the service-station office, Jason found toothbrushes and a disposable razor, but the only beauty product available was a jar of petroleum jelly. Cathy used it to remove her makeup and as a night cream. They both utilized it as hand lotion, smoothed it on their chapped lips and over their arms and faces when they went exploring in the high altitude sunlight—and had enough left to polish their dusty shoes before going to dinner!

FRUITS

Lemon juice or orange juice blended with olive oil is a time-tested keep-it-supple skin moisturizer. Apples contain *malic acid*, a moisturizing agent. Peaches-and-cream complexions have been attributed to smoothing on a blender-whirred mixture of half a peeled peach or apple and a dollop of cream.

> ❧ **Peach moisturizer for dry or normal skin:** In an electric blender, whir 1 chopped, peeled peach with $1/4$ cup almond oil, 3 tablespoons rose water, 4 drops tincture of benzoin, and (if desired) a few drops of orange oil or other perfume. Strain and store in the refrigerator.

❧ **Fruit cream for normal or oily skin:** Mash and squeeze through cheesecloth (or liquefy in a blender and strain) enough chopped fresh apricot, honeydew melon, peach, or strawberries to produce 2 tablespoons of juice. Heat $1/4$ cup almond oil and $1/2$ ounce white beeswax or paraffin in the top of a double boiler until the wax melts. Remove from the heat, beat in the fruit juice and $1/4$ teaspoon tincture of benzoin. Continue beating until the mixture is fluffy, then transfer to a wide-mouth jar with a tightly fitting lid.

GLYCERIN

As described in an 1895 ladies' magazine, "Glycerine Emollient" is justly favored for pulling moisture into dry skin. The instructions call for bringing $1/2$ cup glycerin to a boil, letting it cool, then adding $1/4$ cup rose water.

Glycerin and honey, in the proportions of 3 tablespoons glycerin to 1 teaspoon honey, is recommended by modern skin-care experts as a wear-all-day or leave-on-all-night moisturizer.[99]

LECITHIN

For a multipurpose moisturizer-makeup base-hand smoother, whir $1/2$ cup almond or apricot kernel *or* avocado oil in an electric blender with $1/4$ cup *each* water and water-dispersible lecithin powder. For more night-nourishing benefits, substitute $1/4$ cup honey for the water.

Lecithin yogurt requires refrigeration and has a shorter life span, but it is a wonderful night cream you can whir up in the blender.

> *3 tablespoons water-dispersible lecithin powder*
>
> *2 tablespoons* each *water and plain yogurt*
>
> *2 tablespoons* each *avocado oil and wheat germ oil*
>
> *2 teaspoons potato flour*
>
> *5 drops of your favorite perfume (optional)*

MAYONNAISE

Mayonnaise (see Glossary for homemade recipe) can be massaged into a clean, damp face and throat whenever skin is dehydrated from exposure to sun, wind, or winter cold. With the excess blotted off after a few minutes' absorption time, mayonnaise is also a night cream.

Milk and Cream

Sweet or sour milk or cream, buttermilk, or whey are all moisturizers especially recommended for irritated skin.

Miss Muffet's moisturizer: Add a lemon slice to $1/4$ cup warm milk, cover, and let stand for 2 hours. Strain and discard the curds which will have formed (or sit on your tuffet and eat them), then apply the liquid whey to your skin with a cotton ball.

Vegetables

For centuries, French women and men have moisturized their faces with lettuce juice; our rural ancestors used split fresh cucumbers to revive their dehydrated skins.

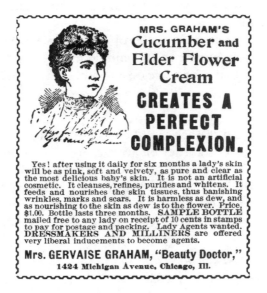

- **Cucumber cream:** Cut a $5/8$-inch slice off one of the 2-$1/2$-inch-by-5-inch-by-$5/8$-inch cakes of paraffin sold for topping home-made jelly. Melt the half-ounce of paraffin in the top of a double boiler or in a a heat-proof glass bowl set in a pan of water over low heat. Stir in $1/4$ cup almond oil a teaspoonful at a time. Puree a medium-size cucumber, chopped but not peeled, in an electric blender or food processor; strain through cheesecloth into the oil-paraffin mixture and blend thoroughly. Let the creamy mixture cool to room temperature, stirring several times to prevent crystals from forming; then transfer to a wide-mouth jar and store in the refrigerator for up to 2 months.

ᴥ **Montmartre Moisturizer:** Simmer lettuce leaves until tender in a lidded pan with just enough distilled water to cover. Let cool, strain off the liquid and apply as is, or blend a spoonful of it with an equal amount of yogurt. Refrigerate the surplus lettuce liquid.

NIGHTTIME NOURISHING: MOISTURIZERS THAT WORK WHILE YOU SLEEP

In sixteenth-century Venice, beauty-conscious ladies slept with milk-soaked veal cutlets secured over their cheeks to moisturize and improve their complexions. We have more comfortable and less costly methods of nighttime nourishing. Besides those previously mentioned, a thin film of white vegetable shortening, soybean margarine, or milk blended with butter will seal in needed moisture. For more sophisticated skin nourishing, try one of these options.

FRUIT AND VEGETABLE NOURISHERS

ᴥ **Artichoke butter,** used nightly, helps tighten crinkled or "crepey" skin. To prepare a week's supply for refrigerator storage, remove the heart from a cooked artichoke, mash it, then gradually work in $1/4$ cup unsalted butter and $1/4$ teaspoon tincture of benzoin.

ᴥ **Avocado.** Mash an avocado slice with a fork until it is the consistency of butter. Massage into your face and throat, let penetrate for 5 minutes, then tissue off the excess.

Avocado cream. Melt 1 ounce white beeswax (or a $1\text{-}1/4$-inch slice of paraffin) in the top of a double boiler, and add one fourth of an avocado (well mashed). Beat in 2 tablespoons apricot-kernel, almond, or coconut oil plus 1 tablespoon lanolin if you are not allergic to wool. Add 2 tablespoons rose water and $1/4$ teaspoon tincture of benzoin. Continue beating until the mixture solidifies, then refrigerate.

Fruitless avocado cream. Melt 1 ounce white beeswax in the top of a double boiler. Beat in $1/4$ cup avocado oil, 2 tablespoons rose water, 2 teaspoons lanolin, and $1/4$ teaspoon tincture of benzoin. Beat until creamy.

• **Strawberries and tea** are a "dream treatment" for normal or combination skin. Mash a few ripe strawberries, squeeze through cheesecloth, then dilute with a spoonful of water and sponge over your face before going to bed. In the morning, rinse off the dried juice with warm chervil tea.

GELATIN-BASED NIGHT NOURISHERS

These miraculous elixirs should be smoothed over clean, damp skin, allowed to penetrate for a few minutes, then blotted with a tissue. If you or your resident male are plagued by tiny under-the-skin bumps, add 1 teaspoon vitamin C crystals and a crushed aspirin to either of the following formulas and share the skin-leveling results. This may be just what the doctor would have ordered: salicylic acid (present in aspirin) is used for prescriptive skin treatments.

How to prepare the gelatin base:

Measure out $1/2$ cup water; place 2 tablespoons of the water in the container of an electric blender and sprinkle with $1 1/2$ teaspoons unflavored gelatin. Allow the gelatin to soften while you bring the remainder of the water to a boil. Pour the boiling water into the blender and whir to dissolve the gelatin.

Nighttime formula for dry-normal-combination skin: To the gelatin base in the blender container, add:

> *$1/2$ cup almond oil (or avocado, olive, peanut, or wheat germ oil)*
>
> *2 tablespoons water-dispersible lecithin powder or liquid lecithin*
>
> *1 tablespoon castor oil*
>
> *$1 1/2$ teaspoons cod liver oil*
>
> *1 teaspoon dried, ground kelp*
>
> *100 IU vitamin E (squeezed from a pierced capsule)*

Blend on medium speed for 15 seconds, or until smooth. Refrigerate in a lightproof container.

- Variation for dry skin: Add 1 teaspoon glycerin and 1 teaspoon sesame oil before blending.

- Variation for combination skin with an oily T-zone: Add 2 tablespoons vodka before blending.

- Variation for skin with large pores, wrinkles, and/or sags: Add 1 egg white, 1 teaspoon sesame oil, and 1 teaspoon vitamin C crystals before blending.

  Nighttime formula for oily skin: To the gelatin base in the blender container, add:

  1/2 cup sparkling mineral water

  1 teaspoon glycerin

  1 teaspoon dried, ground kelp

  1/8 teaspoon vitamin C crystals

  5,000 IU "dry" vitamin A (from a 2-part capsule)

  100 IU "dry" vitamin E (from a 2-part capsule)

  Whir on medium speed for 15 seconds, or until smooth. Transfer to a lightproof container and refrigerate.

- Variation for oily skin with breakouts: Add 2 tablespoons vodka before blending.

- Variation for oily skin with enlarged pores: Increase the amount of vitamin C crystals to 1 teaspoon.

- Variation for oily skin with lines and sags: Increase the amount of vitamin C crystals to 1 teaspoon, and add 1/4 teaspoon alum before blending.

OIL CREAMS

For a night cream that doubles as a body lotion, warm 3 tablespoons *each* corn oil and olive oil with 1 tablespoon almond oil in the top of a double boiler. Add 2 tablespoons distilled water and beat until creamy.

  Wheat germ and honey moisturizer: It takes less than five minutes to whisk up a month's supply of this shelf-stable, anti-aging moisturizer considered the equivalent of a world-famous beauty fluid.

> *3 tablespoons* each *honey and wheat germ oil*
> *2 tablespoons* each *glycerin and witch hazel*
> *1 tablespoon rose water*

Place all ingredients in a glass bowl, whisk to combine, then store in a tightly capped bottle.

5

AT-HOME FACIALS WITH
SALON-LIKE RESULTS

Prestigious salons, now catering to men as well as women, feature herbal steam treatments and natural masques based on formulas that have endured for centuries. At-home salon-type facials can be as sophisticated or as simple as is expedient. You can treat your face to a simple pack without any steamy preliminaries, have a two-minute hot-towel wrap, or indulge in a 10-minute steaming and a two-layer 30-minute masque.

BEFORE YOU BEGIN: THE "BARE" ESSENTIALS

Assembling the components is the first step. Charging out into the world in search of a fresh peach or a container of yogurt can be disconcerting when your pore-cleaned face is enhanced only with a towel turban. The next two steps are every-facial essentials:

1. Pull the hair back off your face with a ribbon or headband, or protect it with a wrapped-around towel.

2. Remove any makeup and cleanse your face as you would normally. Apply a moisturizer around your eyes and over your cheeks if your skin is exceedingly dry.

FACIAL SAUNAS: A COMPLETE GUIDE TO CLEANSING, PURIFYING, AND SOFTENING YOUR SKIN

Facial steaming improves circulation, softens roughness, clears out pores, and imparts a healthy glow to your plumped-up skin. The steaming can be a complete-unto-itself-facial if you follow it with a dousing of cool water or toner, then pat almost dry with a soft towel and smooth on moisturizer. For the ultimate in pore-flushing: the moment you finish steaming, close your eyes and spray your face with mineral water or toner. To incorporate a treatment with your spray:

- *For normal skin*: Mix camomile tea and cold skim milk half-and-half.

- *For dry skin*: Mix cold whole milk and rose water in equal proportions.

- *For oily skin*: Mix $1/3$ cup triple-strength camomile tea with 2 teaspoons *each* lemon juice, skim milk, and witch hazel. Refrigerate the remainder to use as a toning refresher between steamings.

HOW TO STEAM CLEAN YOUR SKIN

Steaming prior to applying a masque is optional; "opening your pores" is a matter of semantics. The American Medical Association states that pores are not controlled by muscles, therefore they cannot either open or close.[159] However, heat does affect the skin to allow free access to the pores and soften their contents. Barbershop hot-moist towels are a case in point. You can follow suit by wringing a lightweight towel out of hot water (with or without herbal enhancements), folding the towel lengthwise, and covering your face (except for nose and mouth) for two minutes. Electrical devices for releasing steam vapor have been used in Europe for over 50 years and are becoming increasingly popular in the United States, despite the fact that they have been charged with several cases of "jungle acne" resulting from overmoisturization.[33] If you have a facial sauna appliance, abide by its instructions. If you don't, there are no-cost methods of achieving similar results without the hazards. Be sure to keep your eyes closed, your face far enough away from the heat to avoid irritating your skin, and never steam for longer than 10 minutes.

To tent or not to tent (by draping a towel over your head to hold in the steam) is a question most experts answer in the affirmative. If you choose to tent, protecting your hair with a shower cap or towel turban before you cover up with the bath towel will prevent the aftermath of an overly curly or damply limp coiffure.

There are two options for do-it-yourself steaming: (1) Fill the bathroom basin with steamy-hot water and lean over it for 2 to 5 minutes. (2) If you wish to incorporate herbs to intensify the benefits, or if your tap water is not that hot, bring 1 or 2 quarts of water (plus herbs, if used) to a boil on the stove. Turn off the heat and either hover over the pot or move it to a table so you can sit comfortably for 5 to 10 minutes.

HERBAL STEAMING SUPPLEMENTS

Plain steam is good, particularly when you merely have blackheads to remove or wish to increase the effect of an exfoliant. Herbal steam is better and more penetrating for cleansing, purifying, and softening. Use the same proportions as for making tea: one tea bag, or the equivalent in dry herbs or herbal oils, for each cup of water. For normal or combination skin, you can mix or match your favorite teas; for special effects, there are special suggestions.

- Acacia, clover, cowslip, elderflower, violet, and yarrow are recommended for dry skin.

- Camomile, eucalyptus, lavender, peppermint, and sage not only soothe and disinfect the skin (camomile is especially recommended for men and for everyone with blemished complexions), they contain aromatic oils beneficial to sinus passages.

- Elderflower, rosemary, and red dock root are suggested for steaming blackheads.

- Lemon, lemon grass, rose, and rosemary teas are especially helpful for oily complexions. To scent the house with lemon freshness while you purify your skin, simply add a few lemon slices to your simmering water and herbs.

- Vacation-simulating steam will rise nostalgically from a mixture of 1 tablespoon *each* camomile, eucalyptus leaves, juniper berries, and dry peppermint tea—or from pine needles or pine or bayberry oils. A tablespoon of kelp generates an oceanside tang.

❧ Double-duty Make-ahead Herbal Mixture ❧
for Dry or Normal Skin

1/4 cup each dried acacia flowers and elderflowers

1/4 cup each dried peach leaves and strawberry leaves

2 tablespoons each camomile, clover, lavender, and peppermint tea

2 tablespoons each crushed anise, caraway, and fennel seeds

2 tablespoons ground licorice root

Combine and store in an airtight container. When you are ready for a facial, place 2 tablespoons of the mixture in each quart of steaming water. For a masque to follow your steam cleaning: strain out the herbs, spread them on a washcloth moistened with the herbal water, then cover your face with the moistened cloth (herb-side-down) for 5 minutes.

❧ Double-duty Make-ahead Herbal Mixture ❧
for Oily Skin

1/4 cup each camomile, lavender, lemon grass, and lemon peel

1/4 cup each dried peach leaves and strawberry leaves

2 tablespoons each crushed anise, caraway, and fennel seeds

2 tablespoons peppermint

Combine and store in an airtight container. For facial steaming: add 2 tablespoons of the mixture to each quart of boiling water. For a masque-after-steaming: strain out the herbs, spread them on a washcloth moistened with the hot liquid, then place the cloth (with the herbs next to your skin) over your face and let it remain until cool.

Stimulating Steaming: How to Give Yourself the "Hot and Cold" Treatment

To bring a glorious glow to a weary complexion, intersperse a cold-towel pack with your hot towels or hot-water-steaming. Place a few ice cubes in a bowl of cold water next to your steam source, saturate a towel in the ice water, then interrupt your steaming once each minute with a 20-second application of the cold towel.

Rosemary, sage, camomile and lavender (1 teaspoon of each) make a stimulating steam to help counteract a muddy or sallow complexion.

Natural Masques: How They Work, When to Use Them

Whether termed masques, masks, or packs, they dislodge cellular debris that can give skin a drab, gray cast, firm and clear skin, plump up wrinkles, and are the "fun" part of a facial. Mother Nature's line is more extensive and exciting than cosmetic-counter offerings, and far less costly. One budding-but-budgeting actress splurged on a "miracle masque," read the fine print on the gilt wrappings as the goo dried on her face, and was more than somewhat disappointed to discover that the product contained nothing more than egg white embalmed with preservatives, perfume, and artificial color. She could have filled her refrigerator with real eggs for the same price.

Intrepid experimenters report that masquing several times each day for months improves rather than harms their skin, and although few of us have time for such frequent indulgence, a brief facial pack before a breakfast meeting, or a 5-minute skin-tightening masque before a dinner engagement can be well worth the effort. Some dermatologists advise a twice-weekly steam treatment for women with average or oily skin, and for men who wear stage makeup or use bronzing gel. Most skin-care experts, however, suggest once a week for all men and women with normal skin, once a month for dry skin, and seldom if ever for those troubled by acne or spider veins because heat may aggravate either of these conditions.

Paying heed to the reaction of your own skin is the best guide to what is right for you. If your face is dry in some areas and oily in others, you may want to apply a different mask on each section (i.e., gelatin or avocado mixture for your cheeks, egg white for your T-zone). Although complexity and time requirements vary, the basic application and removal is similar for all:

1. With hair pushed back off your forehead, smooth or pat the masque over your entire throat and face except for the fragile skin around your eyes.

2. Allow the masque to dry thoroughly (5 to 30 minutes, 20 minutes is the accepted average). Reclining on a slantboard or lolling in bed with your feet propped on pillows and refreshing pads on your eyes while you listen to soft music is sensuously luxurious, and increases the benefits from a masque. Soaking in a scented tub prolongs drying time and enhances the masque's effect.

3. Remove the masque with warm or cool water, rinse well, then tone and moisturize.

Masquing Marvels That Rejuvenate and Nourish Your Skin

Prior steaming, or even a hot shower, will make your skin more receptive to a masque's nourishing treatment, but any of these masques may be applied to a freshly cleansed face.

- **Almond meal.** Two tablespoons *each* almond meal, honey, and whole milk; blended and patted on, makes a masque for all skin types.

- **Cornmeal**, mixed to a paste with egg white, smoothes rough, bumpy skin.

- **Eggs** have been acknowledged skin beautifiers for centuries, probably since the first cavelady improved her appearance with a bit of pterodactyl egg. For all types of skin: Beat an egg until frothy; apply to the face, neck, and shoulders.

  Eggnog masques. Each variation is ample for two or for coating your shoulders, bosom, and face.

  Cognac eggnog for normal or oily skin: Whisk (or whir in an electric blender) 1 raw egg with 2 tablespoons *each* cognac, lemon juice, and fluid milk. Let stand until room temperature before applying.

  Alcohol-free eggnog for normal or dry complexions: Beat 1 tablespoon dry milk into a stiffly beaten egg white, then fold in an egg yolk stirred with 1 teaspoon honey.

Egg white, plain or beaten, smoothed on with the fingertips or applied with a blusher brush, pastry brush, or shaving brush, draws out impurities and refines the pores as it dries.

Egg white, beaten and mixed with 1 teaspoon honey, is a twice-a-day texturizer used by photographers' models. Let it dry on your skin for 10 minutes before rinsing off. Store the remainder in the refrigerator. For additional benefits, add 1 tablespoon of mashed papaya and the contents of a snipped vitamin-E capsule.

Egg-white and alum plus honey pack is an old-fashioned skin rejuvenator. Beat an egg white with $1/_8$ teaspoon alum, smooth on and let dry until your face feels very taut. Rinse thoroughly, blot dry, then pat on a coating of honey and let that remain for 5 minutes. Rinse off the honey and tone your face with rose water.

Egg white, milk, and honey skin tightener. Beat together 1 egg white, 1 tablespoon instant nonfat dry milk, and $1/_2$ teaspoon honey. Mint or sage tea is suggested as a toner after this masque has dried and been removed.

Egg yolk, lightly beaten with a fork, then smoothed on and allowed to dry, is a comfortably gentle skin firmer for dry or normal skin.

Egg-yolk honey is a masque for dry, wrinkle-prone skin: Blend 1 egg yolk and 1 tablespoon honey with $1/_2$ teaspoon almond oil. Adding a tablespoon of yogurt makes it even more effective.

Egg yolk and olive oil. One teaspoon of the oil beaten with 1 egg yolk is an Italian dry-skin treatment. For a variation with zing, blend the egg yolk with 2 teaspoons safflower oil and $1/_2$ teaspoon mint extract.

&. **Fruit masques** are easily prepared skin treats. (To rehydrate naturally dried, unsweetened fruit: soften in hot water or cook until tender.) Puree or mash enough fruit to cover your face and throat. Blend in 1 teaspoon oil, cream, or milk if your skin is dry or normal; 1 teaspoon lemon juice if your skin is oily or normal. For variety, try the following.

Apple. Originally developed as a masculine masque, this combination is equally effective for feminine faces. Core and quarter a small, unpeeled apple. Puree it in a food processor or electric blender with 1 tablespoon honey and $^1/_2$ teaspoon dried sage (or 1 tablespoon snipped fresh leaves) for normal or combination skin; add 1 tablespoon lemon juice for oily complexions.

Apricots or peaches are valuable skin nourishers you can use as often as needed to refresh tired skin or enliven a wan complexion and make it less wrinkle prone. Blend in $^1/_2$ teaspoon lemon juice with the pureed fruit before applying to oily skin; 1 teaspoon of cream, honey, or vegetable oil for dry skin. For a superlative skin-tightening masque, blender whir 1 egg white with the fruit.

Avocado, mashed or whirred in a blender with a few drops of lemon juice, makes a nourishing, gently astringent masque for men or women. If your skin is very dry, add 1 egg yolk, or 1 tablespoon honey, or 1 teaspoon vegetable oil.

Banana, peeled and sliced or mashed, is a Guatemalan favorite for relieving dry skin. When you have time to lie perfectly still for 20 minutes, you can arrange thin slices of banana all over your face and let the banana's oils and vitamins permeate your epidermis. If you anticipate squirming or sneezing, mash the banana to a smooth paste before applying. For very dry skin, add 1 teaspoon olive oil while mashing the banana. For added benefits, incorporate the peel by blender-pureeing half a banana with half its peel (cut up) and 1 teaspoon honey.

Grapes cleanse and moisturize all types of skin. Whir a handful of seedless green grapes in an electric blender, smooth the puree over your face and throat, and wait 10 minutes before rinsing off. For a South American skin-rejuvenating treatment, blend a tablespoon of flour with the grape puree.

Melons—cantaloupe, honeydew, or watermelon, mashed or pureed—make a refreshing masque to cleanse and tighten pores and to help obliterate fine-line wrinkles.

Oranges are said to slow skin aging and erase signs of fatigue. Apply only the pulp, let dry for 15 minutes, remove with a damp washcloth, and rinse thoroughly.

Papaya contains an enzyme, papain, which helps clear impurities and heal blemished skin. The peeled, mashed, or pureed fruit can be smoothed on, allowed to dry for 15 minutes, then rinsed off. For more exfoliating action: Wait only 5 minutes after applying the papaya puree, gently massage your face with a fresh papaya slice, remove the melange with a washcloth, then rinse.

Pears, mashed or pureed with a bit of lemon juice, have astringent properties beneficial for oily skins.

Pineapple with honey is a tropical skin-texturizer. Smooth on a thin coating of honey and let dry for about 10 minutes, or until it feels tacky. Remove with cotton pads soaked in fresh pineapple juice, then apply a second coating of pineapple juice or rub a slice of fresh pineapple over your face. Wait a few minutes before rinsing.

Plums, cooked and mashed with a teaspoon of almond oil, make a rich 10-minute masque for oily skin.

Prunes do more than relieve costiveness, they can regenerate tired, dry skin. Blender-puree 4 cooked, pitted prunes with 1 teaspoon sesame oil.

Strawberries are time-tested skin improvers that clean pores, tighten skin, help clear up blemishes, and postpone wrinkling. Mash fresh or frozen unsweetened strawberries, smooth the puree over your face, and let it dry for 10 minutes before rinsing off with cool water. For more pronounced cleansing and softening: Mix $1/4$ cup mashed strawberries with 2 tablespoons cornstarch or yogurt; or blend the mashed strawberries with cream and/or oatmeal to make a pretty pink paste. This 10-minute after-shave masque is especially for men: 1 tablespoon mashed strawberries blended with 1 teaspoon sour cream.

Gelatin masques are ideal for dry or sensitive skin. Manufacture an easy one by softening a packet of unflavored gelatin in a little cold water, stirring the mixture over boiling water (or microwaving it) to dissolve, then letting it cool for a few minutes before smoothing over your face.

Yellow-Jell-O® refresher. Dissolve 2 tablespoons lemon gelatin dessert in $1/4$ cup boiling water, stir in 2 tablespoons strained fresh lemon juice, and let stand until room temperature.

❧ NOURISHING GELATIN MASQUE ❧

1 teaspoon unflavored gelatin

$1/4$ cup water

$1/4$ cup soybean oil

1 tablespoon each liquid lecithin and sesame oil

1 teaspoon liquid multivitamins or 1 teaspoon each brewer's yeast and cod liver oil, the contents of a 100 IU vitamin E capsule, and $1/4$ teaspoon vitamin C crystals

Stir the gelatin into the water, heat to boiling, stir to dissolve, then pour into the container of an electric blender. Add all other ingredients and blend for 15 seconds. Apply and let penetrate for 10 minutes before rinsing off. Refrigerate the remainder for your next facial treatment.

❧ **Herbs**. Any of the herbs or herbal combinations suggested for facial saunas may be steeped in boiling water, drained, and spread on a washcloth for use as a masque. For additional benefits, the herbs can be mixed to a paste with yogurt and/or lemon juice, then patted over the face.

Fresh bay or eucalyptus leaves, ground to a paste with regular-strength pekoe tea and allowed to stand for 24 hours, are a healing-toning masque recommended by plastic surgeons.[62]

Fresh mint refines pores when $1/4$ cup of the leaves are blender-ground with 2 tablespoons almond meal and enough water to make a paste. Massage into your skin and let dry for 5 minutes. Rinse off; follow with a coating of honey; then let that dry for another 5 minutes before rinsing.

Pizza pack: Place 1 tablespoon dried Italian seasoning (from the spice shelf) in a cup with $1/4$ cup tomato juice. Cover and let stand for 8 hours.

❧ **Honey**, all by itself, is a stimulating, smoothing facial pack when patted on the face and allowed to remain for 5 minutes.

Honey and lemon juice is a French specific for lackluster skin. Mix 1 tablespoon honey with 1 teaspoon strained lemon juice. Apply to your freshly cleansed face and leave on for at least 30 minutes. Remove with rosemary tea or tepid water.

Honey and wheat germ, mixed to a paste, is another nourishing-masque option.

🍃 **Mayonnaise**, either store-bought or homemade (see Glossary for recipe), is a marvelous skin softener and revitalizer that can be used every day. Allow 5 to 20 minutes for it to permeate, then rinse off with warm water. For superbly smooth, rejuvenated skin: Mix 1 tablespoon mayonnaise with 2 teaspoons almond meal and $1/8$ teaspoon alum.

🍃 **Milk**, like honey, not only contributes to other facials, but can masque alone. Skim milk aids oily skin; whole milk helps under-40 skin; half-and half or heavy cream discourages over-40 dryness; buttermilk cleanses and blanches; sour cream soothes dry skin; yogurt is good for every type of skin, has antibacterial properties, and helps thicken other masques.

Four-layer milk masque is a Hungarian treatment for delicate or dry skin. Mix a tablespoon of evaporated milk (or fluid whole milk) with $1/4$ teaspoon of olive oil. Smooth a thin film over your skin with your fingers or a sponge, let it dry for a minute or two, then apply a second layer. Repeat until four layers have dried and your face feels like granite. Remove with lukewarm water and a washcloth.

Instant nonfat dry milk is a 5-minute skin-texturizer when mixed to a paste with water. If your skin is very dry, blend in a few drops of salad oil. If you want a pepper-upper, add 3 drops of peppermint extract. If you want to lighten as well as tighten your skin, use lemon juice to make the milk paste.

Sour cream is a soothing skin-tightener that first found favor with Russian czarinas.

Sweet cream or whipping cream soothes and texturizes dry skin.

Yogurt, plain or mixed with a few drops of lemon juice, makes a skin-toning pack. For a skin-lightening masque: Blender puree a slice of lemon and a quarter of an orange (both unpeeled) with $1/4$ cup yogurt. Pat over your face and let dry for 20 minutes before rinsing off.

🔊 **Milk of Magnesia**, straight from the bottle, neutralizes the fatty acids that accumulate on oily skin. Simply smooth on, let dry for 15 to 20 minutes, then rinse.

🔊 **Mud**. If you don't have access to a natural spring surrounded by pure clay, you can pick up a package of fuller's earth at the corner drugstore. Mud or clay masques require 30 to 40 minutes' drying time to clear off cellular debris, remove excess sebum from oily skin, and also lift out grime, blackheads, and whiteheads. If your skin type is dry or normal-combination, smooth on a protective film of salad oil before applying the masque. Mix the fuller's earth with mint tea, mint mouthwash, or witch hazel for extra zing.

Bret discovered a mud-masque bonus. Running late for a night meeting, he nicked his chin while shaving. With no time to spare, he covered the bleeding spot with a dab of the masque Jane had just prepared for her evening-alone beauty ritual. To their mutual surprise, the mud masque not only staunched the flow of blood; it also concealed all evidence of the mishap.

Alcoholic mud helps in treating super oily skin. Combine 2 tablespoons rubbing alcohol with 2 teaspoons fuller's earth. Add 1 teaspoon peppermint extract, if desired.

Almond mud is a cleansing-toning masque you can prepare by combining 1 tablespoon *each* almond meal and fuller's earth, a few drops of benzoin, and enough witch hazel to make a spreadable paste.

Carrot clay has blemish-healing as well as skin-texturizing qualities: Mix 1 tablespoon *each* carrot juice and fuller's earth with mineral water until you have a thick paste.

Egg-yolk mud sounds dreadful but does delightful things for dry or normal skin. Use a fork to beat 1 egg yolk with 1 tablespoon fuller's earth. Stir in 1 teaspoon honey and add mineral water to make a soft paste.

Herbal mud for oily skins can be prepared by steeping 1 teaspoon each rosemary and sage in $^1/_2$ cup boiling water, straining, and mixing enough of the liquid with 2 tablespoons fuller's earth to make a smooth-on paste.

Muddy oatmeal is great for rejuvenating tired skin. Mix 1 tablespoon each leftover cooked oatmeal and fuller's earth with water to make a paste.

&. ***Yogurt mud*** refines pores and tightens normal or oily skin. Mix 1 egg white, 1 tablespoon yogurt, 1 teaspoon *each* fuller's earth and honey. Or, mix 2 tablespoons yogurt, 2 teaspoons fuller's earth, a few drops of mint extract, and enough water to make a creamy paste. Or, mix 1 tablespoon *each* yogurt and fuller's earth with $^1/_2$ teaspoon honey and $^1/_8$ teaspoon baking soda.

&. **Oatmeal** is given credit for many flawless complexions. Regular or quick-cooking dry oatmeal can be mixed with water or milk and allowed to dry on your face and throat for 10 to 15 minutes to smooth, soften, and remove dead cells. To multiply the benefits, blend 1 egg white, 1 tablespoon of instant nonfat dry milk, and $^1/_4$ teaspoon almond oil with the oatmeal. For sensitive skin, pulverize the oatmeal in an electric blender or food processor; or stir 2 tablespoons oatmeal into $^1/_2$ cup milk and cook it to soft mush.

For a spectacular dry-skin masque: Mix 2 tablespoons uncooked oatmeal with buttermilk or triple-strength camomile tea to make a thick paste. Or, mix 2 tablespoons *each* oatmeal and honey with 1 teaspoon white vegetable shortening. Or, mix 2 tablespoons oatmeal with 1 teaspoon *each* honey and cider vinegar, and $^1/_2$ teaspoon almond meal.

Nutty Mexicali oatmeal improves circulation, conditions and feeds normal or oily complexions, but should not be used on dry or sensitive skin.

2 tablespoons each *brewer's yeast, chopped cashew nuts, honey, and uncooked oatmeal*

1 egg white

$^1/_4$ teaspoon chili powder

Place all the ingredients in the container of an electric blender. Whir until smooth, spread over your face and neck, and allow to dry for 30 to 45 minutes.

- **Oil packs** are the original dry-skin remedy. Coat your face and throat with almond, olive, sesame, or wheat germ oil, or petroleum jelly; cover with a moist hot towel (leave your nostrils exposed); lie down until the towel cools. For even greater benefit, reheat and replace the towel several times. If you are ready for bed, just tissue off the excess oil; if not, remove it with warm water and a washcloth.

- **Sea spa masque**. Mix sea salt with warm water until it is the consistency of moist sand. Pat over your face and let dry for 15 minutes, covered with a hot towel for the full effect. Aficionados claim this masque does more than rejuvenate the surface, it also shapes up droopy sags.

- **Vegetables** are venerated beautifiers.

  Beets make a magenta-hued masque that men and women will appreciate. In a blender or food processor, puree a raw beet with a teaspoon of heavy cream.

  Carrots, grated, ground, or pureed in their raw state, help firm skin and clear blemishes. An exclusive strictly-for-males salon features a masque you can prepare in a blender from 1 tablespoon beer, 2 teaspoons *each* orange juice and grated carrot, 1 teaspoon yogurt, and $^1/_2$ teaspoon lemon juice. If your skin is drier than the housemate with whom you are sharing, add a few drops of olive oil to your portion.

  Cooking the carrots releases more of their vitamin A for added skin benefit. Mash them to a paste with a little of the unsalted water in which they were cooked; apply while still warm.

  Corn, cut or grated from a fresh ear and mashed or pureed, is a soothing, toning masque for dry skin. Let the milky pulp dry on your face for 20 minutes.

  Cucumber, blender-pureed with cream or yogurt, can work wonders for dry skin. For oily skin, blend a 2-inch chunk of peeled cucumber with an egg white or 2 teaspoons lemon juice plus $^1/_2$ teaspoon mint extract. For normal-combination skin, add 2 teaspoons instant nonfat dry milk.

Peas, fresh or frozen, pureed in a blender and patted over face and throat, make a stimulating masque reported to help even out discolored patches of skin.

"Rabbit" Masque is concocted from "rabbit food" and may qualify your skin for a magazine advertisement: Blender-puree $1/4$ cup *each* chopped cucumber, lettuce, and raw white potato with 1 lemon slice, $1/2$ teaspoon dried peppermint, and $1/8$ teaspoon vitamin C crystals. Scoop the mixture onto lettuce leaves, press over your face and throat, cover with hot-moist towels for 20 minutes, then remove with warm water.

Tomato is a mild astringent that refines pores and acts as an exfoliant. Cut a tomato in thin slices to place over your face for 10 minutes; or, drain the juice and seeds from the slices, mash them to a pulp, and pat on. To add curative benefits for blemished skin: Mix in 1 teaspoon lemon juice plus a little brewer's yeast, oatmeal, and dry milk or yogurt. To increase penetration, cover the tomato masque with a hot, moist towel.

- **Wheat masques**. For normal or oily complexions, mix raw wheat germ (or 1 tablespoon whole wheat flour) with $1/2$ teaspoon vinegar plus water to make a paste. If your skin is dry, mix 1 tablespoon wheat germ with 1 tablespoon milk, yogurt or wheat germ oil. Let stand to soften before patting over your face, then extend the drying time by luxuriating in a beauty bath for 20 minutes.

- **Yeast**. *Baker's yeast,* once sold in moist blocks or foil-wrapped cakes, is a perennial favorite for removing impurities and firming oily skin for males and females. Soften a packet of freeze-dried baking yeast in water to make a smooth paste, slather over your face, then let dry before rinsing off.

  Brewer's yeast can be used for circulation-stimulating, texturizing masques. For normal or combination skin: Mix the yeast into a paste with water. For dry skin: Use milk as the liquid and add a teaspoon of honey; or incorporate 1 teaspoon *each* almond oil, honey, and lemon juice with 3 tablespoons brewer's yeast plus enough water to make a thick paste. For oily skin or normal-combination skin: Use rose water, witch hazel or yogurt to make a paste with the yeast. Add a few drops of peppermint extract for extra zing. For wrinkled skin: Use milk as the liquid and add the contents of a vitamin E capsule. If your skin is very dry, use wheat germ oil instead of milk to mix the paste. After the masque has dried and been rinsed off, rub a little of vitamin E oil (or wheat germ oil) into the wrinkled areas before retiring. For best results, apply twice weekly.

AFTER THE FACIAL IS OVER: HOW TO PROTECT YOUR SALON-LIKE RESULTS

Scandinavians plunge into the snow after a sauna; you can give your facial a Finnish finish by splashing on cold water as the final rinse. To reestablish your skin's pH balance, apply your favorite toner or a mixture of one teaspoon cider vinegar or lemon juice and one-third cup water. Then, to seal in all the good things you have done for your now glowing and rejuvenated skin, apply a thin film of oil or your usual moisturizer.

6

SUCCESSFUL STRATEGIES FOR CLEARING UP NAGGING SKIN PROBLEMS

Skin is so closely related to emotional climate that it not only turns pale and clammy from anxiety, blushes in embarrassment, and glows with happiness; it also responds to malnutrition or stress, as well as external care. Complexion imperfections are equally distributed between the sexes and, for each problem, potential or existing, there are natural preventives and remedies.

PARAFFIN HEAT TREATMENT: QUEEN NEFERTITI'S WAX SECRET UNMASKED

Egypt's Queen Nefertiti is credited with originating this hot-wax facial which is now offered by twentieth-century salons as a multi-purpose unisex skin clarifier and rejuvenator, and has been adapted for at-home use. If your skin is very dry, smooth a film of vegetable oil over your freshly cleansed face before beginning the treatment.

Melt half of a four-ounce cake of paraffin in a cup set in a pan of water over low heat. Test to be sure the wax is not hot enough to burn your skin, then paint your face—except for the tender area around your eyes—with a half-inch paintbrush. Apply generously so the wax forms an airtight seal.

Heat the back of a metal serving spoon by holding it close to water in your wax-melting pan; then "iron" your face with the spoon, paying particular attention to any blemishes, lines, or wrinkles the wax coating will have exaggerated. Continue the ironing for 5 minutes, reheating the spoon each time it cools.

61

Peel off the paraffin as soon as it solidifies after the ironing. Dry-skin lines or wrinkles will have softened and, if your face has been harboring impurities, they will have been drawn to the surface and embedded in the wax. Rinse with cool water, then apply your toner and moisturizer.

How to Eliminate Blackheads and Whiteheads Safely and Naturally

Approximately 20 percent of the body's toxic waste is eliminated through the skin,[20] so scrupulous cleansing plus a diet containing a minimum of saturated fat is important for controlling and removing exterior accumulations of waxy oil. When a minuscule globule of sebum collects at the top of a pore, a whitehead develops; when the waxy oil hardens, plugs the pore and is exposed to air, it turns black through oxidation and becomes a blackhead. Called *comedones* by dermatologists, these facial pests can be exterminated by natural means.

Five Home Remedies for Washing Away Blemishes

1. **Baking soda,** slightly moistened and gently massaged over whiteheads, is sufficiently abrasive to remove the thin covering so the sebum can escape.

2. **Almond meal.** Mix to a paste with water, work into the skin with a complexion brush, and rinse off with cool water.

3. **Cornmeal.** Blend half-and-half with white vegetable shortening, massage in, then tissue off before completely removing with soap and water.

4. **Soapy meal.** Combine $1/4$ cup finely grated castile soap with $1/4$ cup *each* almond meal and cornmeal; store in an airtight container. To use: Scoop a spoonful of the mixture into the palm of your hand, moisten with water, and massage into your face with a complexion brush or sponge. Rinse thoroughly, then splash on a toner made from 1 teaspoon cider vinegar and $1/3$ cup water.

5. **Tomato.** Even before "love apples" were deemed fit for human consumption, beauty-conscious damsels were instructed to cut

a slice from one of the red orbs and rub it into areas plagued by "skin worms." (Tomato contains vitamin C plus an acid that removes dead epidermal cells, thus helping to clear whiteheads and prevent blackheads from turning into pimples.)

REMOVING BLACKHEADS—WHAT THE EXPERTS RECOMMEND

Squeezing is frowned upon by some dermatologists; others admit that physical force is the only way to dislodge deeply embedded blackheads and recommend using a "blackhead extractor" (a metal tool with a tiny hole in the end) or pressing out the offenders with tissue-wrapped fingertips. Before attempting either type of removal, soften the blackheads by steaming or with this "loosening solution" preferred by prestigious salons.

Epsom Salt and Iodine: Bring $1/2$ cup water to a boil, stir in 1 teaspoon epsom salt and 3 drops of iodine. Dip strips of absorbent cotton in the slightly cooled solution, place them over infested areas, and cover with a dry washcloth to retain the heat. Repeat two or three times, reheating the liquid if necessary. After popping out the blackheads, go over your face with peroxide or an alcohol-containing astringent.

HOW TO REDUCE ENLARGED PORES

Usually resulting from the overactive sebaceous glands responsible for comedones, enlarged pores most often appear where the glands are most concentrated, such as on the nose, inner aspects of the cheeks, and the chin. Men are especially vulnerable to this problem, but, as all of us age, our skin loses elasticity and pore openings expand. Improving your diet by including more vitamin-A-containing foods (see the Vitamin and Mineral Chart), or augmenting with a supplement, may be helpful. (A deficiency of vitamin A can cause dead cells below the skin surface to clog oil glands and distend the delicate openings.) While nothing short of plastic surgery will permanently alter existing pore size, much can be done to make large pores less obvious.

- **Benzoin.** In the 1890s, men as well as women were advised to sponge their enlarged pores with a half-and-half blend of tincture of benzoin and water.

Benzoin-cucumber lotion is an even more effective modern adaptation. Grate and mash (or whir in an electric blender) 1 cucumber. Strain into 1 cup of rose water and stir in 1 tablespoon tincture of benzoin. Refrigerate and apply with a cotton ball after each daily cleansing.

- **Buttermilk oatmeal.** Stir 2 tablespoons dry oatmeal into $1/4$ cup buttermilk. Cover and let stand overnight. Strain off the liquid and smooth it over your face. Allow 20 minutes' drying time, rinse off with cool water, rub with an ice cube, then blot dry.

  Buttermilk salt is easier to prepare. Make a gritty paste from buttermilk and table salt. Work into enlarged-pore areas, then rinse with warm water. Repeat several times a week.

- **Egg skin** is a poor-folks' pore-shrinker that also helps bring skin eruptions to a head. Break an egg, reserve its contents for other use, then carefully remove the membrane from the inside of the shell. Smooth this egg skin over the enlarged pores; let dry before peeling off.

- **Make-ahead pore reducer.** Pulverize half of a one-pound package of steel-cut oatmeal in an electric blender or food processor. Mix with $1/2$ cup almond meal, $1/4$ cup powdered orris root, and 1 ounce castile soap (grated from 4-ounce bar). Store in an airtight container. Whenever you cleanse your face, moisten 1 tablespoon of the mixture, apply gently with the fingertips, then rinse off.

How to Win the War Against Acne— and Protect Your Skin from Battle Scars

Papules and pustules sound, and are, ugly—but their eruption doesn't necessarily indicate acne. Facial blemishes can occur as a result of illness, emotional stress (witness pimples popping up before prom night or a promotional presentation), dietary indiscretions, or sketchy cleansing. When sebum and dead skin cells seal up a pore-opening, the continuing flow of waxy oils may force the plug (a white head) to protrude as a blackhead, invade and inflame surrounding tissue, harbor bacteria, and erupt as an angry red bump. Pinching at a blackhead without removing it may also aggravate the skin into producing a blemish. The old rule, "never pick at a pimple," is still good advice; the infection may spread and scarring may result. The following treatments, old and new, for acne papules or pustules are equally viable for all pimples—masculine or feminine.

In true acne (*acne vulgaris*), cells in and around follicle openings reproduce at a greater rate than they die and are shed. Combined with excess sebum production triggered by hormones, the pore-clogged results are the scourge of more teenage boys than girls, and the bane of more women than men because of fluctuating hormonal levels due to menstrual cycles. "Allergy" acne, which can result from reaction to anything from facial cosmetics to the feathers in bed pillows, is no respecter of gender, and may appear on masculine chests and backs as well as faces.

Many men have found that giving their skin a mini-vacation by not shaving on weekends lessens acne-aggravating facial irritation; occasionally, however, more frequent shaving is the answer. Alan's acne, which he thought he'd outgrown, reappeared shortly after he began shaving. A dermatologist's examination revealed that each pustule contained, and was instigated by, an ingrown hair. Shaving more often, *with* instead of *against* the grain, resolved Alan's problem. Stubbornly resistant acne may require medical attention, but natural, at-home care usually is all that is needed.

HOW YOUR DIET CAN HELP REDUCE ACNE FLAREUPS

A balanced diet with adequate protein, ample fluids, sufficient vitamins and minerals, and enough fiber to avoid constipation is essential for basic skin health. Eating habits are no longer believed responsible for creating acne (theories regarding sexual activity, or its lack, as a cause have also been debunked), but nutrition, especially during breakout periods, plays as important role in its control. In their book, *Complete Handbook of Nutrition*,[127] Gary and Steve Null suggest two daily glasses of any combination of fresh carrot, cucumber, lettuce and/or spinach juice. Dr. Blaurock-Busch, co-author of *The No-Drugs Guide to Better Health*,[20] advises drinking one-half cup of beet juice (or eating steamed beets) twice each week. Dr. J. Daniel Palm[129] recommends that women substitute fructose for sugar a few days prior to the menses. Avoiding chocolate, nuts and other fatty foods, strong seasonings, and anything containing iodides (saltwater fish, shellfish, iodized salt, bromides) has benefitted some acne endurers.

Personal experimentation is the best policy: eliminating all possible offenders for two weeks, then reintroducing them one at a time will let you know which foods trigger flareups.

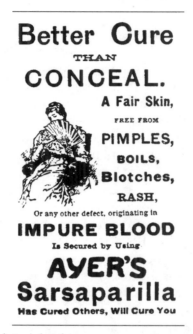
Herbalists advise drinking one or two cups a day of any one of these herb teas to "purify" the blood and clear skin disturbances: burdock, chaparral, chickweed, dandelion, red clover, strawberry leaf, valerian, white oak bark, or yellow dock.

Holistic doctors have found daily doses of up to 100,000 IU water-soluble vitamin A (for brief periods) and 5 grams vitamin C of benefit in some cases of acne.[141] More impressive results have been obtained with the inclusion of a high-potency B-complex tablet, 400 IU vitamin D, 100 to 400 IU "dry" vitamin E, 1,000 milligrams calcium, and 50 milligrams zinc.[19,136] Acidophilus (in supplements or as a serving of yogurt with each meal) is often helpful and is considered essential whenever antibiotics are prescribed. Brewer's yeast or desiccated liver (one to two tablespoons, or the equivalent in tablets, daily) has proven effective for some individuals; and charcoal tablets (two after each meal for two weeks, then two per day) are credited with astounding results.[77]

NATURAL SOAPLESS CLEANSERS

Gentle cleaning, performed several times daily to remove excess oil and surface contaminants, has been shown to successfully manage 25 percent of acne conditions.[141] Harsh scrubbing or the folk remedy of plastering pimply areas with soap and allowing it to remain overnight so irritates the skin that the sebaceous glands secrete even more sebum than they would normally. There are natural, soapless cleansers, but if you prefer soap and live in a hard-water area you can avoid the deposits of greasy sludge (created by soap mingling with water and minerals) by softening each quart of washing-rinsing water with one teaspoon of either baking soda or borax. Follow every cleansing with an astringent toner, then allow the pores to breathe by skipping the troubled areas when applying moisturizer.

- **Buttermilk or skim milk.** Wash your face with the milk, rinse with water, then reapply the milk and allow it to dry on your skin.

- **Lemon juice.** Dilute generously with water and rinse thoroughly.

- **Oatmeal, honey, and egg white.** Mixed to a paste and massaged into the face, this mixture cleanses the skin and loosens blackheads.

- **Rubbing alcohol.** Combine 1 part alcohol with 10 parts water.

Steam cleaning is seldom advised during acne outbreaks but brief steaming or hot-towel packs applied for a few minutes once or twice each day may coax the papules into vanishing, or may bring them to a head so they will open and drain.

COMPRESSES, MASQUES, POULTICES, AND LOTIONS

Unless otherwise directed, follow each of these natural treatments with a tepid-water rinse and an application of 3-percent hydrogen peroxide, a solution of one tablespoon vinegar and half a cup of water, or an astringent.

- **Aloe vera gel and lecithin.** Whir $1/4$ cup aloe vera gel with 1 tablespoon water-soluble lecithin powder in an electric blender. Apply once each day and let remain for at least 15 minutes, preferably several hours or overnight, before rinsing off. Use plain aloe vera gel as a moisturizer for your entire face.

❧ **Bran and baking soda.** Mix 1 tablespoon miller's bran and 1 teaspoon baking soda to a paste with water. Pat over your skin and rinse off after 15 minutes.

❧ **Cabbage.** You can prepare a lotion by liquefying enough raw cabbage to make 1 teaspoon of "juice" and mixing it with an equal amount of tincture of benzoin. It smells terrible but helps clear blemishes.

❧ **Cabbage pack.** Soften cabbage leaves in hot water with a pinch of boric acid. Spread the leaves over your face and let them remain for 20 minutes.

> *White cabbage pack*, consisting of nothing more exotic than the ground or mashed inner leaves of raw cabbage, is a German treatment for skin blemishes.

❧ **Carrot pulp**, blender-pureed from raw carrots or mashed from cooked ones, improves broken-out skin when thickened with instant nonfat dry milk, patted on and allowed to dry.

❧ **Cornstarch and alcohol.** Mix rubbing alcohol with a teaspoon of cornstarch to make a paste. Dab a bit on each pimple with a cotton-tipped swab, leave in place for 30 minutes to 8 hours before rinsing off.

Gerald had wonderful success with this drying-out remedy suggested by his barber; his occasional pimples disappeared after a few overnight treatments. Suddenly, however, the pustules began multiplying so noticeably that the barber asked if he had been trying a new treatment. "No, I'm still daubing on the cornstarch and alcohol every night," Gerald said. "The only thing 'new' is the shaving brush I bought last month. First time I've ever used one, and, if it wasn't for these pimples, I'd really enjoy shaving every morning." After the barber explained that shaving brushes can become contaminated with bacteria from existing pustules and spread the infection, Gerald went back to lathering up with his hands. By the time he went in for his next haircut, the acne was once again under control.

❧ **Cucumber and rum.** Blend 2 tablespoons grated raw cucumber with 2 teaspoons rum. Pat on and let dry before rinsing. Refrigerate the remainder to apply as the next treatment.

🖎 **Dock root**, also called yellow dock, is a centuries'-old cure for skin eruptions. You can mash the hot, cooked, roots, spread them on gauze squares and apply them to your face for 30 minutes (replacing the compresses when they cool); or blender-puree the dock with the water in which it was cooked, strain, and use the liquid as a clearing-toning lotion each time you wash your face.

🖎 **Eggs.** Smooth on a film of vitamin E (from a pierced capsule), wait 30 minutes, then apply a coating of whisked egg white.

Egg yolk, despite its fat content, often brings improvement when lightly beaten, patted over the skin, and allowed to dry.

🖎 **Garlic.** Rub a slice of fresh garlic over the pimples several times each day.

🖎 **Honey.** Use plain or mix with raw wheat germ to kill germs and draw out blemishes. Apply with tapping motions, wait 5 minutes before rinsing off.

🖎 **Milk of magnesia** is not only a "drawing" masque, it is, according to makeup expert Paula Begoun,[13] a more effective acne medication than those prescribed by doctors. Smooth over your clean skin, let dry, then rinse off. Repeat several times daily but never leave on your face overnight.

🖎 **Oatmeal.** Cook in milk and apply daily as a 10-minute masque.

🖎 **Papaya mint tea**, brewed double strength and applied as a hot compress for 15 minutes twice daily, often brings immediate improvement and clears skin within two or three days.[33]

🖎 **Pears** have a disinfectant, drawing action when peeled, cored, mashed, and used as a 10-minute facial pack.

🖎 **Potato lotion.** Grate a raw potato into a sieve over a bowl and let stand until the "juice" drips out. Apply this liquid with a cotton ball, let dry before rinsing.

🖎 **Tomato pulp** helps heal blemishes. Mash or puree tomato slices and blend with nonfat dry milk to make a paste. Smooth on and let dry for 10 minutes.

🖎 **Valerian tea.** Prepare double strength and apply as a hot compress several times a day.

᠊᠊ **Witch hazel.** Saturate gauze or cotton pads with witch hazel straight from the bottle, and cover the affected areas for 5 minutes at a time at least once a day.

SUNLIGHT

Exposure to the sun helps kill pimple-causing germs on the skin, instigates the body's production of vitamin D to assist with the assimilation of skin-improving vitamin A, and encourages the upper epidermal layer to peel off and unplug the oil-gland ducts. Moderation is essential, however, to prevent provoking a pimply condition with a sunburn or with the mineral salts from perspiration. If you're using an acne medication containing retinoid acid, be forewarned that when exposed to ultraviolet light it can increase the danger of burning and the risk of skin cancer. A 60-watt light bulb in an unshielded base offers an alternative to sunlight. It won't do anything for your vitamin-D supply, but, when positioned a foot away from the pustules for 15-minute periods, may help dry them up.

ALL-NATURAL TREATMENTS FOR DEALING WITH SKIN DISCOLORATIONS

ACNE ROSACEA: THE RED-FACED FLUSH

No respecter of skin type or sex, acne rosacea's red-faced flush is aggravated by extreme temperatures, emotional stress, eating highly spiced foods, or imbibing alcoholic beverages. In severe cases, more common among men than women, small acne-like pimples appear and the skin may thicken, become purplish-red over the cheeks and chin, and create the bulbous-looking nose associated with chronic alcoholism. Usually, however, the dilated blood vessels responsible for the unattractive rosiness will shrink back to normalcy with proper care.

Here are some preventive measures you can take:

᠊᠊ Protect your face from inclement weather, wind, and fireplace or open-oven-door heat.

᠊᠊ Cleanse gently with mild cleansers and tepid water. Use non-tingly toners or after-shave lotions; refrain from exfoliating scrubs, facial saunas, or icy chillers.

🍃 Eat and drink wisely. Supplement your daily multivitamin with a B-complex tablet at each meal; up to 300 milligrams per day of each of the "major" B's is considered safe for periods of a few weeks.[115] (Alcohol destroys vitamin B, which may account for acne rosacea being dubbed "grog blossoms" in colonial times.)

BLOTCHINESS

In addition to the treatments described for dealing with a fading tan in Chapter 9, ingesting two tablespoons of brewer's yeast daily, including fresh peas and fish in your diet, and frequently splashing your face with a solution of one tablespoon vinegar plus one-half cup water, may help obliterate the blotchiness. Masques of mashed fresh peas or raw wheat germ blended with honey have also proven beneficial.

SPIDER VEINS

Fair skins are most susceptible to these little red lines (technically termed *telangiectases*) that wander over cheeks and noses, but anyone can acquire them from a variety of causes. Overzealous scrubbing or blackhead squeezing, dilation from overexposure to sunlight, or the sudden contraction and expansion necessitated by wintery cold and indoor heat may rupture close-to-the-surface capillaries. Vitamin deficiencies can so weaken them that blood seeps out into surrounding areas and/or they lose their elasticity. With tender care, the tiny veins become less obvious and may shrink back into oblivion. The *don't*s are the same as those for acne rosacea: avoid irritation from extreme temperature changes, harsh physical treatment, or overindulgence in spicy foods or alcohol. The *do*s are also similar, with a few additions.

Foods and Supplements: To augment your basic good-skin diet (sufficient protein, lots of fiber-rich fruits and vegetables, ample fluid), take a multivitamin-mineral and at least one B-complex tablet each day. To strengthen capillaries and connective tissues, eat foods high in vitamin C (see the Vitamin and Mineral Chart) and take supplements of C plus bioflavinoids.

Herbal Treatments:

🍃 **Camomile and white oak bark**: Simmer $1/2$ teaspoon white oak bark in 1 cup water for 10 minutes, add $1/2$ teaspoon camomile, turn off the heat and let stand, covered, until comfortably warm. Strain. Saturate pieces of cotton cloth in the liquid and place them over the veins for 5 minutes at a time once each day.

- **Parsley**: Cook half a bunch of freshly washed parsley in water to cover, or whir the raw parsley and water in an electric blender. Strain. Stir a teaspoon of honey into the liquid and smooth it over the spidery veins several times a day.

- **Shave grass**: This is a folk remedy for alleviating splotchy veins and improving the elasticity of connective tissue. Place 2 tea-spoons dried shave grass in 1 cup cold water. Bring to boiling, cover, and let steep for 10 minutes before straining. Drink two-thirds of the tea, then saturate cotton cloth in the remainder and cover the affected area for 5 minutes. Repeat the treatment every other day.

HOW TO PERK UP PALE FACES

Medieval beauties aspired to skin so pale that a swallow of red wine could be seen flowing down their throats. This about-to-faint look is no longer desirable. If your physician has verified that your wan appearance is not due to internal dysfunction, you can restore a healthy glow by:

- Exfoliating your face every few days to dispense with dead-cell debris and revive natural color.

- Getting more fresh air and exercise to stimulate your circulation.

- Getting more rest and sleep to counteract the exhaustion that might be responsible for your weary appearance.

- Icing the skin surface to stimulate blood flow. If you are not trou-bled with broken veins, crush a few ice cubes, wrap them in a thin towel, spritz with witch hazel from a spray bottle, then rub the frosty bundle over your face and throat with uplifting motions. Repeat several times a week.

- Rubbing a cube of fresh watermelon over your face and letting the liquid dry before rinsing. (You can stash a cache of small chunks of watermelon in a plastic bag in the freezer for retrieval during out-of-season months.)

- Masking your face with soy powder and yogurt mixed to a paste, rubbed in and allowed to remain for 30 minutes before removing with a wet washcloth.

- Supplementing your diet with copper, folic acid, and iron (see the Vitamin and Mineral Chart for food sources).

- Trying the folk-healers' advice for "pallid women": Bathe your face in water to which a few drops of tincture of benzoin have been added. If this is not sufficient, follow with an application of $1/_8$ teaspoon benzoin mixed with 1 tablespoon rose water and allow it to dry on the skin. If all else fails, mix 1 tablespoon rose water with $1/_2$ teaspoon each ammonia and glycerin, rub into your face after the benzoin wash, let dry for 3 minutes, then blot with a soft towel.

How to Smooth Rough, Bumpy Skin

Sometimes appearing as "goose flesh" on the backs of upper arms as well as on male and female faces, small bumps at the base of invisible hair follicles are called *folliculosis*. They, and rough-textured skin, may indicate a deficiency of vitamin A that can be corrected by daily supplements of 25,000 IUs of A plus 400 IUs of vitamin D. Here are some other suggestions:

- Facial scrubs and steams help to depose any accumulation of dead cells or pore-clogging soil which might be responsible for the roughness.

- Pat on some honey and allow a few minutes of skin-softening-time before rinsing off.

- Massage mayonnaise (store-bought or made from the recipe in the Glossary) into your face, let permeate for 5 minutes or leave on as a skin-smoothing night cream.

- Rose water and brandy, combined half-and-half and sponged over the face several times daily, is an 1890's suggestion for combating windburn or persistent roughness.

- Rosemary egg white is a skin smoother that should be stored in the refrigerator and applied every other day: Steep 1 teaspoon dried rosemary in 2 tablespoons boiling water for 15 minutes.

Strain, then blend with 1 egg white and 1 teaspoon instant non-fat dry milk.

ꝗ Watercress water is a time-proven remedy for rough skin. Boil a cup of freshly rinsed, chopped watercress leaves and stems in a cup of distilled water. Let cool, strain, and apply several coats of the liquid. Allow each layer to dry before the next application, then rinse with cool water. Store in the refrigerator and use daily until improvement is noticeable. Prepare a fresh supply every seven days and continue biweekly treatments as preventive maintenance.

MANAGING MATURING SKIN: HOW TO HELP OFFSET—AND PREVENT—UNSIGHTLY LINES, SAGS, AND WRINKLES

No one wants the expressionless face of an android or a store manikin; the goal is to maintain a youthful appearance by postponing or lessening the lingering lines from smiles and scowls that herald what we regard as "maturing skin." Our adversaries are the biological reduction of glandular activity which dries skin and deteriorates its connective tissues so lines and wrinkles form; and gravity, whose downward pull creates baggy eyes, saggy jowls, and double chins. Mother Nature is the ally who will assist our nurturing efforts, diminish the signs of time, and slow their advance.

TIPS ON NOURISHING MATURING SKIN

What you ingest affects facial muscles and supportive tissues as well as the epidermal surface. To compensate for the body's gradually slowing cell production and less efficient metabolism of foods, it is important to provide it with ample protein (meats, eggs, dairy products, legume-grain-milk combinations), and with a generous supply of vitamins.

Manufacturers offer higher-potency multiples for the "chronologically advantaged"; nutritionists often advise adding individual supplements:

- Taking a daily B-complex tablet (and/or a tablespoon or so of brewer's yeast) is good insurance. Laboratory tests have shown that a deficiency of any one of the B's causes young animals to develop the wrinkled aspects of old age.[79]

    • Vitamin C is good for collagen and elastin, the intertwining fibers
supporting your face. Collagen cannot be absorbed from even the
most convincingly advertised cosmetic, it is produced and maintained by the body from ingested protein and vitamin C with the
assistance of the B complex.[159] Taking 1,000 to 5,000 milligrams of
vitamin C in divided doses each day helps preserve and rejuvenate collagen's ability to prevent lines, sags, and wrinkles.[7]

Ｈｏw to Control Expression Lines

The 55 muscles in your face, each "wired" to nerves connected to your
brain, react to everything you do, eat, or think. Except for those around
your eyes and mouth, these muscles are not bound to the bones as
they are on the rest of the body; they are attached to the skin by wisps
of fibrous tissue that gradually lose their elasticity and allow your skin
to become set in its ways. Facial tenseness, squinting, frowning in concentration or displeasure all pull at the skin, bunching it up to create
little furrows which can become permanent expression lines.
Although considered "character lines" on masculine faces, they are an
aging-skin giveaway men as well as women are eager to postpone.
These lines are so commonplace that remedies abound. Facial massage, gently performed on clean, lubricated skin is one solution.
Isometric exercises are considered ideal for improving facial muscles
(laboratory tests show that tensing muscles for six to ten seconds each
day increases their resistance to our expression lining and gravity's
efforts[141]). Smoothing out the lines with surface reminders is another
option.

"Label" Your Lines

Trim stationery-store gummed or peel-and-press labels to fit your
lines. Cleanse and dry your face, then gently rub the lines against
the grain to flatten the skin before pressing the label in place. For
normal training, leave in place for 30 minutes at a time, three times
a week. For an accelerated course, sleep with your labels one or
two nights a week. Peel off carefully (after moistening mucilage-
backed labels), rinse with warm water, then use your toner and
moisturizer.

LEARN TO WATCH YOURSELF

Keeping a mirror by your telephone is a tricky way to catch yourself frowning or wrinkling your brow as you talk. Once you are aware of how these expressions "feel" on the inside, you can avoid them.

Smiling at yourself also pays handsome dividends. You have to experiment. You don't want to look like Mona Lisa or the Cheshire Cat—just a hint of a smile. After you practice for a while, it becomes automatic.

PSYCHOCOSMETICS: DO-IT-YOURSELF PHYSICAL AND MENTAL FACE CONTROL WITH THE HELP OF A MIRROR

Based on the premise that radiant external beauty can be developed through physical and mental face-control in front of a mirror, Psychocosmetics is a European science you can practice without a license.

1. Slowly bend your head backward, then forward until your chin touches your chest. Relax your lower jaw and shake your head for a minute.

2. Raise your head, place your palms over your cheeks, and bend your head back as far as possible for a few seconds.

3. Lift your head, look yourself in the eye (in the mirror), and give your facial muscles some positive autogenic suggestions: "The corners of my mouth rise, my forehead is smooth" . . . whatever reinforcement your face may require. Conclude the treatment with a deep yawn.

RELAXING YOUR FACE

1. Lean back, tense your face by squinching your eyes shut and clenching your teeth, then relax. Imagining warm water flowing over your face may assist relaxation efforts. Relaxing your hands by shaking them vigorously before dropping them limply in your lap also encourages facial relaxation.

2. Mentally visualize yourself in a calmly pleasant setting. Once you establish this feeling of untensed muscles, maintain it for five minutes by luxuriating in your imagination and rejecting any interfering, stressful thoughts; then yawn deeply.

FLATTENING FOREHEAD AND FROWN LINES

1. Banding your forehead increases circulation and helps break unconscious habits of brow wrinkling. Make your headband by sewing or pinning a 3-inch-wide elastic bandage so it fits snugly. Prepare a medicated lotion by dissolving $^{1}/_{4}$ teaspoon epsom salt in 1 tablespoon hot water, then stirring in 2 teaspoons glycerin and 1 teaspoon 10-percent menthol solution. Use a cotton ball to smooth the liquid over your forehead, position the band, and leave it in place for an hour once each day.

2. Massaging, plumping or stroking minimizes both horizontal and vertical lines. Sit with your elbows resting on a tabletop, apply cream or oil to your forehead.

   Massage by pressing your left hand firmly on the hairline on the right side, then using the fingertips of your right hand to rub the area below your left hand with circular motions for 10 seconds. Move your left hand to the center of your hairline, then to your left side, repeating until your entire forehead has been massaged.

   Plump by creating suction between the heel of one hand and the lines, then vigorously "pumping" at least 10 times.

   Stroke your forehead gently, with upward-outward motions starting between your brows, until you feel a soothing sense of relaxation.

3. Exercising your forehead requires working the muscles against resistance because there is such a thin layer of tissue supporting the skin.

   a. Press the heels of your hands against each temple. Intermesh your fingers over your forehead, hold them stationary while attempting to first pull your forehead up toward your hairline, then down toward your eyes. Maintain each position for 10 seconds, repeat 5 times.

b. Press the heel of one hand over your scowl lines to flatten them out. Try to move the skin by attempting to frown against the pressure, then try to stretch the frown muscles toward your temples. Repeat each movement 5 times.

NEGATING NOSE TO MOUTH FURROWS

Exercise can help avoid or abolish the parenthesis-shaped lines between nose, mouth, and cheeks.

1. Puff out your cheeks as far as you can, then use your fists to press out the air. Repeat 10 times.

2. Simulate a kiss by puckering your lips. Move them in a circle from right to left, then left to right. Repeat 8 times for each side. Follow by opening your mouth wide, then puckering up again. Repeat 10 times.

3. Smile toothlessly by slowly opening your mouth and turning the corners up as you keep your teeth covered with your lips. Hold until you experience tension, then slowly form an "O" with your mouth. Relax and repeat.

4. Squeeze your eyes shut, wrinkle up your nose, hold for 10 seconds. Relax, then repeat 10 times.

   ⮞ Masque the furrows. To decrease line depth, make a thick paste of brewer's yeast and water. Pat it over the lines and let dry. Rinse off with warm water, blot, then smooth on moisturizer. Repeat 3 times each week.

   ⮞ Soften the lines by massaging them with a dab of moisturizer each time you cleanse your face.

HOW TO SAFELY MINIMIZE WRINKLES

Product-promises for producing more youthful skin probably predate Cleopatra, but none, so far, has proven reliable. *The Harvard Medical School Health Letter* of December 1987 states that estrogen-containing cosmetics have no long-lasting results; and the anti-wrinkle food supplement *SOD* (superoxide dismutase) can't even reach the skin because its enzymes are destroyed by digestive juices in the stomach.[22] The exciting news about wrinkle-removing *tretinoin* (a derivative of vitamin A marketed as Retin-A) has been tempered by the results of further study; the *University of California, Berkeley Wellness Letter* (April 1988) reports that four months of treatment were required before even subtle improvements were apparent, and that most of the subjects tested suffered skin inflammation lasting from two weeks to several months. *Alpha hydroxy acids* are another recently unveiled "fountain of facial youth." *Prevention* (March 1988) describes these acids as natural compounds which, when used under the guidance of a dermatologist, can change the structure of the skin to reduce existing wrinkles. While waiting for these miraculous cures to be perfected, there are many natural methods for regenerating our maturing faces.

THREE WAYS TO REVITALIZE DRY SKIN

Heredity is only one factor in the onset of after-30 dryness and lack of resiliency besetting most women and many fair-skinned men. Exposure to ultraviolet rays or smoking (which impairs circulation by constricting blood vessels) hastens the process. You can forestall drying, collagen collapse, and premature wrinkling by:

- Humidifying your rooms during the heating season to add moisture to your skin's environment.

- Including two tablespoons of unsaturated oil in a balanced diet containing adequate protein; counting your drinks to be sure you imbibe the equivalent of six to eight glasses of water each day; and taking a daily multivitamin-mineral supplement, a B-complex tablet, and at least 1,000 milligrams of vitamin C (more, if you smoke).

- Pampering your skin with gentle cleansers, toners, moisturizers, and masques, including this herbal-oil treatment: Empty the contents of 2 camomile tea bags into a jar. Add $1/4$ cup sesame oil and 2 tablespoons wheat germ oil. Shake to combine, let stand for 24 hours. Shake again, strain the oil, and store it in the refrigerator. Smooth over dry-skin areas after your morning cleansing, let permeate for 5 minutes, then rinse off with lukewarm water. Repeat before bedtime, but instead of rinsing, blot the excess oil with a tissue and leave the remainder for an all-night treatment.

EIGHT WRINKLE-PREVENTION TREATMENTS

Cheeky is what wrinkles are, and where they usually make their first appearance. As reported in *University of California, Berkeley Wellness Letter* (February 1989) women are more prone to wrinkling than men because most males have a thicker dermis (the layer just under the skin's surface), which remains elastic longer than a woman's. Sleeping on your back to avoid skin-tugging-and-wrinkling by your pillow is one method of prevention and treatment, and there are others:

- Castor oil, cocoa butter, and coconut oil, the most revered wrinkle chasers, may be applied as frequently as desired.

- Egg white. Daily use of any of the egg white masques described in Chapter 5, or merely covering your face with raw egg white (with or without a few drops of lemon juice) each morning before you brush your teeth and rinsing it off as you shower, can produce dramatic results.

- Egg yolk and mayonnaise. Use a "blush brush" to paint your face with raw egg yolk, applying it thickly over wrinkled or lined areas. While the egg is drying, mix 2 tablespoons mayonnaise with $1/_2$ teaspoon *each* fuller's earth and powdered kelp. Apply this paste over the egg yolk; rinse off after 10 minutes.

  Mayonnaise, bottled or homemade (see Glossary for recipe), has transformed "prune faces" into "peaches and cream" when applied several times daily for several months.[41] For speedier results, blend an egg yolk with $1/_4$ cup of the mayonnaise.

- Ironing out the wrinkles is a before-the-party treatment. Cleanse your face, smooth on a generous coating of petroleum jelly or vegetable oil, then "iron" the lines and wrinkles with the bowl of a metal spoon heated in a cup of hot water. Go over your face several times, reheating the spoon when it cools. Tissue off the excess oil and sponge your face with a mild freshener.

- Lecithin granules, dissolved in warm water, mixed with cold-pressed vegetable oil and rubbed into the skin for all-day or all-night treatments reduce wrinkles when used religiously over a period of months.

- Oatmeal masques soften skin, making it less prone to wrinkle. For a no-bother, daily regimen: Reserve $1/_4$ cup leftover breakfast oatmeal in the refrigerator. Every evening, mix 1 tablespoon of the oatmeal with $^1/_2$ teaspoon each cream and vegetable oil. Gently massage over your face and throat, and rinse away after 20 minutes.

🍂 Olive oil, lemon juice, and salt improve skin as well as salad. Twice each day, rub olive oil into your clean face. Pat on lemon juice, drop by drop, until your skin feels "tacky," then briskly rub sea salt (or a half-and-half blend of epsom salt and table salt) over your face. Rinse off with warm water and blot dry.

🍂 Yogurt and vitamin E are aging-skin fighters. Blend 2 teaspoons yogurt and $^1/_2$ teaspoon *each* honey and lemon juice with the contents of a 400 IU vitamin-E capsule. Smooth over your face, let penetrate for 15 minutes, then rinse.

EGG WHITE: NATURE'S UNIQUE WRINKLE-ERASER

Egg white can make wrinkles disappear for a few hours. Stir a raw egg white with a fork, then use a fine camel's hair brush to carefully paint each visible wrinkle. For around-the-eyes lines, pat on a thin-as-possible coating of the egg white. Let dry, then apply a makeup foundation with equal care, using tapping rather than stroking motions.

Tom watched Martha painting out her wrinkles and was so astounded by the results he decided to try egg white on the fine lines around his eyes. Rather than resort to painstaking brush strokes, he simply rubbed his finger around the inside of an eggshell, then smoothed on the thin film of egg white. The effect was almost instantaneous. Now, each time Martha cracks an egg, Tom applies his wrinkle eraser.

COPING WITH CROW'S FEET

🍂 **Exercise** tones muscles to prevent or diminish crow's feet and eye crinkles.

1. Open your eyes as wide as possible. Look up, down, to the left, and to the right, holding each position for 6 seconds.

2. Close your eyes, scrunch up your face, and hold that position for 6 seconds. Then open your eyes and raise your eyebrows for 6 seconds.

3. Place your palms on your cheeks, your fingers at the outer corners of each eye. With the fingers, draw the eye muscles toward your temples. Hold for 6 seconds, relax, then repeat.

❧ **Massage** stimulates circulation to strengthen muscles and revitalize skin. Without stretching the skin, run your fingers around the bony edge of your eye sockets. Begin at the bridge of the nose, move under the eyebrows, then across the top of the cheeks. Repeat until you have made 6 complete trips around your eyes. To stimulate the under-eye area, fingertip-tap the circular area from the top of your ears to the bridge of your nose.

❧ **Vitamin E.** Doctors Evan and Wilfred Shute[166, 167] who pioneered vitamin E research, discovered that alpha tocopherol molecules penetrate the epidermis to reach supporting skin tissues, and demonstrated that when applied regularly, vitamin E's firming and tightening action postpones and lessens wrinkles. Independent clinical studies verify that four weeks of under-eye treatment with vitamin E can make fine lines less noticeable.[47]

Snip a capsule of d-alpha tocopherol (not a "dl" synthetic or "mixed" tocopherol). Pat the slightly sticky liquid under your eyes and let it dry. If you treat your face twice a day, use 200 IU capsules; if only once each day, use 400 IU capsules.

De-LINING YOUR MOUTH: HOW TO OFFSET SURROUNDING LINES

A variety of remedies are offered for abolishing, or at least reducing, vertical or cross-hatched lines between the upper lip and nose, and the tiny crevices that cause lipstick to bleed into skin surrounding the mouth. Patience is a necessary virtue in these treatments; it took years for the "whistle marks" to develop, and it may take months to reduce or obliterate them.

❧ Vitamin E (from a snipped capsule), or wheat germ oil, sometimes dispenses with these sunburst lines when rubbed across-the-grain to flatten and fill in cracks and crevices.

❧ Do-it-yourself skin peels, performed twice weekly on the area between nose and upper lip, help smooth out these lines.

Experiment with the exfolients in Chapter 2; or heat a table-spoon of bottled mineral water, stir in $1/2$ teaspoon sea salt, rub it in and let it dry, then rinse off and follow with a moisturizer.

&. Exercises are especially effective around the mouth because the muscles are directly attached.

1. Form an "O" with your mouth. Tense the muscles for 6 seconds. Relax for 6 seconds. Repeat 5 times.

2. Open your mouth as wide as possible by simulating a yawn, then pull your lips over your teeth and smile toothlessly. Hold for 6 seconds, relax, then repeat 5 times.

3. Push your lips out as far as possible and suck in your cheeks. Hold for 6 seconds, then relax. Repeat 5 times.

FIRMING UP: HOW TO SABOTAGE GRAVITY'S SAGS AND BAGS

Movie makeup artists pad young faces with wads of cotton to portray aging visages. In real life, gravity and flabby muscles produce the bulgy sags, while firming the muscles with massage and exercise preserves (or restores) youthful contours. In addition:

&. Apply creams or oils with upward strokes on the face and with gentle taps around the eye area to avoid pulling or stretching the fragile skin.

&. Munch chewy nibbles such as carrot and celery sticks to improve your jawline as well as your middle.

&. Eat a well-balanced diet to provide Mother Nature with the ingredients for cell production, and don't succumb to yo-yo dieting which can shrink and stretch skin tissues almost beyond repair.

&. Recline on a slant board for a few minutes each day to reverse gravity's pull and increase blood circulation to the face.

HOW TO MASSAGE YOUR FACE AND THROAT

Giving yourself a facial massage is fundamentally a matter of lubricating your skin and working your way up from throat to forehead with firm-but-gentle movements. Skin specialists advise a more precise method of manipulating your face after you have coated it with petroleum jelly, vegetable oil, or either of these two lotions to help your fingers glide over the skin.

Almond-castor oil lotion: In a wide-mouth jar, combine $1/4$ cup *each* almond oil and castor oil with 2 tablespoons petroleum jelly and $1/2$ teaspoon peppermint extract (optional). Refrigerate if it is not all used within 2 weeks. Warm in a pan of hot water if it becomes too thick to spread.

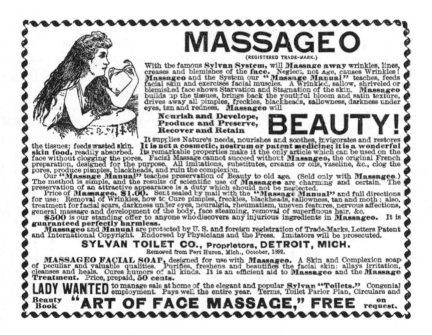

❧ GINSENG-GELATIN LOTION ❧

$1/2$ cup bottled mineral water (divided)

1 teaspoon unflavored gelatin

$1 1/2$ teaspoons ginseng powder or crushed ginseng tablets

$1/2$ teaspoon each glycerin and powdered kelp

1 capsule each natural vitamin A and vitamin E

Place 3 tablespoons of the mineral water in the container of an electric blender. Sprinkle with the gelatin and let it soften while bringing the remainder of the water to a boil. Pour in the hot water and whir to blend. Add remaining ingredients—squeezing in the contents of the capsules—and blend on medium speed. Decant into a wide-mouthed jar and refrigerate if not used within a week or so.

Here's how to massage your face and throat:

1. Pull your hair away from your face with a headband or towel turban. Sit comfortably at a table and rub a generous amount of your massage lotion between your palms.

2. Point your chin toward the ceiling. Using rapid strokes, smooth your palms upward and outward from collarbone to chin on each side of your neck. Repeat 5 times. Then apply lotion to the heel of one hand and use it to massage the tensed muscles under your chin.

3. Starting at the chin line on either side of the mouth, lift upward and outward from mouth to cheekbone, using your palms with firm, gliding motions. Repeat 10 times.

4. Apply lotion to the backs of your fingers. Make a fist with each hand and use your coated fingers to make firm, upward movements from your jawline to the tops of your ears. Repeat 10 times.

5. Dip your fingertips in the lotion. Place your fingers in the center of your forehead and sweep toward the temples. Repeat 10 times. Arch your fingers and press the entire forehead from brow to hairline, allowing 5 seconds for each pressure area. Follow by firmly pressing your thumbs over your scowl lines.

6. Form a "V" with the index and middle finger of each hand. Make 8 firm, upward strokes from the corners of the mouth to the tops of the ears, then start at the edge of the nostrils and repeat.

7. Extend the fingers of both hands and go over your entire face 5 times with small, circular motions. If you encounter any painful spots, pause and apply direct pressure for a few seconds to relieve tension and ease the discomfort.

8. Conclude the massage by tapping your fingers over your skin, beginning at the base of the throat and ending at the temple pressure points. Remove the lotion with tissues and a warm-water rinse.

In his late forties, George was still regarded as the "fair-haired young man" of his company, and maintaining this image was vital to his climb up the corporate ladder. When his wife began a regimen of before-bed facial massage and exercise, he decided to join her. Within two weeks George realized that his face-lifting endeavors had produced a bonus—his skin's increased smoothness and elasticity made shaving much easier!

FACE-LIFTING EXERCISES

Practiced persistently on a daily basis, exercise can restore lost strength to facial muscles and elasticity to their supporting tissues. Devise your own regimen from the following options, with or without an application of this stimulating cream applied to the jowl and under-chin area: 1 egg white, 1 tablespoon milk, 1 teaspoon each honey, liquid camphor, and mint extract; whisked to blend. Smooth on the mixture and let it dry. After completing your exercises, rinse with cool water and apply a moisturizer.

- Press the heels of your hands firmly against the crow's feet area, elevate your chin slightly, and open your mouth about an inch. Wrinkle your nose, contract your neck muscles, and smile as broadly as you can. Hold for 6 seconds. Relax and repeat 10 times.

- With your head thrown back, try to bite an imaginary apple. Relax and repeat 10 times.

- Open your mouth wide and try to contract your neck muscles at the same time. Repeat 10 times. Then open your mouth again and pull your lips in over your teeth. Pretend you are chewing by closing and opening your mouth 10 times.

- Stick out your chin and position your lower teeth over the upper ones. Nod your head up and down as you turn from far left to far right. Relax and repeat for a total of 10 left-to-right swings, then repeat the sequence from right-to-left.

- With your lips slightly parted, move your jaw from side to side as far as possible. Relax a few seconds between 10 repetitions. Then press your tongue against the roof of your mouth as forcefully as you can for a slow count of 6. Relax and repeat 3 times.

- Close your mouth but keep your teeth a quarter of an inch apart. Suck your cheeks between your teeth and hold for 6 seconds. Relax and repeat 3 times.

- Clench your back teeth, hold for 6 seconds, then release and drop your jaw. Slowly bring your jaw up again and bite down on your back molars for another 6 seconds. Relax and repeat for a total of 10 clenchings.

- Without lifting either shoulder, try to touch your left shoulder with your left ear and your right shoulder with your left ear. Repeat 3 times for each side. Follow this exercise by slowly circling your head 5 times to the right and 5 times to the left.

- Play turtle by pushing your neck out as far as it will go without moving your shoulders. Hold for 6 seconds, then slowly pull your chin in as far as you can toward your throat. Hold that position for 6 seconds, then relax and repeat several times.

- Wring a lightweight terry towel out of warm water, twist it into a rope and firmly but gently seesaw it under your chin with upward, outward motions.

- Lie on your back across a bed. With shoulders supported, let your head hang over the edge, then slowly raise and lower it 10 times.

- Squat with your buttocks resting on your heels, hands on your knees, and back straight. Thrust your hands out in front of you with fingers spread. Look up toward the ceiling with eyes wide open. Stick your tongue out and down as far as possible, then up to try to touch your nose. Hold this ungainly pose for a few moments; exhale deeply and relax. Repeat 5 times. (This Oriental yoga position, called "The Lion," tones muscles in both face and throat.)

DOUBLE-CHIN LIFT

European salons espouse this doubly potent method for disposing of double chins. You can achieve the same results, and save airfare to Paris, by contriving a strap from a strip of 3-inch-wide elastic bandage placed under your chin and tied at the top of your head. To duplicate the salons' secret solution: Dissolve $1/2$ teaspoon epsom salt in 2 tablespoons hot water, stir in 1 tablespoon glycerin and 1 teaspoon 10-percent menthol solution. Store tightly covered.

Saturate gauze-covered cotton rectangles or eye pads in the liquid, tuck them between the elastic strap and your chin, and wear the contraption for an hour a day. If the solution irritates your skin, rinse it off and dilute the mixture with water. Use it as strong as bearable to stimulate circulation and help strengthen weakened muscles.

❧ PECTIN INSTANT FACE-LIFT SOLUTION ❧

Cover your hair with a shower cap or towel turban; apply an egg-white masque from Chapter 5, or blend the following ingredients for a pectin face-lift solution:

> *¹/₂ cup mineral water*
>
> *1 tablespoon liquid pectin*
>
> *¹/₂ teaspoon each alum and lemon juice*
>
> *¹/₈ teaspoon vitamin C crystals*

Smooth a thin layer over your face, then dip the gauze in the remaining pectin mixture. Wind the saturated gauze (use dry gauze if you have egg on your face) around your face and head by looping it under your chin, then making several slightly overlapping layers before tying the ends together on top of your head. The gauze should be tight enough to feel firmly comfortable. Leave the mummy-mask in place for 20 minutes while it stiffens to mold facial contours. Remove the gauze and rinse off the residue.

8

BATHING BEAUTY:
THE LUXURIOUS WAY
TO CLEANSE AND BEAUTIFY
YOUR BODY

Dry bathing, accomplished by rubbing the body with a coarsely textured mitt or friction glove, is a European favorite for removing surface debris and leaving skin looking like polished marble. Sponge baths suffice for invalids, or when no other facilities are available. Showering is a fast, efficient method of coping with body-cleaning chores. Tub bathing is a stress-relieving mini-vacation, the luxurious way to cleanse and beautify.

From ancient Roman baths accommodating 20,000 to California hot tubs with room for eight, sociable soaking has been part of almost every culture. Fourth-century aristocrats had their own private baths (as well as indoor latrines with stone troughs for free-flow of sewage into the streets). Cleanliness, however, has not always been regarded as virtuous. Early Christian saints considered dirtiness an insignia of holiness, philosophers' filthy beards were proof of their austere lifestyle. During the Middle Ages and well into the nineteenth-century, European society consisted of the unwashed working class who stank of sweat, and the equally unwashed nobility who reeked of cover-up scents. Our present-day penchant for odor-free cleanliness makes daily ablutions a required ritual.

How TO CONTROL PERSPIRATION AND BODY ODOR

Men sweat. Women perspire. Regardless of terminology, evaporation of this natural moisture is essential for dissipating excess body heat accumulated from metabolic processes, muscular exertion, and external sources. *Eccrine* sweat glands (widely distributed over the body) are stimulated by heat, physical activity, or nervous tension. The *apocrine* sweat glands do not develop until puberty, are activated by pain, sexual excitement or emotional stress, and are concentrated under the arms and around the genitals, with additional outlets on men's backs. Males perspire more profusely than females, although excessive perspiration may be caused by hormonal fluctuations, then wane as glandular activity decreases with age. Studies reported in *American Health* (July 1987) found that aging skin cells contract to partially close off sweat ducts; women between 52 and 62 perspire 30 percent less than younger women.

Normal perspiration is odorless when secreted; "body odor" is produced by bacteria growing and decomposing in the liquid. Only in our well-scrubbed society is this natural fragrance deemed unpleasant; it once was considered so sexually appealing that "love philters" filled with sweat were worn as aphrodisiacs. There is no firm evidence relating the aluminum in commercial deodorants and antiperspirants with the high aluminum levels found in patients with Alzheimer's disease, but for those who prefer Mother Nature's alternatives, there are many.

How Dietary Control Can also Control Perspiration

What we ingest can affect the amount and the scent of our perspiration.

- Caffeine or other stimulants in coffee, tea, chocolate, soft drinks, or over-the-counter medications may be responsible for excess perspiration due to nervous tension.

- Garlic and other pungent seasonings can produce odiferous perspiration.

- Sage. Experimental studies in Germany show that drinking a cup of sage tea every day reduces excessive perspiration;[20] tomato juice blenderized with a handful of fresh sage leaves is even more effective.

- Vitamins and minerals. Dietary supplements of B-complex and magnesium often help reduce the amount of odor-forming perspiration, and a 30- to 50-milligram tablet of zinc each day can perform a dramatic odor-disappearing act.

  ❤ Water. Drinking enough water to dilute as well as replace the pints of liquid the body pours out through the skin each day helps diminish perspiration odor.

Four Natural Deodorants and Antiperspirants

Removing dead skin cells and existing bacteria by washing the armpits with a sudsy loofah during daily bathing usually forestalls odor problems. For additional freshness-security:

1. **Alcohol** is a deodorant and temporary antiperspirant. Apply rubbing alcohol, let dry, then dust with cornstarch.

2. **Baking soda and cornstarch.** Mix equal amounts of soda and cornstarch, or use cornstarch by itself—with a pinch of cloves, if desired. Apply to clean, dry armpits for a deodorant and mild antiperspirant.

3. **Clorophyll.** Chrysanthemum leaves, romaine or other leaf lettuce will produce a few drops of chlorophyll when the leaves are bruised and squeezed. Applied to the armpits, this liquid destroys odor-forming bacteria.

4. **Lavender oil.** Applying a single drop under each arm helps eliminate odor.

Six Natural Solutions for Internal Bathing

Advertisements notwithstanding, a certain degree of odor in the vaginal area is normal and, unless there is an infection or other physical dysfunction, daily douching is not only unnecessary but unwise.[159] When you do want a cleansing, refreshing douche, herbal infusions or other natural solutions are safer, and often more effective, than perfume-and-chemical-laden over-the-counter products.

  ❤ Aloe vera gel is noted for its healing properties. Mix 2 to 4 tablespoons with a quart of water.

  ❤ Baking soda. Dissolve 1 tablespoon in each quart of water.

  ❤ Garlic is helpful for yeast infections. Blender-puree 1 garlic clove with 1 cup water; strain, then add water to make 1 quart.

  ❤ Herbal combinations. For a cleansing-healing combo: Steep 1 teaspoon *each* horsetail and white oak bark in 1 cup boiling water. Strain, stir in 1 tablespoon aloe vera gel and 1/4 teaspoon garlic powder, and add 3 cups water.

Make-ahead deodorant combo: Mix $^1/_2$ cup each dried comfrey, myrtle, peppermint, and spearmint. Store in an airtight jar. When ready to use, bring $^1/_4$ cup of the mixture to a boil in 2 cups water. Cover and steep for 15 minutes. Strain, then add 2 cups water.

&. Individual herbal infusions. Prepare 2 cups regular strength tea from any of the following herbs: barberry, bistort (specific for vaginal bleeding), black walnut, blue cohosh, comfrey, fenugreek, ginger, golden seal, horsetail, marshmallow (specific for vaginal irritation), mint, myrrh, plantain, red raspberry, rose geranium, rosemary, slippery elm, uva ursi, white oak bark (specific for yeast infections), witch hazel bark. Strain through a fine sieve if not using tea bags, then combine with an equal amount of water before using as a douche.

&. Vinegar. Add 1 tablespoon of either white or cider vinegar to 1 quart water, or use 2 tablespoons of any of the Cosmetic Vinegars described in Chapter 3.

Tub Time: Tips on Bathing in Bliss

Body cleansers vary from pure soaps (which leave a residue on both body and tub) to synthetic detergent-deodorant bars (which don't create any scum but may irritate sensitive skin). When tub bathing, the suggested procedure is to soak for 5 to 20 minutes, pull the plug, lather up and scrub while the water drains, then refill the tub with fresh water or turn on the shower to rinse. Loofahs slough off dead skin cells and long-handled brushes are handy for hard-to-reach areas. Men need to pay particular attention to the center of their backs where they have a high concentration of oil glands. To avoid the necessity for fresh-water rinsing, try one of these body-cleansing alternatives you can place in cotton bags or tie in cloth squares to use as scrubbers.

> $^1/_2$ *cup dry oatmeal*
>
> $^1/_2$ *cup each cornmeal and powdered orris root*
>
> *2 tablespoons each almond meal, cornmeal, and crushed elderflowers*

Adding herbs, oils, or other enhancers turns bathing into a bliss-ful interlude whether the purpose is to unwind tense nerves, relieve sore muscles (even the Spartans indulged in warm baths after athletic contests), soften and smooth rough or irritated skin, or simply refresh and invigorate. To transform a prosaic bathroom into your oasis of tranquility: dim the lights or turn them off and light a few candles, then tuck an inflatable bath pillow (or a rolled-up towel) under your head while you luxuriate.

TIME AND TEMPERATURE: DON'T OVERDO

Water has an almost magical ability to either soothe or stimulate, depending on its temperature. A warm bath before bed summons the sandman, a 10-minute tepid soak followed by draining out half the water and refilling the tub with cool water energizes you for an evening engagement or for facing a new day. The vibrant beauty of hearty Scandinavians is not diminished by their practice of charging out of steamy saunas into snowbanks, but our health and beauty experts rec-ommend no such extremes unless prescribed as medical treatment. Piping hot baths increase heart action and expand tiny capillaries into potential spider veins. Icy cold water constricts blood vessels and bru-tally jolts the nervous system. From comfortably warm to briskly cool is the temperature range most beneficial and beautifying. Although Benjamin Franklin reportedly read for hours while reclining in a tub he brought back from England, 15 to 20 minutes is considered sufficient wallowing time. Immersion for longer than 30 minutes can actually leech moisture from your skin, leaving it dry and uncomfortable.

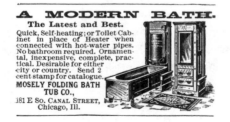

PREBATH TREATMENTS FOR DRY SKIN

- **Oil massage.** Stand in the empty tub. With deep, circular motions, coat yourself from neck to toe with cold-pressed vegetable or nut oil. Let it permeate for 2 to 3 minutes, then fill the tub and proceed with your bath.

🍂 **Steam-heated treat.** Close the shower door or curtain and turn on the hot spray. While steam collects inside the shower, stand beside it on newspapers or an old towel and slather vegetable or nut oil over your face and body. Allow a few moments for it to penetrate before scraping off the excess with a rubber spatula or the back of a table knife. Turn off the water and stand in the closed shower until the steam dissipates, then fill the tub with warm water and soak for 10 to 20 minutes.

With Jeremy's promotion had come the opportunity for midday workouts, and the extra showers were taking their toll. Flaky patches, impervious to lotions, appeared all over his body and he came to the conclusion his skin was either washing off or wearing out. Hesitant about tub bathing (he visualized trying to wash while sitting in a few inches of water with his knees drawn up under his chin), Jeremy agreed to try this steam-heated combination only to save his skin. Which it did. And it was enjoyable. He actually looks forward to his relaxing Saturday-night bath but he can't resist the caustic comment: "You might know . . . I finally rate a key to the executive washroom, and now I have to stand on newspapers outside my own shower!"

BOTANICAL BATHING: HOW TO ENHANCE YOUR BATH WITH HERBS

Marie Antoinette, who bathed in a gilded tub, and Ninon de Lenclos, who scandalized seventeenth-century France with her entourage of avid male followers until she was in her eighties, attributed their beauty to herbal baths. Archaic directions for herbal bathing call for steeping the botanicals in boiling water for 20 minutes, then emptying solids as well as liquids into the bathwater. Today's plumbers might welcome service calls for herb-clogged drains, but emerging from a tub with a coating of soggy seeds and leaves has little appeal. For problem-free botanical bathing:

🍂 Toss a dozen tea bags in the empty tub, run an inch or so of steamy hot water over them, then wait 10 minutes before filling the tub and joining the tea bags.

&. Steep a minimum of $1/2$ cup (ideally, 10 ounces) dried herbs in boiling water for 20 minutes. Strain. Pour the liquid in the tub, then spread the solids on a washcloth for a facial pack or use them as a cloth-encased scrubber. One young man, who is into herbs but not into tub bathing, scrubs with the herb-filled washcloth, then uses the strained liquid as an after-shower rinse.

&. Fill a drawstring cloth bag with the herbs; or place them in the center of a square of doubled cheesecloth, pull up the corners and secure the bag with string, rubber bands, or grocery-store twisters. Hang this pouch over the tub spout waterfall as the tub fills; or, place the bag in a few inches of very hot water in the bottom of the tub for 10 minutes, then fill the tub and soak and scrub with the bagged botanical. If neither you nor your favorite fellow have time for boiling water before bathing, simply anchor the giant tea bag to the shower spout for an herbal waterfall, then detach it for a final rubdown.

25 HERBS AND THEIR UNIQUE BENEFITS

For voluptuously velvety skin, swish a teaspoon of avocado oil in your bath after the herbs have been added, or include half a cup of miller's bran in your herbal bath. You can steep and strain the bran right along with the botanicals; or bag it separately or with your choice of herbs.

&. **Bergamot** is used for relaxing and inducing sleep.

&. **Blackberry leaves,** dried, crumbled, steeped and strained, invigorate the body and relieve sore muscles.

&. **Camomile** is a comforting herb; soothing and relaxing, it has an anti-inflammatory effect on muscles.

&. **Cloves** should be used sparingly, too much can numb the skin.

&. **Comfrey,** used once or twice weekly, rejuvenates the skin.

&. **Elderflowers** are mildly astringent and stimulating.

&. **Eucalyptus leaves** make a body-stimulating bath especially enjoyed by the masculine contingent.

&. **Ginger** is another bath pleaser; adding $1/4$ cup of powdered ginger will chase a wintry chill and help rid the body of toxins. For a mid-summer zinger with male appeal, grate a large ginger root into boiling water and let it steep for 20 minutes. Strain the liquid into a tubful of tepid water, then wrap the solids for a spice-sponge to rev up circulation.

ও **Hops,** basically a beer ingredient, calms the nerves to prepare you for sleep.

ও **Jasmine** can be used for tropical scent plus skin smoothing.

ও **Juniper berries,** the secret ingredient in gin, relieve pain and stimulate circulation to promote a rosy glow. (Adding a few drops of juniper oil is said to have the same effect as $1/_2$ cup of the dried, crushed berries.)

ও **Lavender** is used for fragrance, relaxation, and a clear complexion.

ও **Mint** provides mental as well as physical soothing.

ও **Mustard** soothes sore, tired muscles. Place 1 teaspoon dry mustard in a tub of water.

ও **Oat straw** (the herb) has such a calming effect it is used as a remedy for insomnia.

ও **Orange blossoms and leaves** have both been favorites for all-over skin beautifying since ancient Roman times.

ও **Peppermint** is a tonic for oily or irritated skin, a before-bed nerve calmer, and a terrific cooler for hot days.

ও **Pine needles** relieve nervous tension, especially if you fantasize about bathing in a peaceful primeval forest.

ও **Plantain leaves** have healing properties. Steep the dried, crumbled leaves in boiling water, strain the liquid into your bath, then apply the solids to ailing skin.

ও **Raspberry leaves** are astringently cleansing and refreshing.

ও **Rosemary** soothes skin and regenerates the nervous system.

ও **Sage,** when taken internally as a tea, aids mental alertness; as a bath additive it is a sleep inducer.

ও **Thyme and valerian** are soporifics, great for "unwinding" at any time of day or night.

ও **Yarrow** inhibits infections and is recommended for oily or blemished skin.

    Yellow dock relieves itchy skin. Steep and strain before adding to the tub.

You can individualize your beauty bath by blending two or more of the following aromatic herbs: acacia, angelica root, cinnamon, cloves (no more than 1 teaspoon per tub), lavender, lemon peel, lovage root, marigold, myrtle leaves, orange leaves, pennyroyal, rose geranium, rosemary, sandalwood, verbena.

SIX ADVANTAGES OF USING DRIED HERB MIXTURES IN YOUR BATH

Specific combinations of dried herbs are especially effective for:

    Deep cleansing. Steep 2 or 3 tablespoons *each* hibiscus, lemon grass, peppermint, rosemary, and witch hazel leaves or bark in boiling water. Strain. Add the liquid to your bath, wrap the solids in a washcloth to use as a scrubber.

    Dry, itchy skin. (See also the sunburn-relieving baths in Chapter 9.) Prepare equal amounts of camomile, fennel, lovage, peppermint, rosemary, sage, and yarrow by any one of the herbal-bath methods.

Or, mix $1/4$ cup *each* almond meal, cornmeal, oatmeal, and orris root. Secure the mixture in a cloth bag or washcloth; squeeze out the milkiness while you are soaking, then rub your skin with the bag.

    Rejuvenating and energizing. Mix equal parts of alfalfa, comfrey, orange peel, and parsley; or of basil, bay leaves, fennel, and mint (a masculine favorite); or of lavender, orange blossoms, and rose petals; or of juniper, lavender or rosemary, and rose geranium. Or, combine $3/4$ cup jasmine with $1/4$ cup orange blossoms.

    Relaxing. Mix equal amounts of camomile, horsetail, rosemary, pine needles, and valerian; or of camomile, peppermint, and rosemary; or of comfrey, lavender, mint, and rosemary (with thyme added if desired); or of comfrey, marigold, and yarrow.

    Relieving stiff muscles. For best results, massage the sore muscles while you are soaking with strawberry leaves and sage, mixed half-and-half; or with equal amounts of agrimony, camomile, and mugwort.

Spicy luxuriating. For a Parisian extravaganza, steep 2 tablespoons *each* bay leaves, lavender, marjoram, rosemary, and thyme in 2 cups of boiling water for 15 minutes. Strain and add to your bath with $1/2$ cup cognac.

NINE NATURAL ADDITIVES FOR PAMPERING YOUR SKIN WHILE YOU BATHE

1. **Glycerin** silkens your skin while it prevents "ring around the tub." Swish a tablespoonful into the water; add rose water for fragrance, if desired.

   Cucumber glycerin: For a skin-rejuvenating treatment, simmer an unpeeled, sliced cucumber in unsalted water until tender. Strain off the solids and add the liquid to your bath with 2 tablespoons of glycerin.

2. **Honey.** Add 1 tablespoon to your tub to soften your skin.

3. **Lemon.** To reduce the oils on your skin, and to unjangle your nerves, swirl a cup of fresh lemon juice in the bathwater.

4. **Milk.** The words "milk bath" evoke a vision of Cleopatra lolling seductively in her swan-shaped tub, surrounded by a procession of Nubian slaves decanting ornate jeroboams of camel's milk. Between that exotic scene and the simplicity of swishing a cup of powdered milk into the tub as it fills, lie 2 000 years of experience with its skin-softening, soothing benefits. The recent revival of interest in milk bathing has led several cosmetic companies to include packets of scented "milk" in their lines, but the predominance of preservatives and chemicals in commercial products makes their virtue questionable. Mother Nature still knows best. Whether fluid or dry, whole or skim, just-plain-milk added to your bath water produces the sensation of floating in a soft, warm cloud—without leaving a sticky residue.

   Two to three cups of fluid milk, or one cup of instant dry milk (noninstant powdered milk turns into lumpy globs if not first dissolved in water or encased in a cloth bag) will soften hard water, smooth, and firm your skin. For even more spectacular results, indulge in one of these combos.

Oil and milk pamper your skin and dispense with dry flakies. Reverse the usual procedure by cleansing before entering your beauty bath—milk and oil may mix with water, but soap gets scummy—and be cautious when exiting from any bath containing oil, as both you and the tub will be slippery. Depending upon how dry you are, add $1/2$ teaspoon to $1/2$ cup almond, avocado, wheat germ, or other unsaturated oil and 2 to 6 cups fluid milk (or the equivalent in instant dry milk) to the tub as it fills. Swish to combine, then luxuriate for at least 15 minutes before polishing off dead skin with a loofah or bath brush.

Salty milk is a potent solution for transforming rough, scaly skin into silky smoothness. Dissolve 1 cup of table salt in a pan of boiling water. Pour it into your tub and mix in 4 cups of instant nonfat dry milk (or 3 quarts of fluid milk). Soak, then scrub with a washcloth or loofah.

Simulated milk bath: To reap the skin-smoothing benefits of a genuine milk bath, stir 1 cup cornstarch with mineral oil to make a thick liquid; mix into the water as the tub fills.

Super-soother for skin-pampering nourishing: Simmer $1/2$ cup barley in a quart of water until tender. Place $1/4$ cup *each* almond meal, oatmeal, and orris root (if available) in a cloth bag or a square of doubled cheesecloth and fasten securely. Strain the barley liquid into the bathtub as it fills. Add the filled cloth bag and 1 cup instant dry milk. As you soak, gently rub your skin with the squishy bag.

Tea with milk and honey makes a milk bath good enough to drink. Mix 2 cups double-strength camomile tea with $1/2$ cup honey. Stir into your bath water with 4 cups instant dry milk (or 3 quarts fluid milk).

5. **Oatmeal with bran and bay leaves** are perfect post-sports bath enhancers. Combine $1/4$ cup *each* dry oatmeal and miller's bran with 2 tablespoons crushed bay leaves; simmer for an hour in 2 quarts of water before straining the liquid into the tub. For a more femininely scented version, substitute 2 tablespoons of lavender for the bay leaves.

6. **Oils**. Olive and sesame oils were the ancient Roman and Egyptian favorites; tropical-island inhabitants utilized coconut oils. Here's how to manufacture your own coconut oil:

Drain and reserve the milk from 2 coconuts. Grate the meat, add $1/2$ cup of the coconut milk, and squeeze the mixture through your fingers for several minutes. Strain into a nonmetal cooking container and simmer the liquid for an hour. Strain again and bottle. If you are a perfectionist, you can clarify the oil by adding 3 times as much water as you have oil, boiling the mixture for 15 minutes, pouring it into a glass bowl, and cooling it until you can skim off the clarified product before discarding the water.

Bathing in an emulsion of oil and water helps restore the moisture lost through the assaults of detergents, counteracts chemical dyes from clothing, repairs skin damage from exposure to heat and cold, and relieves dry, itchy skin. The soft film of oil clings, even after toweling, to leave you sleek and smooth. Any vegetable or nut oil produces equally beautifying results when one-fourth teaspoon to one-fourth cup is swirled in the water. For fragrant silkiness, you can dilute the homemade Attar of Roses from Chapter 3 with almond or olive oil.

Almond bath oil. Emulsify 1 cup almond oil and 1 tablespoon detergent shampoo with an electric blender or a rotary egg beater. (Include $1/2$ teaspoon of your favorite perfume, if desired.) Bottle and shake well before pouring 2 tablespoons into your tub. The shampoo breaks the oil into fine globules, making it cling to all seven million of your pores.

❧ Apricot Bath Soak ❦

2 tablespoons wheat germ oil

1 tablespoon melted butter

3 large, ripe apricots

1 cup whole milk, divided

2 small eggs or 1 extra large egg

$1/3$ cup yogurt

2 tablespoons witch hazel

1 teaspoon apple cider vinegar

Combine the wheat germ oil and butter. Let stand while liquefying the pitted apricots with $1/2$ cup of the milk. Strain. Return the liquid to the blender, add all other ingredients and whir until emulsified. Use $1/3$ of the mixture for a luxurious, skin nourishing bath. Store the remainder in the refrigerator.

Floral bath oil. The Charitable Physitian, written in 1639 by Philbert Guibert, Esq. & Physitian Regent in Paris, recommends the "enfleurage" method of procuring rose oil:

❧ TO MAKE OYLE OF ROSES ❧

Take a pound of red Rose buds, beat them in a marble morter with a wooden pestle, then put them into an earathen pot, and pour upon them four pound of oyle of olives, letting them infuse the space of a month in the Sunne, or in the chimney corner, stirring of them sometimes, then heat it, and press it and strain it, and put it into the same pot or other vessel to keep.

Dr. Guibert's method must have been effective and might apply to producing other floral oils, but there is a less time-consuming way to transform a bottle of salad oil into an exotic bath enhancer.

For your floral oil you will need a 9-by-12-by-2-inch glass pan; a roll of absorbent cotton; clear glass to cover the pan; a pint of oil; tincture of benzoin; and gardenia, heliotrope, honeysuckle, jasmine, magnolia, rose, stock, verbena, violet, water lily, or other scented flower petals.

Place a layer of cotton in the bottom of the pan. Blend 1 teaspoon benzoin with 2 cups almond or other natural oil; drizzle $1/2$ cup of it over the cotton. Arrange a thick layer of unsprayed, dust-free flower petals over the oil-saturated cotton, cover with another layer of cotton, and pour in the remaining oil. Top with clear glass and place near a sunny window. Once each day, for at least three days, lift the top layer of cotton, remove the old flowers, and replace with fresh petals. When the scent reaches the desired strength, squeeze the oil out of the cotton, strain out the flower petals, and funnel your perfumed oil into a lightproof, airtight bottle.

7. **Salts**. As sold commercially, "bath salts" are water softeners. To manufacture your own: Place 2 cups borax in a jar. Stir in $1/4$ teaspoon of your favorite perfume. Cover and let stand 24 hours. Stir in another $1/4$ teaspoon perfume and store tightly closed. Use 2 or 3 tablespoons for each bath.

   Epsom salt has a reviving effect on the body when $1/2$ cup is added to the bathwater. A solution of 1 pound per tub is a restorative for overworked muscles and ligaments if you alternate underwater massaging with relaxing.

Sea salt (or table salt mixed half-and-half with epsom salt) also has a beneficial effect on sore muscles, cleanses pores, and revs up weary bodies. Use 1 or 2 cups for each bath.

Sea salt scrub is an allover exfoliant to depose dead skin cells and restore rough skin to seductive smoothness. Mix 1 cup sea salt with enough water, milk, or oil to form a paste. Stand in a partially filled tub while vigorously rubbing the salt mixture over your wet body. Fill the tub with warm water, then soak and bathe as usual.

Table salt is said to help guard against vaginal infections when $1/_2$ cup is dissolved in the bathwater.[137]

8. **Vinegar** can help relieve achy muscles or flaky, itchy skin. It will both relax and invigorate your body when 1 cup is added to your bath. For pizzazz plus fragrance, use one of the cosmetic vinegars from Chapter 3.

9. **Wheat flour** doesn't sound glamorous, but when it is encased in a muslin bag, or heaped on an old handkerchief and tied into a packet, it is a wonderful skin softener. Hang your bag or packet over the spout as the tub fills, then remove it to gently massage your body as you soak.

For dry skin, put 2 tablespoons *each* whole wheat flour and powdered milk in the bag.

For oily or blemished skin, use 2 tablespoons *each* whole wheat flour, camomile, and lemon balm.

ENTICING AFTER-BATH MOISTURIZERS

To seal in your skin's newly acquired moisture (the January 1988 issue of *Health* reports that a 20-minute soak creates temporary skin hydration of up to 40 percent), smooth on one of the facial moisturizers from Chapter 4, petroleum jelly, your own floral bath oil, or either of these harem-favorite lotions.

Morocco Moisturizer: Combine $1/_2$ cup *each* almond oil, honey, and strained, fresh lemon juice in the top of a double boiler or small saucepan. Heat and stir until thoroughly blended. Bottle and refrigerate.

Sultan's Secret: Pulverize a handful of sesame seeds in an electric blender. Continue blending while gradually adding water until you have a milky lotion. Strain and store in the refrigerator.

How TO MAKE YOUR OWN NATURAL BATH POWDER

Commercial dusting powders and talcs may contain chemical additives or perfumes that irritate sensitive skin and can cause allergic reactions or internal damage.[33] For the delight without the danger, try these natural options:

Arrowroot, cornstarch, or old-fashioned laundry starch are perfume-free and as absorbant as talcum powder.

Fuller's earth is a harmless, basic-beige dusting powder.

Rice flour, sifted until fluffy, was a preferred powder for bodies as well as faces until twentieth-century cosmetology became a profitable industry.

SCENTED POWDERS

- **Gardenia**. If you harbor fond memories of your senior prom, and have access to a gardenia bush, fill a pint container with fresh gardenias, add as much cornstarch (or other talc substitute) as possible, and cover tightly. Shake the mixture each 8 hours and replace the gardenias every other day until the powder is as fragrant as desired.

- **Herbal dusting powders** require either a mortar and pestle or a spice-coffee grinder to pulverize the dried botanicals before combining with any of the talc substitutes.

    Floral: Mix equal amounts of powdered lavender, orris root, and rose petals. Stir in cornstarch to double the total quantity.

    Spicy: Blend equal parts of powdered cloves and sage. Match their combined amount with orris root, then stir in arrowroot to double the volume.

    Springtime essence: Combine equal amounts of powdered lilac blossoms, orris root, and violet blooms. Add cornstarch to triple their total volume.

Hოw TO MAKE SPLASH-ON COLOGNE

In a glass jar, combine 1 pint ethyl alcohol or 80 proof vodka; 2 tea-spoons oil of lavender; and 1 teaspoon *each* oil of balm, oil of lemon, oil of orange, and oil of rosemary. Keep tightly covered and shake three times a day for one week. Strain through moistened coffee-filter paper into an attractive bottle with an airtight stopper.

❧ *9* ❧

SUN SMARTS:
HOW TO HAVE FUN
WITHOUT THE BURN

The ancients paid homage to the sun as a god but only during this century have sun worshippers prostrated themselves beneath its rays to darken their skins. "Sun bronzed" replaced "alabaster white" as a status symbol when laborers moved indoors from fields to factories, and the discovery that sunshine is the primary source of vitamin D encouraged sun exposure. According to the March 1988 issue of *Men's Health*, sunlight is sexually stimulating and may improve the odds of child conception by increasing ovulation in women and sperm production in men. Along with appreciation of its benefits, however, has come awareness of sunlight's potential dangers.

HOW TO AVOID THE HAZARDS OF SUNNING

Frequent misting with water is no longer advised as a tanning aid. The water cools your skin as it evaporates, enabling you to prolong your sunning without discomfort, but it increases the potential for skin damage. As explained in *Health* (January 1988), skin cells flatten out when they are wet and allow more of the burning rays to permeate. Sun damage accumulates slowly, often requiring years to overpower the body's natural defenses. This cumulative overexposure is now being held responsible for premature aging of the skin, most skin cancers, and many cataracts.

PHOTOAGING

Differing from normal aging, *photoaging* results from ultraviolet rays penetrating the epidermis, dilating dermal blood vessels, and clumping the elastin and collagen which support the skin—thus creating skin sags and wrinkles, plus other problems such as:

- *Liver spots/age spots*. Byproducts of photoaging, not liver dysfunction, these small, flat, liver-colored spots on the skin are medically identified as *senile lentigines* (from the Latin "old" and "brown spots") because of the years of accumulated sun exposure required to produce them.

- *Droopy noses*. In the December 1987 issue of *Prevention*, Dr. Albert N. Kligman states that noses react to sunlight with more than temporary redness; long-term exposure can damage the cartilage and make the tip of your nose droop.

PHOTOSENSITIVITY

Interaction between the sun's ultraviolet rays and cosmetic ingredients, drugs, or foods may cause brown splotches, an itchy rash, or other unpleasantries. Shaving immediately before sun exposure magnifies the sensitivity of male faces or female legs.

- Colognes, perfumes, and after-shave lotions may leave semipermanent brown spots on your skin if you apply them before going out in the sun.

- Deodorants and deodorant soaps containing hexachlorophene can bring out an itchy, red rash if used before sunbathing.

- Drugs and medications, such as tetracycline and other antibiotics, diuretics, and tranquilizers can make you especially prone to sunburn. Oral contraceptives cause some women to develop a *pregnancy mask* (a pattern of dark blotches around the eyes) from exposure to the sun.

- Foods that can be photosensitizing include celery, citrus fruits, figs, parsnips, and vanilla.

CATARACTS AND SKIN CANCER

Even more disturbing than rashes, blotches, or premature wrinkles is the possibility of eye damage or skin melanoma. Studies have demonstrated that excessive exposure to the sun results in cloudy vision with increased incidence of cataract,[138] and the *University of California, Berkeley Wellness Letter* (June 1988) reports that approximately one-tenth of the million cataracts removed each year in the United States are sun related.

Statistics given in the *Journal of the American Academy of Dermatology* (December 1987 issue) show that between the years 1980 and 1987 new melanomas in the United States increased 83 percent, while the population rose by only 10.6 percent. Doctors and researchers attribute these skin cancers to cumulative effects from the sun-worshipping 1960s and 1970s because of the 15 to 20 years required for melanomas to develop; and, as reported in the October 1987 issue of *Trends*, it is estimated that at least one out of every seven Americans eventually will have one or more skin cancers.

TANNING WITHOUT THE SUN

Bronzing gels for sunless tans are presumed harmless but are still undergoing safety tests. Tanning salons are touted as being safer than the sun because their high-intensity light sources emit fewer of the burning UVB rays. However, according to reports in *Health* (June 1987) and *University of California, Berkeley Wellness Letter* (February 1989), man-made ultraviolet rays are from 5 to 100 times more powerful than those of the midday sun, penetrate the skin more deeply, and are proportionately more likely to cause premature aging or melanomas. The American Academy of Dermatology has requested that health warnings be mandated in tanning parlors as they are on cigarette packages.

If you can't deal directly with the sun, you might try this natural skin bronzer with astringent properties that offers a beautifying bonus of pore refining and skin tightening: Brew strong black pekoe tea by steeping 3 tea bags in 1 cup boiling water until comfortably warm. Stand in the bathtub and sponge the tea over your face and body with the tea bags. Let the liquid dry for a few minutes, then blot (do not rub) with a soft towel. Repeat daily until as dark as desired, then twice a week for maintenance.

PLAYING SAFE IN THE SUNSHINE

Lurking indoors during daylight hours is not the only option. You can apply a sunscreen, wear sunglasses, and, for prolonged exposure while working or playing in the sun, a hat with a brim wide enough to shade your nose. To test your clothing for sun safety, hold the garment up to a light. Loosely woven fabrics offer scant protection, tightly woven cloth such as blue denim is excellent.

SUNSCREENS

Sunscreens absorb, reflect, or scatter the ultraviolet radiation that causes sunburn, yet permit some of the less-dangerous, tanning rays to travel through to the skin. Moisturizing substances are incorporated to replace tanning lotions and help prevent an aftermath of flaky dryness. They are rated from 2 to 35 according to their SPF (sun protection factor), with 2 providing twice the natural skin protection, and 35 presenting an almost impenetrable barrier under laboratory conditions, but diffusion by perspiration or swimming can reduce their potency. The official recommendation is to apply the sunscreen 15 minutes before going outside and reapply it several times during sunbathing.[26] This consistent protection allows your skin to begin repairing existing photoaging damage by building a new network of collagen, connective tissue, and elastin fibers.[27] For tanning with a sunscreen:

> If you are in a hurry to obtain a tan, and do not burn easily, use SPF 4.

> If you tan normally, start with SPF 15, then reduce to SPF 10 after establishing a base tan.

> If you burn easily, use SPF 15 to 35 and do not overindulge in sunbathing.

SUNGLASSES

Eyes, too, need protection from the sun. Eyelids are subject to skin cancer, and, in addition to the increased potential for cataracts, unprotected eyes lose 50 percent of their night vision after a day at the beach or on the ski slopes; it may be a week before your eyes recover from a two-week holiday in the sun.

Eskimos wear gogglelike pieces of bone carved with narrow slits to shield their eyes, and Nero watched the Christians versus lions arena-entertainments through an emerald lens. However, neither shields nor color can provide the protection our eyes need; they require specially ground lenses to filter out the rays that damage eyes and the tender skin surrounding them. When you shop for sunglasses, make sure they are designated "Z-80.3" or have an SPF rating of 15. For protection against sun reflection from water or snow, experts advise opaque side pieces on the glasses.

TIPS FOR PROTECTING EXTRA-SENSITIVE AREAS

Eyes, ears, nose, and throat. These are especially sensitive thin-skinned areas. While your sunscreen-lotioned body is soaking up direct sunlight, covering your eyes with gauze pads dunked in cool water, pekoe or slippery-elm tea can prevent puffy-eyed evenings and future wrinkles. If you remain in the sun very long, your ears, too, may need the protection of cotton pads. A plastic nose cover can keep you from looking like W. C. Fields, and extra slatherings of sunscreen should avoid the possibility of becoming a "red neck."

Hair, natural or tinted, may redden or blanch from exposure to the sun's rays; permed hair can be further weakened. The combination of sun and perspiration, especially when compounded with ocean salt or swimming-pool chlorine, can be disastrously destructive. For shiny, manageable hair—instead of a headful of discolored, strawlike strands—comb in a bit of conditioner; cover your head with a scarf, terrycloth turban, or hat while sunning; wear a bathing cap when swimming; and rinse or shampoo your hair after each exposure.

Hands and feet deserve their fair share of attention and lotion; sun-blistered feet and blotchy, sun-puffed hands can spoil the effect of an otherwise perfect tan.

THIRST QUENCHERS: WHAT TO DRINK WHILE SUNNING

Replenishing the fluid your body loses through perspiration is essential. What to drink while sunning? Water, lemonade, and diluted fruit juices are ideal choices. If you feel faint or nauseous, stir $1/4$ teaspoon baking soda and $1/2$ teaspoon salt into a glass of lemonade or water, then sip about half of it. The salt and soda provide quick replacement of critical minerals lost in the perspiration. If your internal unease lingers, drink the rest of the mixture.

> Alcoholic beverages are mild diuretics that deplete the body of water and make you more thirsty. They also constrict blood vessels (making you feel hotter) and rob you of B vitamins required for the tanning process . . . saving them for the shade is suggested.

🍂 Caffeine increases skin sensitivity and the chances of burning before tanning, so caffeine-containing coffee, tea, and soft drinks are not recommended while sunning.

How to Cultivate a Healthy Tan

Suntanning is a complex process. Pigment cells in the skin undergo an immediate biochemical change that darkens them within a few hours. Exposure to ultraviolet rays also triggers a delayed reaction which stimulates the production of more pigment cells, and continues to deepen the tan for up to 96 hours.

You can acquire a light tan just by watching the sun worshippers. Fifty percent of the sun's tanning rays bounce off pavement, pool decks, sand, and water to reach you under a beach umbrella, boat canopy, or shaded lanai; and they penetrate lightweight clothing. Spectacular tans must be carefully cultivated. Your geographical location, chronological age, and how brown you want to be determines the best way to go about achieving your goal.

🍂 If you're tanning while traveling, it's wise to bear in mind that the sun's rays are more intense in equatorial regions and at high altitudes than they are in your own backyard.

🍂 The body's metabolic balance changes with age; your tolerance for sunshine may be much less when you are 50 than it was when you were 15.

🍂 Clouds can't be counted on; approximately 80 percent of the sun's burning rays seep through smoggy cloud cover.

Dark-haired Lorna had no trepidation about sunbathing. She had tanned beautifully in the high-altitude Colorado Rockies and on the Arizona desert—and she never burned. The vacation day she scheduled for California sunbathing, however, proved to be a disastrous learning experience. The sky was overcast, the fog didn't roll out, the smog didn't lift, and an almost chilling breeze blew across the sand. Disappointed, Lorna read the book she had brought along, and waited for the sun to appear. It didn't. But prickling, burning sensations commenced on the drive back to the hotel. Lorna subdued the discomfort of her beet-red skin with cool baths and vitamin-E oil . . . but well remembers the burn-with-blisters resulting from a sunless day at the beach.

How to Time Your Tanning

The sun's rays are the most powerful when directly overhead; less penetrating in the early morning and late afternoon. Besides adhering to the old dictum of "not between 10 A.M. and 2 P.M.," you can take advantage of modern technology to monitor your tanning time. There are solar-powered meters that give a digital readout of the ultraviolet level, and adhesive strips that change color according to your level of sun exposure. Watching your watch is a less expensive alternative.

Starting with two brief sunning sessions a day is the recommended approach. Blondes and redheads with fair skin and blue eyes have little defense against the sun. Their beginning exposure time should be limited to no more than 20 minutes. Brunettes with darker, less sensitive skin have more natural protection, and may be able to double that time. Deep olive to black skin provides a built-in sun shield against burning but is not immune to the hazards of sun-induced skin cancer and aging.[160]

As your tan develops, your skin thickens and you can gradually lengthen your time in the sun. The moment you notice signs of redness, feel nauseous, or have cold, clammy skin, however, go indoors to avoid a sunburn or the possibility of sunstroke.

Enhancing Your Tan with Natural Lotions

To pamper your skin and enhance the golden glow acquired with sunscreen protection, slather on any of the natural substances once used as tanning lotions.

- ❧ Aloe vera gel or petroleum jelly.

- ❧ Vegetable oils, singly or in combinations such as avocado or almond oil mixed with wheat germ oil.

- ❧ Cocoa-butter cream made by blending $1/4$ cup coconut oil with $1/4$ cup melted cocoa butter.

- ❧ Yogurt cream, prepared by placing the following ingredients in a blender container and whirring them until smooth:

    3 tablespoons water-dispersible lecithin

    2 tablespoons yogurt

    2 tablespoons each avocado oil and sesame oil

    1 tablespoon water

    1 teaspoon potato flour

🍂 Tea lotion, an old favorite that can be stored in the refrigerator for up to three months.

    $1/_2$ cup water

    4 tea bags of regular pekoe tea

    $3/_4$ cup wheat germ oil

    $1/_2$ cup sesame oil

    $1/_4$ cup apple cider vinegar

    1 teaspoon iodine

Bring the water to a boil, add the tea bags, cover and let steep until room temperature. Whisk the oils with the vinegar, then beat in the tea and the remaining ingredients.

TANNING SUPPLEMENTS

🍂 *Vitamin A*: Studies indicate that additional vitamin A plus a bone-meal supplement increases the protection provided by sunscreens.[139] A daily capsule of 25,000 units of beta carotene (which the body converts to vitamin A as needed) helps reduce night blindness resulting from exposure to bright light.

🍂 *B Complex*: B vitamins are necessary for the production of tanning pigments, so your body may rob its stores to pay for your bronzed beauty, or you may burn instead of tan. Eating more B-vitamin-containing foods (see Vitamin and Mineral Chart) and/or taking a B-complex supplement helps your system assist the sun.

According to nutritionist Adelle Davis, persons who sunburn readily and those who are susceptible to skin cancers have unusually high B-vitamin requirements and can increase their sun-tolerance by taking 1,000 milligrams of PABA plus a 30-milligram tablet of zinc daily.[50,51]

🍂 *Vitamin C*: A lack of this vitamin may be responsible for a spotty tan. Eating vitamin-C-rich foods (see Vitamin and Mineral Chart) and taking supplemental C also strengthens skin tissues to help prevent photoaging.

WHAT TO DO WHEN YOU'RE OVERDONE: TIPS ON RELIEVING SUNBURN PAIN

Overexposure to the sun causes tiny blood vessels in the dermis to dilate. Within a few hours blood serum from these dilated vessels seeps into skin tissues and distends the surface. Blisters erupt from a severe sunburn and, eventually, the top layer of skin peels off. Besides the temporary discomfort, repeated sunburns can instigate an assortment of skin problems. As reported in *Prevention* (May 1988), blistering sunburns double the chances of developing skin cancer. Skin may become leathery, the underlying tissue lose its elasticity (a degenerative change called *solar elastosis*), and wrinkles form. Tiny red spots from burst capillaries may appear on fair skins; spider or splotchy veins may worsen from being expanded by the heat; and existing freckles and little brown blotches become more obvious.

Underestimating the power of the sun is what usually leads to a sunburn. Overcast skies present no barrier to its burning rays, and neither does water. In addition to allowing penetration by ultraviolet rays, water acts as a prism to concentrate the sun's heat—in the same way that a magnifying glass can be used to start a fire with solar power.

HOW TO RELIEVE SUNBURN PAIN

Hardy souls may swear by a hot shower to extinguish sunburn fire, turn the red into tan, and prevent blistering, but most of us prefer gentle cooling as the first step. The force of water from a shower can be painful; soaking your sizzling body for 15 minutes in a tub of cool water eases the burning and replaces some of the moisture in your dehydrated skin. While you lie there soaking and vowing never again to overexpose, placing moist tea bags or thin slices of raw potato or cucumber over your sun-puffed eyelids helps reduce their swelling. Adding one of these naturally soothing and healing substances to your bath will make the total relief more immediate, and more long lasting.

- Swish 2 cups of apple cider vinegar, or 2 cups of fluid milk, or $2/3$ cup of instant nonfat dry milk in the bathwater. To further pamper your mistreated skin, add a tablespoon of almond oil.

ख Place 2 cups of cornstarch in the tub; mix with the water while the tub fills.

ख "Old-tyme receipts" say to place 1 cup of oatmeal in a drawstring bag or a muslin diaper with the corners tied together. If you don't happen to have either item, encase the oatmeal in doubled cheesecloth or in a nylon knee-hi. Let the container soak with you in the tub, then squeeze it to drizzle the oatmeal juices over your skin. If sharing your bath with a cup of uncooked porridge in a snagged stocking offends your sensibilities, simply swish in $^1/_2$ cup of *colloidal oatmeal* (a commercially available mixture of powdered oatmeal, lanolin, and mineral oil).

ख Place 2 ounces of dried rosemary in 2 cups of water and bring to a boil. Cover and let steep for 30 minutes. Strain, then pour into the filling tub. To save time, substitute rosemary tea bags: let the water run until steamy, put the plug in the tub and toss in a handful of the tea bags. Shut off the water as soon as the bags are covered, let them "steep" for 10 minutes, then fill the tub with tepid water and join the floating tea bags.

DOUSING OR COMPRESSING

If a tub bath is not feasible, you can cool your sun-abused skin with any of these liquids—sprayed, splashed, or smoothed on, or made into cloth compresses.

ख **Alcohol.** Add 1 tablespoon rubbing alcohol to 2 cups cold water.

ख **Almond milk.** In an electric blender, whir 1 cup water with $^1/_4$ cup almond meal. Strain before applying.

ख **Alum.** Dissolve 1 teaspoon alum in 2 cups of water.

ख **Apple cider vinegar.** It doesn't smell any better than it ever did, and you may have to repeat the application every 20 minutes, but splashing on vinegar does bring relief, just as it did hundreds of years ago.

ख **Baking soda.** Dissolve 3 tablespoons soda in 1 quart cold water.

ख **Milk.** Saturate cloths with cold milk and apply to the burned areas.

- **PABA lotion.** Dissolve 1 teaspoon crushed PABA tablets in $^1/_4$ cup water. Sponge over burned areas.

- **Pekoe tea or sage tea.** Make a strong infusion from 4 tea bags in 1 cup of boiling water. Add ice cubes to cool, then pat the liquid over your skin with the moist tea bags.

- **Potato juice.** Liquefy raw potatoes in an electric juicer or blender, then douse your skin to help remove the heat and relieve the pain.

PAIN-HALTING COATINGS FOR YOUR SKIN

After the initial cooling, coat your sunburned areas with one of these air-excluding substances because, as Dr. Goodenough explains in his 1904 book of home cures,[70] the oxygen in the air coming in contact with the skin is what produces sensations of smarting and burning.

- **Aloe vera gel.** This ancient remedy for burns is cooling, soothing (one of its constituents is a chemical cousin of aspirin), and healing.

- **Baking soda or equal parts of baking soda and cornstarch.** Blend with water or milk to make a paste. Cover the burned areas and do not rinse off for an hour.

- **Cream or yogurt.** Apply over the burned areas. Leave on until dry, then rinse off and reapply to reap all of the pain-relieving, healing benefits.

- **Cucumber.** Puree a chopped cucumber in an electric blender with 1 tablespoon witch hazel and 1 teaspoon honey. Pat over your sunburn and leave on for 15 minutes before rinsing off.

- **Egg yolk.** Folk healers advise smearing raw egg yolk over sunburned areas and letting it dry for 30 minutes before washing off.

- **Honey.** Plain honey is recognized as one of the best ointments for burns. Mixing it half-and-half with wheat germ oil incorporates the healing benefits of vitamin E. For severely burned areas, try whirring honey and wheat germ oil in a blender with dry comfrey tea to make a thick paste.

- **Laundry starch.** Old-fashioned laundry starch, prepared as for starching shirt collars, brings radical relief to sunburned skin.

🍃 **Mayonnaise.** Cover the sunburned parts with mayonnaise, store-bought or made from the recipe in the Glossary.

🍃 **Oils.** Referred to as *sweet oil* in the 1800s, olive oil was applied to sunburned skin and covered with a light bandage. Polyunsaturated vegetable oils have greater skin-penetrating power and don't require bandaging.

To make an oil and vinegar dressing: Cover the burned areas with vinegar-saturated cloths for 10 minutes, then remove the compresses and gently coat your skin with oil. For one-step application: Mix equal amounts of oil and vinegar in a shaker bottle.

🍃 **Petroleum jelly.** Apply directly from the container or heat in the top of a double boiler until runny. If your skin is parched as well as sun-struck, place several layers of gauze over the petroleum jelly and cover with a heating pad (on its lowest setting) for 10 minutes to increase absorption.

🍃 **Vegetable shortening.** In the 1940s, a standard remedy called for slathering a sunburn with white vegetable shortening and then turning round-and-round in the breeze from an electric fan.

🍃 **Vinegar lotion** is a super-soother you can make ahead and store in the refrigerator.

> *1 cup white vinegar*
> *$1/3$ cup each salt and yogurt*
> *2 tablespoons aloe vera gel*
> *400 IUs vitamin E from a snipped capsule*

Whisk or blenderize until creamy, transfer to a pump-dispenser bottle, then smooth over your uncomfortable skin every hour of so.

🍃 **Vitamin E,** squeezed from punctured capsules or purchased in a bottle, is credited with relieving pain, transforming beet-red skin to bronzed-brown, and preventing the formation of blisters.

HOW TO HEAL THE BLISTERS

When blisters erupt, the skin's protective barrier is damaged, and bacteria normally present on the outer skin quickly multiply in the plasma that leaks from the dilated blood vessels. The three cardinal rules for guarding against infection are

1. Wash blistered skin gently with mild soap and water.

2. Blot dry rather than rub with a towel.

3. Never attempt to deliberately open the blister by pricking or squeezing.

Covering the blisters with a protective coating of any of these substances speeds healing:

❧ Aloe vera gel or petroleum jelly.

❧ Avocado oil or wheat germ oil. To add healing benefits, blend 50,000 units of vitamin A and 1,000 IUs of vitamin E (obtained from punctured capsules) with 4 tablespoons of the oil.

❧ Honey or a half-and-half mixture of honey and wheat germ oil.

❧ Vitamin C (made into a liquid by dissolving 1 tablespoon of vitamin C crystals in $1/2$ cup of water), or vitamin E from snipped capsules.

DEALING WITH THE LEFTOVERS: SUN SPOTS AND A PEELING TAN

Freckles and age spots often darken after exposure to the sun and become more obvious as a tan fades. Nutritionists and holistic doctors have found that the following supplements will help fade existing sun signs and prevent new ones from forming: B-complex vitamins with additional B-2, to lighten the spots;[79] vitamin C to build strong collagen that will prevent the pigment clumping that results in brown spots;[174] and vitamin E (100 IU with each meal) to forestall the instigating accumulations of melanin.[51]

Regardless of the care with which you cultivate a suntan, its demise is seldom a pretty sight. Filmy skin fragments detach themselves, departing blisters disclose pale patches, and you feel like a reptile shedding its skin. Fortunately, there are natural ways to speed a return to attractive normalcy.

How to Wash off Unsightly Sun Signs

Fifteen-minute tub-bath soaks followed by gentle rubbing with a washcloth or a loofah help to "wash off" no-longer-perfect tan by removing some of the darkly pigmented surface skin. Any one of these bath additives will hasten the process.

- ❧ *Milk or vinegar.* Add 2 cups of fresh milk (or $^2/_3$ cup instant dry milk), or 1 cup of vinegar, to the bathwater to soften your skin, get rid of the dry flakies, and ease the separation of old, peeling skin from its fresh new replacement. Including a tablespoon of vegetable oil will leave your skin feeling satiny.

- ❧ *Lemon juice.* Add $^3/_4$ cup strained lemon juice to your tub to lighten your skin and get rid of that flaky, last-rose-of-summer look.

- ❧ *Oatmeal.* Taking an oatmeal bath (as described for soothing a sunburn), then using the squishy bag as a scrubber leaves you with sleek, emollient-pampered skin.

Natural Remedies for Bleaching Out Uneven, Fading Tans

Centuries of insistence upon pale skin as an essential attribute of beauty have left us a legacy of natural remedies for bleaching out fading tans and brown sun signs.

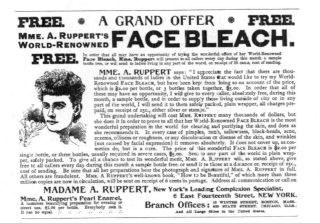

During the 1890s, cosmetic preparations such as Mme. Ruppert's Face Bleach were popular.

❧ **Borax** is a skin-lightening favorite from the nineteenth century. Dissolve 2 teaspoons of borax in 1 cup of water. Add 1 cup of rubbing alcohol and 2 more cups of water, then sponge over your skin several times a day.

For a more potent remedy, mix $1/4$ cup borax with $1/2$ cup granulated sugar in a glass jar. Cover and let stand for 48 hours. Once each day, stir the mixture and rub a spoonful on your discolored skin.

"Glycerinated Lotion of Borax" was used as a daily wash to render the skin exquisitely soft and white. Mix 1 teaspoon powdered borax with 2 tablespoons glycerin and $3/4$ cup rose water.

❧ **Botanicals** have a well-established reputation for skin lightening.

Aloe vera gel. Smooth over sun-darkened freckles or brown spots at least twice a day.

Dry comfrey root tea. Mix to thick paste with water and apply to brown spots or splotches for 15 minutes each day. Rinsing off the paste with fresh lemon juice hastens the bleaching process.

Dandelion leaves. Liquefy a handful of the fresh leaves with three ice cubes in an electric blender. Strain before applying to discolored skin.

Dandelion flower and parsley lotion is reported to be even more effective. Bring 1 cup *each* dandelion blooms and chopped, fresh parsley to a boil in 4 cups of water. Cover and let steep until cool. Strain, refrigerate, and use the liquid as a wash two times a day.

Horseradish. Grate into buttermilk, vinegar, or water, then steep for several hours before straining and applying.

Watercress. Place a freshly washed bunch of watercress in 2 cups cold water. Bring to a boil, cover, and simmer for 10 minutes. Strain and store in the refrigerator. Each morning and evening, sponge the chilled liquid over your fading tan, allow it to dry, then rinse with tepid water.

❧ **Fresh apricots, strawberries, and green grapes** all have skin-bleaching properties. Use one of the apricot masques from

Chapter 5, or simply mash the fruit and pat it on. For a more complex, but supposedly infallible fading-tan remover: Rinse a bunch of green grapes, sprinkle with a mixture of powdered alum and salt, wrap in parchment paper, and bake until tender. Squeeze out the juice and sponge it over your skin.

ๅ **Cranberries** contain acids that bleach and clear the skin. Once or twice each day, crush a handful of fresh or frozen cranberries. Rub the extracted juice over tanned areas, allow it to remain for several hours, then rinse off.

ๅ **Lemon juice** can be used in a variety of ways: Blended with an equal amount of glycerin, it can be sponged on to remove a tan. When mixed to a paste with salt or sugar and allowed to remain on the skin for half an hour once each day, lemon juice may lighten brown splotches caused by the sun.

Lemon juice and egg white. The 1870's instructions call for combining the juice of a lemon with the unbeaten white of an egg in an earthen bowl, placing it at the back of the stove for half an hour, and stirring constantly with an ivory spoon while taking care not to let the bowl get hot enough to crack. With modern appliances you can "cook" the mixture in a custard cup resting in a pan of boiling water over low heat on the rangetop, or microwave it on "defrost" until congealed. However prepared, it should be smoothed over the skin and allowed to remain for several hours.

ๅ **Milk**, in its many guises, is a time-tested skin lightener. Marie Antoinette bathed in buttermilk and spread sour cream over her face and shoulders to maintain her porcelain-white skin. In the 1890s, a tan-removing lotion was prepared by blending 1 cup milk, $1/4$ cup lemon juice, 2 tablespoons *each* brandy and heavy cream, 1 teaspoon sugar, and a pinch of alum. The mixture was then brought to a boil, skimmed, and allowed to cool before being applied to the skin. (If this fails to do great things for your mottled tan, you might substitute nutmeg for the alum, omit the heating stage, and drink the concoction to improve your disposition!)

Yogurt, plain or blended half-and half with buttermilk, can be used as a night cream to ameliorate a fading tan.

ஓ **Potato water** is an old German cure for fading tans and summer freckles. Simply sponge on the water in which potatoes have been cooked.

ஓ **Tomatoes**. Mash ripe tomatoes and apply the pulp to your fading tan. Let dry before removing with water.

HEAD-TO-TOE
BEAUTY

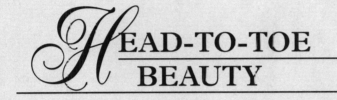

⚓ *10* ⚓

HANDLING YOUR HANDS: GUIDELINES FOR NATURAL NURTURING

Exposed to public view more than any other part of your anatomy except your face, hands should be attractive as well as functional; they can be disastrously revealing. Scarlett O'Hara's alluring "drapery dress" was a futile sacrifice; Rhett Butler discerned her subterfuge the moment he saw her work-worn hands. You needn't go to such extremes as sleeping with them tied above your head (an eighteenth-century Austrian method of maintaining small-veined, lily-white hands); natural nurturing can keep them at their best.

THE FIVE-MINUTE DAILY WORKOUT FOR EXERCISING AND MASSAGING YOUR HANDS

A brief daily workout increases blood circulation to your hands, strengthens their muscles, and improves their flexibility.

1. Stand with your feet 12 inches apart; arms raised straight above your head. Keep your hands stiff while swinging your arms in windmill motions for a count of 20.

2. Sitting or standing, extend your arms parallel with your shoulders. Let your hands dangle loosely and shake them in a circular motion for 30 seconds.

3. With your elbows resting on a table, raise your hands and clench your fists. Open your hands, fan out your fingers, and bend them backwards as far as possible. Repeat 7 times. Slather on a generous coating of lotion. Grasp your left hand with your right, place

your right thumb in the palm of the left hand, and the fingers of your right hand against the back of the left hand. Using deep but gentle circular motions, massage the palm, knuckles, and each finger. Change hands and repeat.

Tip: Gloves provide protection from dirt, detergents, and water as well as cold temperatures. Unless you have coated your hands with lotion to give them a skin-softening treatment while washing dishes, waterproof gloves (even if fabric lined) should be removed every 15 minutes to allow your hands to breathe and to prevent trapped perspiration from inducing chapping.

NATURAL CLEANSERS FOR SOOTHING PROBLEM HANDS

After removing any snug-fitting rings, moisten your hands, wash with a mild cleanser, rinse thoroughly, pat or blot dry. Neglecting these basics can result in "ring rash" or "ring rot," regardless of your jewelry's pedigree. A vacation shopper almost panicked when the skin under her new, half-inch-wide, sterling silver ring turned into a painful, leprous-looking, spongy white mass from an accumulation of public-restroom soap powder and lack of air. A film of vitamin E from a pierced capsule, plus air exposure, produced a quick cure, though prevention would have been more pleasant.

SENSITIVE OR CHAPPED HANDS

- Work a natural makeup-remover into your hands, tissue off, then rinse and blot dry. Or, smooth a facial masque over your hands and rinse off as soon as it dries.

- Mix dry mustard (from the spice shelf), miller's bran, or oatmeal with water to make a paste. Rub it into your hands, then rinse off. If your hands are extremely sensitive, wash with oatmeal paste, then rub dry oatmeal over them to absorb the moisture.

- Soak your hands in a bowl of buttermilk, fresh milk, or rehydrated dry milk; or in a solution of mild shampoo and water; or in a mixture of sugar and water. Add a little uncooked oatmeal or miller's bran for additional soothing and softening.

GRUBBY, ROUGHENED, OR STAINED HANDS

The harsh abrasives in commercial heavy-duty cleansers often leave hands dry and irritated. Men and women will appreciate the gentle effectiveness of these natural cleansers.

❧ **Almond meal, cornmeal, or uncooked oatmeal,** mixed with water, heal as well as cleanse.

> *Almond meal and honey,* mixed half-and-half, massaged into hands and arms, steamed with hot towels for 5 minutes, and then covered with plastic wrap for 10 minutes before being rinsed off, provides cleansing plus soothing.

> *Almond meal dairy cream* is an eighteenth-century unisex cleanser-smoother you can store in the refrigerator for a month or so. Whip $1/4$ cup almond meal with 2 cups milk. Bring to boiling over low heat and stir in a beaten egg yolk. Beat in 1 tablespoon almond oil and $1^1/_2$ teaspoons tincture of benzoin.

> *Cornmeal* is a great grease remover. Thelma was proud of Stan's ability to take care of maintaining their cars but objected to the aftermath of greasy doorknobs and "dirty" soap. Keeping a container of cornmeal in the garage solved their difficulties. Before he goes in to wash up, Stan wipes off as much of the grease or oil as possible, then removes the remainder by rubbing his hands with cornmeal.

> *Cornmeal and lemon juice or vinegar,* blended to a paste, is an old stand-by for cleaning grimy hands that are roughened or chapped.

❧ **Ammonia water** (1 teaspoon ammonia per cup of water) is a highly recommended hand cleaner, but it must be followed by a moisturizer to prevent dryness.

❧ **Granulated sugar,** mixed to a gritty paste with water, is especially good for removing oil stains from hands.

❧ **Lemon juice or citrus peel** (scratched to allow the oils to seep out) removes surface discolorations.

❧ **Super Scrub:** If your hands are frequently grubby, keep a tightly covered jar of this mixture on hand. Combine $1/_2$ cup cornmeal with half of a grated 4-ounce bar of white castile soap, 2 tablespoons almond meal (or 2 tablespoons dried lemon or orange peel from the spice shelf), and 2 tablespoons almond oil or corn oil. Add more oil if needed to make a semisolid paste.

NATURAL HAND LOTIONS AND CREAMS THAT MOISTURIZE AND PROTECT

Hands have so few oil-secreting glands that the assistance of moisturizers is necessary to prevent dryness. To enhance the benefits of lotions and creams, smooth them on while your hands are slightly damp.

- **Glycerin**, applied full strength, can draw moisture from the skin to dry it even further. Mixing the glycerin with rose water obviates the problem, as does blending 1 tablespoon tincture of benzoin with $1/4$ cup glycerin, or stirring up a half-and-half combo of glycerin and fresh lemon juice.

  Glycerin and hydrogen peroxide in equal proportions work miracles for abused hands.

  Glycerin and rose water, the most widely known natural lotion, can be purchased from pharmacies or custom-made at home. The basic formula calls for 1 part glycerin shaken with 3 parts rose water. For a more potent mixture, combine $1/2$ teaspoon borax with $1/2$ cup rose water, then gradually stir into $1/2$ cup glycerin. For a milder variation, blend $3/4$ cup rose water, $1/4$ cup glycerin, and $1/4$ teaspoon *each* honey and apple cider vinegar.

  Vinegar-flaxseed lotion is another time-tested remedy for uncomfortably dry hands: Soak $1/4$ cup flaxseed in 2 cups water for 8 hours. Bring to a boil and simmer 5 minutes. Strain. Add $1 1/2$ cups apple cider vinegar and $1/3$ cup glycerin to the liquid. Return to boiling and beat with a rotary beater to emulsify the mixture.

- **Grapefruit peel.** Quarter half a grapefruit rind, rub the inner side of one piece over your hands; reserve the remainder in a plastic bag in the refrigerator.

- **Herbal lotions** can be as simple as squeezing on the liquid from a chamomile tea bag that has been soaked in 2 tablespoons boiling water for 2 minutes, or as complex as this *Herbal Unguent*: Combine equal amounts of angelica, basil, mint, pennyroyal, valerian, and stinging nettle in a small pan. Pour in white wine to cover the herbs; cook until they are tender and the wine almost boiled away. Mix in melted beeswax to make a thick salve.

- **Honey** is a proven skin softener. For use as a hand lotion, reduce its stickiness by combining the honey with rose water and/or vegetable oil.

- **Lemon** counteracts the alkalinity of soaps. Cook a chopped lemon in water to cover, whir the mixture in an electric blender, strain out any particles of peel, then smooth on the thick liquid. Or, place a lemon slice in a small dish with 1/4 cup warm milk, cover, and let stand for 3 hours. Strain off the liquid to use as a skin-smoother for hands and arms.

  Or, blend 1 tablespoon *each* lemon juice, honey, and salad oil to smooth rough elbows as well as hands.

- **Milk,** warmed and rubbed into the hands each night, dispenses with redness and soothes sore hands.

- **Oil lotion.** Melt 1 tablespoon cocoa butter, stir in $1/2$ cup almond oil, 2 tablespoons *each* olive oil and wheat germ oil, then blend in $1/4$ teaspoon tincture of benzoin.

- **Petroleum jelly** relieves roughened skin and is acceptable to males who resist fragrant cosmetic creams and lotions.

- **Vegetables.** European peasants and American pioneers softened their hands with slices of raw cucumber or potato.

- **Vinegar.** To restore the acid mantle and prevent parchmentlike dry skin, rub a few drops of apple cider vinegar into your damp hands after each washing.

INTENSIVE CARE TREATMENTS: TIME-TESTED SECRETS FOR BEAUTIFUL HANDS

The age-old practice of applying a soothing unguent at night and wearing gloves to bed still works wonders for mistreated hands. White cotton gloves are as effective as the once-advised white kid.

Wear them over a slathering of olive oil, petroleum jelly, any of the ointments described above, or one of these time-tested "secrets" for beautiful hands:

- **Banana butter.** Mash half a ripe banana with 2 teaspoons butter.

- **Egg-yolk salves.** Blend 1 teaspoon rice flour with a raw egg yolk. Stir in 2 teaspoons almond oil, 1 teaspoon rose water, and $^1/_4$ teaspoon tincture of benzoin. Or, try this seventeenth-century chapped-hands remedy: Mix 1 tablespoon *each* honey, lanolin, and tincture of benzoin with 1 egg yolk and sufficient dry oatmeal to make a paste.

- **Lanolin,** originally called "wool fat," was prized as a cure for cracked and bleeding hands even before its prowess was praised in the writings of Ovid and Herodotus. Now stocked by pharmacies, pure lanolin can be used alone or mixed with almond or sesame oil in a ratio of 3 parts lanolin to 1 part oil. For an ointment, stir 2 tablespoons lanolin with 1 teaspoon petroleum jelly and $^1/_2$ teaspoon tincture of benzoin. For a hand cream, mix equal amounts of lanolin and petroleum jelly. To smooth hands and elbows, and to overcome the ashy patches often besetting those with dark skin, blend 2 tablespoons each lanolin and vegetable oil with $^1/_2$ teaspoon lemon or lime juice.

- **Mayonnaise,** either store bought or homemade (see Glossary for recipe), includes hand-soothing in its repertoire.

- **Potato cream.** Cook a small potato in its skin. Peel and mash with almond oil and glycerin to make a soft paste.

HOW TO HAVE FABULOUS FINGERNAILS

Fingernail infatuation is not a recent foible; long, beautifully groomed nails have been a status symbol in almost every period and culture. In 500 B.C., Queen Hetepheres was entombed with her manicure kit of seven golden knives and a metal "orange stick"; ancient Mandarins, who could barely lift a chopstick with their four-inch talons, guarded their nails with sheaths of gold, silver, or bamboo. Wearing today's artificial nails constantly can promote soft, peeling nails or trap moisture to cause moldy infections. Helping Mother Nature grow your own is safer and less expensive.

TIPS ON NOURISHING YOUR NAILS

Nails appear bonelike but are composed primarily of protein (one-fifth of their structure is fluid, another fifth, fat) and derive their nourishment from blood vessels in the dermis. The *matrix* (growth portion) extends beneath the exposed nail bed, produces nails at the rate of about $3/16$ inch per month, requires up to six months to grow a new nail, is speedier in summer than in winter, slows with age, and is influenced by nutrition and general health as well as external care. Studies of nail texture as a means of detecting marginal malnutrition have led to the discovery that internal nail-nourishment requires a daily minimum of 60 grams of protein[33]—much more than an occasional infusion of gelatin (which is helpful if its missing amino acids have been supplied with milk or meat broth) plus a well-balanced diet and supplements when needed.

- **B-complex combination.** Taking a B-complex stress tab plus garlic perles and a zinc supplement each day is said to duplicate the fantastic fingernail improvement achieved by a month of treatment at a European health spa.[20]

- **Brewer's yeast,** 1 or 2 tablespoons per day, encourages nail growth—especially when accompanied by calcium supplements.

- **Calcium,** 1,200 milligrams per day (the amount in a quart of milk), is a healthy-nails essential.

- **Iodine** is another requisite for nail health and strength. Salmon, tuna, iodized salt, or kelp salt-substitute are natural sources.

HOW TO CARE FOR YOUR NAILS

Six to eight daily glasses of water (or their equivalent) are vital for nail health. (As explained in *Health,* January 1988, brittle, flaky nails can result if their moisture level drops below 18 percent.) Too much external water, however, leads to a variety of nail problems. To avoid over submersion, rest your hands on the sides of the tub while luxuriating in your beauty bath, and wear rubber gloves for dishwashing or household cleaning. When your nails are water-logged, applying hand lotion or petroleum jelly will help seal in the moisture to prevent damage. If you are about to embark on a gloveless project, plan ahead by digging your nails into a bar of soap. After your chore is concluded, remove the soap and grime with a nailbrush. Other external encouragements include:

❧ **Buffing** with a chamois buffer to improve circulation, promote growth, and add sheen. Buff gently from cuticle to tip; buffing too vigorously, or with back-and-forth motions, can build up heat and harm your nails. Massage a bit of petroleum jelly or wheat germ oil into your nails before buffing to help strengthen them. For a conditioning treatment that imparts an amber tint, try the "hennicure" once favored by Egyptian royalty. Make a paste from 1 teaspoon dry henna and water. Rub a thin coating into your nails and let it dry before buffing. If you would rather not have the coloring, use neutral henna.

❧ **Exercising** them by playing the piano, embroidering, doing needlepoint, typing, even tapping your fingers to stimulate. Just don't abuse your nails by assuming they are screw-tighteners or tile-grout cleaner-outers.

❧ **Filing** your dry nails from the outside toward the center with an emery board or diamond file. (A steel file or vigorous see-sawing may trigger nail splitting.) Use nail clippers or scissors only after your nails have been softened by soaking.

❧ **Nourishing them from the outside.** Soak your unpolished nails for 10 minutes in a bowl of warmed almond oil (or other natural oil) to which you have added the contents of a vitamin E capsule. Wipe off the excess but do not wash your hands before going to bed.

Or, mix 1 tablespoon wheat germ oil with 1 tablespoon honey, 1 egg yolk, and $1/_8$ teaspoon sea salt. Massage into your nails each night and wash off each morning. Store the mixture in the refrigerator between treatments.

FOUR WAYS TO CARE FOR YOUR CUTICLES

Cuticles help prevent bacteria from attacking the nail base. Protect them by rubbing in a dab of petroleum jelly before swimming or putting your hands in soapy water, cut them only if a hangnail develops, and keep them attractive by:

❧ Pushing them back with a towel, cotton-tipped swab, or orange stick each time you clean your hands.

❧ Massaging them every night with cocoa butter, petroleum jelly, or vitamin E from a snipped capsule.

ಎ Removing roughness by soaking them in warm oil for 5 minutes, then rubbing them with almond meal or cornmeal.

ಎ Trimming off the loose skin of a hangnail, then coating the area with fresh lemon juice, petroleum jelly, or vitamin E from a pierced capsule.

NATURAL REMEDIES FOR NINE COMMON FINGERNAIL PROBLEMS

Nails, although hard, are extremely permeable to water or other fluids. According to the *Harvard Medical School Health Letter* of May 1984, water moves through a fingernail 100 times faster than it penetrates the outer layer of skin. Lengthy immersion disrupts nail structure by causing them to expand with moisture, then shrink as they dry; and may instigate ridging, splitting, or breaking. When detergents or household chemicals are added to the water, nails are further weakened and damaged; studies in Great Britain confirm actual loss of fingernails due to detergents.[33] If nail problems have developed, there are natural remedies and treatments.

1. **Brittle, splitting nails** can result from prolonged exposure to water; insufficient dietary protein, calcium, sulfur, zinc, or vitamins A, B, and C; chronic illness or stress; oral contraceptives; nail polish or polish remover (adding a few drops of olive oil to the remover, and washing your hands immediately after its use, helps counteract the drying effect).

   Brewer's yeast and choline. Taking 2 tablespoons of brewer's yeast in a glass of juice or milk plus 1,000 milligrams of choline each day improves nail strength.

   Iron. A deficiency can cause dry, brittle fingernails. Increasing your intake of iron-rich foods (see Viatmin and Mineral Chart) and taking vitamin C to boost assimilation of the iron may resolve the problem.

   Oil treatments are a standard remedy. Soak your polish-free nails in warm wheat germ oil (or other natural oil) for 5 to 10 minutes each day, then massage from the tips toward the cuticle. Dr. Robert W. Downs, writing in *Bestways* (January 1986), suggests gently breaking the nails' surface tension with an emery board to allow better penetration of the oil.

Soda. Once each day, dissolove 1 tablespoon baking soda in 1 cup of water for a 10-minute fingertip soak. Follow with an application of air-excluding oil or lotion.

Vinegar. Nightly soaks in a half-and-half mixture of apple cider vinegar and warm water are a folk remedy for splitting nails.

White iodine, applied over the tops and under the nail tips twice a day, does more than discourage nail nibling—it helps restore fingernail flexibility and strength.

2. **Discolorations and stains** can be caused by illness, prolonged stress, or by contact with chemical contaminants such as carbon paper, hair dye, nail hardeners or polish, or cigarette smoke. If the nail plate is deeply stained, it will remain so until the new nail grows out. To remove surface stains: Rub them with a cut lemon, or wiggle your fingertips in a lemon half, then rinse dry.

3. **Misshapen nails.** Artificial fingernails have been found responsible for upward curving nails.[171] Spoon-shaped or flattened nails can result from long-term protein or iron deficiencies, and may be remedied with improved diet.

4. **Opaque nails** with a wavy pattern may indicate a lack of protein, a shortage of vitamin A or B, or a mineral imbalance. Improving your diet and supplementing it with a multivitamin plus extra B-6 and 15 milligrams of zinc each day may correct the problem. Totally white nails may indicate a liver disorder; check with your physician.

5. **Pale nails** may be a sign of low zinc and B-6, or can be caused by anemia. See your doctor if the condition persists after you've upgraded your diet.

6. **Pitted fingernails** may indicate a deficiency of calcium, protein, or sulphur (available from eggs, garlic, and meats).

7. **Ridges, grooves, and furrows** can result from careless cuticle trimming or from wearing artificial nails, but usually are caused by illness or nutritional deficiencies.

Horizontal ridges (Beau's lines) often occur following severe stress or illness. Eating an adequate diet with ample protein, and taking supplements of vitamin C plus 15 milligrams of zinc each day, speeds their growing out and disappearing.

Vertical furrows can indicate a deficiency of vitamin A, calcium, or iron. Sometimes they simply begin to develop after the age of 40 because of reduced cell reproduction and are no cause for concern as long as your annual checkup reveals no anemia or lack of vitamins and minerals.

8. **Soft, weak nails.** Excessive contact with water or the chemicals in nail cosmetics are the most common cause; stress and faulty diet come next. Munching on sunflower seeds, increasing your intake of vitamin A (see Vitamin and Mineral Chart), taking 5,000 milligrams of dolomite (a calcium-magnesium supplement reported to restore thin, fragile nails to normalcy in three weeks[188]) and a 15-milligram zinc tablet daily, or swallowing 1 teaspoon of apple cider vinegar three times a day are other successful remedies. Although formation depends on internal nourishment, beveling your nails so there are no blunt edges discourages peeling. There are other strengthening treatments:

Apple cider vinegar or white iodine. Smooth over polish-free nails with a cotton-tipped swab.

Henna. Prepare the neutral shade for a conditioning naildunk. Soak your fingertips for 5 minutes, then rinse, dry, and apply hand lotion or a vegetable oil.

Horsetail. Steep 1 tablespoon of the dried herb in a cup of boiling water until comfortably warm. Use as a nail-soak for 10 minutes each day. To increase the benefits, herbalists advise swallowing a tablespoonful of the hot brew each morning and evening.

Oat straw. Drinking a cup of oat straw tea every day is the folk healer's prescription for improving fingernails.

Oil soaks restore fingernail strength by providing or reinforing the fat content of the nails. Any vegetable or nut oil may be warmed for the purpose; the addition of vitamins A and D, or E (from snipped capsules) makes the soak more effective. Whenever possible, indulge in a 10-minute oil soak at bed-time, tissue off the excess, then refrain from washing your hands until the next morning.

9. **White spots** are the most intriguing nail problem because they are attributed to everything from telling fibs or acquiring a new sweetheart to being deficient in zinc and vitamin B-6. Folklore utilizes them as a fortune-telling medium with this rhyme for counting the white spots

   A gift, a ghost, a friend, a foe,

   A letter to come, a journey to go

Injuries, particularly from cuticle removing, have been known to cause white spots; so have estrogen medications, extreme cold, fasting, fungus infections, and menstrual cycles.

Dr. Pfeiffer[136] and other holistic practitioners correlate all of these occurrences (except for the recent boyfriends, falsehoods, future prognostications, and blows to the nail matrix) to low levels of zinc—so a daily 15-milligram zinc supplement may be worth a try if you have white spots in your fingernails. Or, you can experiment with Dr. Jarvis's folk-medicine remedy of stirring 1 teaspoon *each* apple cider vinegar and honey into a glass of water to accompany each meal.[90]

11

PUTTING YOUR BEST FEET FORWARD: SPECIAL REMEDIES AND EXERCISES FOR YOUR SOLE PROTECTION

Feet are less vulnerable to signs of aging than other body parts, and don't acquire bulges if you gain a few pounds, but they do grow weary. And they are entitled to. During a lifetime they travel a distance equaling three times the circumference of the globe, withstand 1,000 tons of pressure each day as the average worker or homemaker walks a daily ten miles, and support 200 tons of stress when a 125-pound person runs one mile.[137] Until our Cro-Magnon ancestors forsook walking on all fours, body weight was more evenly distributed; the millenia required for evolutionary adjustments, plus almost constant use, account for the tiredness radiating from our overworked feet.

HOW TO FEED YOUR FEET

To perform their amazing feats, the 26 bones in each foot (one-fourth of all our bones are in our feet) must be nourished internally by calcium (at least 1,200 milligrams per day plus accompanying magnesium, phosphorus, and vitamin D), and the muscular structure of our pedal extremities must be maintained with adequate protein, vitamin C, and potassium. (See Vitamin and Mineral Chart for food sources.)

PROTECTING YOUR FEET: PRACTICAL TIPS FOR SELECTING SHOES

Foot traffic in prehistoric villages tamped walkways into unyielding surfaces that were uncomfortable for bare feet accustomed to grassy meadows, so shoes were designed solely for sole protection. By 2000 B.C., Egyptians were cushioning their feet with sandals woven from reeds. Ancient Romans wore leather half-boots or wooden shoes; Northern Europeans enclosed the toes with fur for warmth. Practicality, however, soon gave way to the dictates of style. In the fifteenth century, courtiers supported the 18-inch turned-up toes of their slippers with chains attached to their waists, and aristocratic ladies elevated themselves on 30-inch-high platform-soled shoes called chopinnes. (So many miscarriages resulted from pregnant women toppling off these "stilts" that a law prohibiting such dangerous footgear was passed in Venice in 1430.)

Fortunately, current fashion lacks these extremes. *Footwear News* reports that sales of walking shoes rose 72 percent during 1988, and comfort has become a major concern. Witness the numbers of businesswomen wearing sneakers to commute to work!

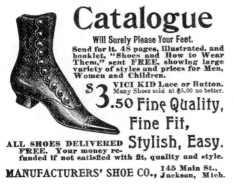
American gentlewomen of the 1890s compressed their feet into stylishly pointed shoes, then stuffed the toes with crumpled paper to prevent rubbing holes in their stockings.

Statistics appearing in *Hippocrates* (November/December 1988) reveal that 45 percent of women wear uncomfortable shoes, and, according to the American Podiatry Association, improperly fitting shoes are the most common cause of the over 30 million podiatric visits made annually.[6] Here are some sensible guidelines to follow:

❧ Don't go shoe shopping in the morning. That perfect fit at 10 A.M. may put frown lines on your face by 5 P.M. because feet expand by as much as half a size during the day.

❧ While standing with your weight on one foot, check the space in the "toe box" by wriggling your toes and pressing down on the shoe. There should be a quarter to a half inch of space beyond your longest toe.

❧ Boot heels should slip a little, shoe heels should neither slip nor sag. Calf-hugging boots should not be tight enough to restrict circulation after a few hours of wear.

❧ When trying on shoes, wear hosiery suited to the footwear (sports socks require shoe space) and be sure the clerk understands your intended use of athletic shoes. The steel-plated soles of biking shoes can do you in if you wear them for jogging; aerobic-dance shoes will not provide the support you need for hiking.

❧ Double check the fit of your new shoes when you get home by pulling a pair of old socks over them (to avoid soiling the soles) and walking around for an hour. If you notice any discomfort, exchange the shoes. Otherwise your feet may break down before the shoes are broken in.

EXERCISES THAT BENEFIT YOUR FEET AND ANKLES

Physical activities that benefit the rest of the body usually involve the feet and ankles, yet provide them little relief.

HI-HEELED COMPENSATION

Mother Nature never intended for us to walk on tiptoe with our feet thrust forward by the force of high heels—the higher the heel, the more unnatural the position. Besides instigating possible postural problems, wearing high heels can cause the hamstring muscles behind your calves to atrophy from not being stretched as far as if your heels were touching the ground.

Ellie was so conscious of her diminutive height that she wore 4-inch heels to work and high-heeled bedroom slippers at home. Enrolling in a fitness program brought her down to earth. She was ready to cancel during the first session; performing the required movements on tiptoe was impossible, and lowering her heels to the floor was too painful. Ellie's coach suggested she gradually stretch her calf muscles with these exercises:

1. Stand 3 feet away from a wall, lean in and place your hands against the wall, stretching them as high as possible. Holding your arms straight and your heels flat on the floor, push into the wall for a count of 15. Repeat 10 times.

2. While standing with your feet 12 inches apart, rock back and forth by lifting first your toes and then your heels off the floor. Intensify the effect by raising your arms high over your head as you rise on your toes, lowering your arms as you rock back on your heels.

3. Fold a towel lengthwise to a 4-inch width. Sit on the floor with legs straight out in front, knees stiff. Loop the towel under your toes and pull back to stretch each calf 6 times.

After a few weeks, Ellie was able to walk comfortably in athletic shoes and rejoin her class. To forestall future difficulties, she stretches her hamstrings each evening, and wears low-heeled shoes or slippers during her hours alone.

RELAXATION AND STRENGTHENING TECHNIQUES

Regardless of shoe-heel-height, if foot muscles are not in shape, inflammation and ankle sprain can result. Walking helps improve circulation and prevent nighttime cramping. To help prevent other foot and leg problems, elevate your feet whenever possible, vary heel height from day to day, and exercise your feet regularly.

- Sit in a chair, hold your feet above the floor with heels down, then make arcs from left to right like windshield-wiper blades.

- Spread a towel on the floor. Stand on it and scrunch it up with your toes.

- Use your toes to pick up pencils or marbles, or to turn the pages of a phone book, one at a time.

ᵃ Climb the walls. Lie flat on the floor with the soles of your feet propped against a wall. "Walk" slowly up and down the wall by grasping with widespread toes.

ᵃ Stand with feet turned out to approximate 10 minutes to 2 on a clock face. Walk forward for 10 steps, backward for 10 steps. Repeat with the toes turned inward like clock hands set at 20 minutes before 4.

ᵃ Walk barefoot on a yielding surface—beach sand or thick carpeting—as often as possible. Barefoot trodding of city pavements or public swimming-pool decking is not recommended. Besides being uncomfortable, these surfaces are rife with contaminants that can lead to foot infections.

ARCH SUPPORTERS

ᵃ Roll a rolling pin, a 12-ounce beverage can, or a tennis ball under your bare feet for several minutes each day.

ᵃ Stand on tiptoe, throw your weight to the outside of your feet, and come down slowly. Then walk on the balls of your feet for 30 seconds. Repeat the routine three times.

ᵃ Each morning, before putting on your shoes, stand with feet flat on the floor, then rise on your toes with a springing motion. Repeat 10 times.

ᵃ When you get home at night, take off your shoes and tiptoe around the house for 3 to 5 minutes. If truly "foot weary," reduce the walking time to 2 minutes, then sit on the edge of the bathtub and run warm water over your feet for 2 minutes; follow with 1 minute of cold water.

FLAT-FOOT FOILERS

ᵃ To prevent or relieve the pain of flat feet: Squat with your weight on your toes, then slowly rock backward until your weight is on your heels. Repeat several times. If necessary, steady yourself by holding onto a stable object.

ᵃ Stand with toes pointing inward in a pigeon-toed position. Go up and down from toe to heel 15 to 20 times.

Hⁱⁱ OW TO REVITALIZE YOUR FEET WITH A MASSAGE

Foot massage stimulates blood circulation, which is important not only for your feet, but also for facial attractiveness and the well-being of the rest of your body. You can use a hand lotion (see Chapter 10) for massaging your feet, or mix up a jar of this *Lubricating Massage Oil* to share with your tired-footed mate: Melt 1 tablespoon lanolin in the top of a double boiler. Stir in $3/4$ cup peanut oil and $1/4$ cup olive oil. Add $1/4$ cup rose water and emulsify with a rotary beater.

Malcolm's first day as a letter carrier was too much for his feet. He hobbled to the parking lot, removed his shoes, and was sitting with his feet propped up on the dashboard when a co-worker paused to initiate him into the rites of foot massage. "Rub some life into those dead dogs," advised the kindly veteran.

1. Grasp the sole of one foot with both hands, thumbs against the heel, and gradually massage toward the toes.

2. Place your thumbs on top of the foot next to the ankle and massage forward to the toes.

3. Play "this little piggy" by gently rotating and pulling each individual toe.

4. Repeat with the other foot.

The relief was so miraculous that Malcolm repeated the massage at lunchtime for a few days. Now, a veteran himself, he merely revives his feet each evening.

For a traditional Chinese massage to revitalize your feet:

1. Rotate your ankles while massaging each toe.

2. Massage the soles of your feet with your fists.

3. Rub the tops of your feet from ankles to toes in circular motions with the flat of your hand.

For a pressure massage to relieve swollen, tired feet:

1. One at a time, hold each toe with your thumb and index finger and apply firm pressure on three spots: the cuticle, the toe joint, and the base of the toe.

2. Massage the spaces between the toes, then move up the instep toward the ankle.

3. Place both thumbs under one heel and massage forward to the ball of the foot, then back to the Achilles' tendon. Repeat with the other foot.

For a quick massage to stimulate your feet: Place a layer of dried peas or beans in a pair of low-heeled oxfords and walk a few steps—very few, any more would be painful.

HOW TO SOAK OUT THE WEARIES: FIVE NATURAL SOLUTIONS FOR ADDING TO YOUR FOOTBATH

When you don't have time for a beauty bath, invigorate your feet by rubbing them with a lemon wedge or by sitting on the edge of the bathtub and running cold water over them for a few minutes. Better yet, soak them for 10 minutes in a foot tub or dishpan that will hold enough of one of the following solutions to reach your ankles. Rinse if necessary, dry thoroughly, then lightly massage with peanut oil or a moisturizing lotion.

- **Coffee grounds**. Refrigerate your coffee grounds so they won't sour, then utilize their remaining tannic acid to revive your feet. Boil 1 cup of the grounds in 2 cups water for 5 minutes. Strain into your footbath and add cool water.

- **Epsom salt**. Place $1/2$ cup epsom salt in your footbath. Swish with hot water to dissolve, add lukewarm water for a comfortable soak, then rinse with cold water.

- **Herbs**. Brew double-strength tea with camomile, comfrey (dried leaves or roots), horsetail, lavender, mint, or sage, then strain into the footbath.

- **Salt**. Using 2 foot basins and alternating soaks of hot salt water ($1/2$ cup table salt in an ankle-high basin) for 3 minutes with 1-minute cold-water soaks for 2 repetitions (conclude with the cold) gives exhausted feet a new vigor.

  Salt and soda, $1/4$ cup *each* table salt and baking soda, dissolved in warm water, soothe and smooth.

ঌ **Vinegar and lemon**. Swish $1^1/_2$ cups cider vinegar and $^1/_2$ cup fresh lemon juice with tepid water.

H OW TO TAKE THE HEAT OUT OF BURNING FEET

Burning sensations on the soles of the feet may be due to a deficiency of B-complex vitamins. Taking extra B-5, B-6, and B-12 along with a daily multivitamin often resolves the problem within a few weeks.

For instant relief, try a circulation-stimulating mustard footbath prepared with dry mustard, or cook up an old-fashioned *Bran Bath*: Stir 3 cups miller's bran into 4 cups cold water. Bring to boiling, cover, and let stand for 10 minutes. Strain into your footbath. Add cool water and $^1/_4$ cup baking soda. Soak your feet for 15 minutes. You can reserve and reuse the bran-soda solution each night for a week.

G OOD OLD-FASHIONED CURES FOR THOSE ACHING FEET

1. **Bandage them with onions**. Roast whole onions until soft; discard the outer layers; mash or puree the onions and apply to the feet on a cloth bandage.

2. **Bury them in sand**. Fill a deep pan with sand; add boiling water to make it moist and warm; bury your feet for 30 minutes and add more hot water if the sand cools too quickly.

3. **Soak them in oak bark tea**. Steep double-strength tea from red or white oak bark. Soak your feet for 15 minutes each night and morning.

4. **Wrap them in cabbage**. Remove the hard central ribs from a dozen large cabbage leaves. Soften the leaves in the top of a double boiler or in a covered container in the oven. Fold the warm leaves around your feet and cover with towels or plastic bags for 15 minutes.

NATURAL REMEDIES FOR CORRECTING SEVEN COMMON FOOT PROBLEMS

ATHLETE'S FOOT

Medically referred to as *tinea pedis*, the term "athlete's foot" was coined in the 1930s to glamorize a foot-powder promotion. The problem never was limited to athletic males (a university survey shows that 15 percent of the female students have athlete's foot[141]) and it is not so contagious as formerly believed. It can, however, be transmitted via shed fragments of affected skin, and can spread to moist skin folds in the pubic area or armpits, to the nails, or the scalp. The infection may be caused by any of several species of fungi or by various types of bacteria that thrive on moist warmth, and are triggered or worsened by emotional stress, physical illness, or air-excluding footwear which can increase the cup-per-day of moisture normally excreted by the feet. Daily cleansing with thorough drying (particularly between the toes), and wearing "breathable" shoes, are both preventives and treatment. If the painful "itchies" have established a foothold, try a natural remedy:

- Supplement your daily diet with a multivitamin, a B-complex tablet, 1,000 milligrams vitamin C, and 400 IU vitamin E; and take 2 acidophilus capsules or eat a serving of yogurt with each meal.

- Wear silk hosiery or acrylic socks to draw perspiration away from your feet. The once-advised white cotton socks absorb moisture and hold it close to the skin.

- Remove athletic shoes immediately after perspiration-producing activities; wear leather sandals whenever possible.

- Bathe your feet with a mild alcohol or vinegar rinse twice a day to restore the pH balance disturbed by the infection.

- Soak your feet once daily in a solution of 1 tablespoon salt per quart of water; or in a footbath of golden seal tea, thyme tea, or a combination of camomile and thyme tea.

- Powder your feet with cornstarch to help absorb moisture and reduce friction; or dust them with powdered golden seal as a curative.

ɣ Apply aloe vera gel every morning and evening, or smooth on yogurt at bedtime and wash it off in the morning. Or, try a B-vitamin ointment made by mixing pulverized B-2, B-3, and B-5 tablets into a paste with brewer's yeast and sesame oil.

ɣ Coat the affected areas twice daily with this variation of the "Wonder Cream" used by Russian soldiers: Blend 2 tablespoons lanolin and 1 tablespoon cod liver oil with $1^{1}/_{2}$ teaspoons *each* garlic powder and honey.

ɣ Expose your feet to sunlight for a total of 1 hour each day in 20- to 30-minute sessions.

BLISTERS

Massaging your feet with glycerin before wearing new shoes may help prevent blisters. Experienced hikers recommend wearing ankle-high silk or nylon hose under thick orlon, cotton, or wool socks. If a blister does form: Avoid the source of injury, protect the blister from further harm with a cushioned bandage, then allow it to heal naturally without pricking. Applying garlic oil (squeezed from a garlic-perle supplement) under the bandage is a modern folk remedy for relieving the pain of a blister and speeding its healing.

BUNIONS AND BUNIONETTES

Bunions (projections from the base of the big toe) and bunionettes (on the little toe) may be hereditary, but customarily result from a combination of loosening ligaments and constricting footwear. If the bunion does not push out too far, it may be corrected by eating a nutritious diet to strengthen the supportive muscles, padding with protectors, rubbing with a little pulverized saltpeter dissolved in olive oil, or with this 1890's treatment: Add 1 tablespoon ammonia per quart of hot water for a footbath. After a 10-minute soak, grasp your foot with one hand. With the other hand, pull your big toe away from your foot and gently rotate it under the water. Reheat the water and soak for another 10 minutes. Dry your feet, then paint the bunion with iodine.

CALLUSES AND CORNS

Dietary deficiencies may be responsible for a proclivity toward calluses (thickened areas of skin formed by the body to protect the flesh over bony prominences) and corns (conical overgrowths with hard, central cores resulting from abrasion or pressure). Including more vitamin A and potassium in your diet (see Vitamin and Mineral Chart) may help circumvent them. Eliminating friction and pressure by wearing well-fitting shoes should prevent their regrowth. Padding around calluses or corns offers temporary relief from the pain they engender; removal usually can be accomplished by one of these natural methods.

1. Soak your feet in soapy water or a solution of hot water and baking soda or dry mustard or salt, or in any of the footbaths suggested for other foot problems. After the soak, gently rub the callus or protruding corn with a pumice stone (smoothing on a coating of glycerin before using the pumice makes it more effective). Blot dry and coat with lotion, petroleum jelly, white vegetable shortening, or a mixture of 2 tablespoons vegetable oil and 1 teaspoon cider vinegar.

2. Massage aloe vera gel, castor oil, or vitamin E from pierced capsules into the calluses or corns twice each day; or, rub them with a paste of baking soda and water.

3. Walk on sand. Joanne's job as a sales rep required a lot of pavement pounding in fashionably high-heeled, thin-soled shoes, and the calluses her feet developed in self-protection were becoming painful. When she realized that walking barefoot on the sandy shore while vacationing had restored her feet to callusless comfort, Joanne put a beach in her bathtub for year-round "foot vacations" to prevent a discomforting recurrence. She keeps a shallow container of sand in the bathroom, places it in the tub after each bath or shower, and "marches in place" for a few minutes. Then she rinses and dries her feet and massages them with lotion.

4. Try a folk remedy for removing corns: Make a paste with breadcrumbs and cider vinegar, or with baking soda and petroleum jelly; apply to the corn each night until it can be lifted out.

   Or, each night for a week, cover the corn with the cut half of a raw cranberry, a slice of raw garlic, the pulp side of a small piece of lemon, a bit of raw onion, or a paste of onion cooked in vinegar.

Or, bind cotton over the corn and saturate it three times daily with turpentine.

Or, every other day, soak the corn-containing foot in a solution of hot water and dry mustard, rub the corn with vinegar, then dry and apply a touch of white iodine.

5. Soft corns between the toes may be mollified and prepared for removal by sponging with rubbing alcohol or castor oil, then wrapping the adjoining toes with wisps of wool yarn; or by scraping a piece of common white chalk, placing a pinch of the powder on the corn, and binding it in place with a strip of soft cloth.

DRY, ROUGH, OR FLAKY FEET

Before going to bed, soak your feet for 15 minutes in warm, sudsy water (use your favorite soap or shampoo) to which you have added baking soda or oatmeal. Rinse and dry; massage with castor oil, peanut oil, or petroleum jelly; then sleep in a pair of old socks.

Linda's feet were neither callused nor corned, but her heels felt rough and had a dirty gray cast. The night before the beach party, she decided something must be done. After her beauty-bath-soak, she scrubbed her heels with a nail brush, thoroughly dried them, rubbed in vitamin E from pierced capsules, and covered them with bed socks. The gray roughness disappeared, and, to her delight, stays away as long as she gives her heels a weekly vitamin E treat.

If only the bottoms of your feet are afflicted: Sprinkle a layer of table salt in a shallow pan, dampen it slightly, and slide your feet back and forth. Rinse, dry, and massage with lotion or oil.

If your legs as well as your feet are flaky, transform them into glossy gams with one of these treatments: Sit on the edge of the bathtub and run warm water over your legs and feet. Blot off the excess water, coat the skin with honey or molasses, then read or meditate for 30 minutes. After rinsing and drying, rub in a half-and-half mixture of lanolin and olive oil.

Or, exfoliate your legs and feet with one of the facial scrubs from Chapter 2. Rinse, dry, apply a moisturizing oil or lotion, then cover with plastic wrap for half an hour.

FOOT ODOR

Try supplementing your diet with 30 milligrams of zinc every day, placing a spoonful of dry oatmeal or miller's bran in your socks, or experimenting with one of these naturally deodorizing, moisture-absorbing foot powders.

- Baking soda and cornstarch, mixed half-and-half.

- One-fourth cup *each* cornstarch and fuller's earth, mixed with 2 tablespoons zinc oxide.

- One-half cup cornstarch mixed with $1/4$ cup zinc oxide and 1 tablespoon powdered orris root. Sprinkle 1 teaspoon of the mixture in each shoe.

INGROWN TOENAILS

To avoid toenail edges growing into adjoining soft tissue, cut the nails straight across and smooth them with an emery board or diamond file. Do *not* cut a "V" in the center of the nail. Besides being ineffectual and painful, this self-inflicted torture can instigate additional problems.

If an ingrown nail is caught before it becomes infected, home treatment is usually effective. After each shower, tub bath, or footbath, gently insert a wisp of cotton under the offending nail corner. To increase the benefit, soak your foot in a solution of hot water and epsom salt, then saturate the cotton with castor oil or vitamin E from a snipped capsule before tucking it under the nail edge. A folk-remedy alternative is a salve made from laundry soap, thick cream, and granulated sugar.

$\approx 12 \approx$

SMILING PRETTY:
HOW TO CARE FOR YOUR
MOUTH AND TEETH

What with food consumption and oral communication, mouths are in motion even more than feet. As sources of beauty and expression as well as functional necessities, they are justifiably entitled to a fair share of any beauty and health regimen.

PROTECT AND SOOTHE

Although lips are constantly being stretched, puckered, and exposed to moisture and extreme temperatures, they contain no oil glands. To prevent (or to heal) dry, chapped lips, follow the beauty experts' advice to "never let your lips go naked" by coating them with honey, lemon juice mixed half-and-half with glycerin, oil, petroleum jelly, or one of these lip protectors and soothers.

NATURAL LIP GLOSS AND POMADE

In the top of a double boiler (or in a heat-proof dish in a pan of boiling water), stir $1/4$ cup petroleum jelly into 2 tablespoons melted beeswax or paraffin. Or, beat 5 tablespoons vegetable or nut oil into 1 tablespoon melted beeswax or paraffin. Or, blend 1 tablespoon honey with $1^1/_2$ tablespoons melted beeswax or paraffin, then beat in 2 tablespoons vegetable oil. Remove from the heat and stir until cooled. Store the pomade in tiny pillboxes or jars. If it becomes too hard, reheat over hot water and stir in a few drops of vegetable oil.

You can add color to your lip gloss while it is still warm by stirring in food coloring or a teaspoon of alkanet root (which produces a lovely burgundy shade but should be strained through gauze after mixing).

Do-it-yourself Remedies for Lip Problems

❧ **Chronically dry, sore lips** may be due to a cosmetic allergy, a deficiency of dietary fatty acids, or to an internal yeast infection. If going without lipstick (or switching to a hypo-allergenic brand), including two tablespoons of vegetable oil with your daily meals, and experimenting with Mother Nature's lip smoothers fail to bring relief, check with your physician.

Coat your lips with honey or petroleum jelly after every washing and before bed each night. Or, blend 4 teaspoons glycerin with 1 teaspoon tincture of benzoin and smooth over your lips several times a day.

Sponge triple-strength white oat bark tea over your lips 3 times a day.

❧ **Cracks at the corners of the mouth** (*cheilosis*) may result from an allergy to commercial mouthwash or toothpaste, from overindulgence in alcohol or spicy foods, or from B-vitamin or fatty-acid deficiencies. A shotgun-approach of avoiding questionable foods and products, taking a high potency B-complex tablet with each meal, and drizzling a tablespoon of vegetable oil on each salad should resolve the problem.

❧ **Cold sores and fever blisters** are caused by *herpes simplex virus 1*, which lurks in a dormant state and can be activated by stress, menstrual difficulties, sunburn, or any illness with a fever. The sores and blisters may spread to the inside of the mouth as canker sores. Toothbrushes are a haven for the virus. If you have a cold sore, switch to a new toothbrush when the blister breaks and again after it has healed. Rather than wait for these unappealing abominations to run their course, try a natural remedy:

Acidophilus, ingested in the form of capsules or tablets taken with milk 4 times a day, or as a generous serving of acidophilus yogurt with each meal, usually relieves local soreness within 24 to 48 hours.[24]

Aloe vera gel from a freshly cut plant contains antibacterial, anti-fungi substances that are lacking in the commercially stabilized gel. Application of the gel at the onset often forestalls cold sores.

B-complex vitamins, taken in high-potency tablets twice daily, may abort an incipient cold sore. Early cures and shortened durations have been achieved by adding 100 milligrams of niacinamide; by taking 500 milligrams of B-5 every two hours; or by combining the B-5 treatment with twice-daily doses of 50 milligrams B-6, 350 micrograms B-12, and 500 milligrams vitamin C with bioflavonoids.

Herbal treatments. Sponge triple-strength red clover tea over the cold sore several times daily. Or three times a day, sip a cup of hot sage tea into which you have stirred a teaspoon of powdered ginger.

Ice. Holding a chip of ice against an erupting sore may halt its development.

Lysine (an amino acid available without prescription) is credited with rapid cures when 1,000 milligrams are taken daily. Lysine is even more miraculous when combined with the acidophilus therapy described above.

Salt water and brandy. At the first sign of a fever blister, dissolve all the salt possible in $1/4$ cup of boiling water. Apply to the sore with a cotton ball every hour, then sponge with brandy.

Vitamin C, accompanied by a calcium supplement and taken in 150 to 1,000 milligram doses each hour, helps clear cold sores.

When Gordon's cold sore erupted the weekend before he was to present the ad campaign he'd worked on for months, he had to do more than speed its recovery—he had to make it disappear. Hoping to augment the effectiveness of the vitamin-C therapy, he coated the blister with vitamin E from a pierced capsule before patting on the powdered C. Every hour, after taking his tablets of calcium and vitamin C, Gordon reapplied the topical treatment. The strategy worked. His lip was still tender, but no lip-puffing sore marred his successful presentation.

Zinc, ingested daily as a 30- to 50-milligram tablet, or pulverized and applied directly to cold sore, is another blister-banisher.

How TO NOURISH YOUR TEETH

Inert as they seem, teeth are alive. Composed principally of calcium, phosphate, and protein, they constantly renew themselves with nourishment from their roots in the bloodstream and the minerals washed over them by saliva. They, and their support, must be strong and healthy to withstand the up to 200 pounds of pressure exerted by the jaw muscles when we chew. A well-balanced diet, including adequate protein and calcium, is essential; a daily multivitamin-mineral supplement provides insurance against possible deficiencies.

- Lack of vitamin A can lead to tooth decay.
- Vitamin C deficiency can cause degeneration of tooth enamel, weakened supporting tissues, and bleeding gums.

Extremely hot or cold foods or drinks can cause dental enamel to suffer "thermal fatigue," which can lead to the formation of fissures in the teeth, and, not only what we eat but when we eat it, affects dental health:

- Chewable vitamin C, sweets, or sweetened beverages should be indulged in at mealtimes (not between meals) so the acids left in your mouth will be neutralized.

- Starches and fats can be as harmful as sweets. An enzyme in saliva transforms starch into sugar; fat makes food stick to the teeth. Raisins and peanut butter are among the worst offenders; most damaging of all is the folk practice of taking a spoonful of blackstrap molasses as a before-bed sleep-inducing nostrum.

- Chocolate, nuts, and certain cheeses (Cheddar, Monterey Jack, Swiss) help neutralize the decay-causing acids.

- Eating a quarter of a raw apple after a meal removes 30 percent more food debris from the teeth than an immediate brushing.[107]

- Taking 1 teaspoon of apple cider vinegar stirred into a glass of water at each meal is a folk remedy for reducing plaque and strengthening gums.

- Chewing sugar-free gum or ginger root, or rolling your tongue around your mouth to simulate tooth brushing, activates the salivary glands to protect the teeth and relieve a dry mouth.

🍃 Drinking generous amounts of tea (which contains flouride) provides as much protection from tooth decay as flouridated water. In *The Food Pharmacy* (Bantam, 1988), Jean Carper recommends using tea as an anti-cavity mouthwash.

Sturdy foods such as crispy salads, nuts, seeds, and whole-grain toast not only provide excellent nourishment; they also stimulate blood circulation to the teeth and gums, and lessen the risk of periodontal disease (which affects 90 percent of adults, accounts for all but 2 percent of tooth loss, and gives rise to bad breath and bleeding gums). Munching hard candy, ice chips, or popcorn kernels can crack your teeth. Chewing unchewable substances can wear them down; witness ancient skulls with teeth abraded to half their original length by the grit included with flour ground on stone metates.

How to Massage Your Gums and Protect Against Gum Disease

The friction of direct massage helps preserve a tight collar af gingival tissue around the teeth to protect against gum disease.

🍃 Lightly brush the gums with a soft-bristled toothbrush, or use the flexible rubber tip on the handle of your brush.

🍃 Make a paste of baking soda and 3 percent hydrogen peroxide. Rub this into the gums with a fingertip, then rinse your mouth with a saline solution of $1/4$ teaspoon table salt in $1/4$ cup water.

🍃 Massage your gums with table salt, then rinse with water.

🍃 Several times each day, practice the Oriental pressure-massage of pressing the corners and the center top and bottom of the lips with a firm, rotating motion.

How to Cleanse Your Teeth

An inmate of England's infamous Newgate Prison devised the first toothbrush by inserting tufts of hair into a piece of bone drilled with tiny holes. Prior to this ingenious invention, teeth were cleansed by chewing on twigs, rubbing with cloth, or by having the debris poked out of their crevices with toothpicks of porcupine quills, ivory or gold, or with the pointed ends of eating knives. The origin of our round-tipped dinner knives is attributed to Cardinal Richelieu's edict prohibiting the sharp tips that so often drew blood when seventeenth-century diners picked their teeth.

Directions for which direction to brush with what type of bristles at which angle have undergone radical changes since "up and down with stiff bristles" was eulogized. The most recent advice from the American Dental Association is to use a brush with soft, rounded bristles, hold it at a 45-degree angle to the gum line and brush in a slow circular motion, covering about three teeth per circle. To reach the inside of the front teeth, insert the brush vertically and gently push it up and down; then brush the chewing surfaces with short back-and-forth strokes.

For controlling plaque and removing debris between the teeth, correct flossing is as vital as brushing. Curve the dental floss around each tooth and scrape up and down several times, then employ a gently sawing motion between the gums and the neck of each tooth.

When to Clean Your Teeth

Concluding each meal with a few bites of fibrous food (apple, orange, raw carrot, or celery) and a "swish and swallow" mouth-rinsing of plain water is considered as effective as brushing every time you eat. In fact, according to a report in *Health* (October 1987), one thorough cleansing per day may be all that is necessary because mouth bacteria require 24 hours for recolonization. Periodontists, however, still advise brushing every 12 hours for plaque control. The most important time to clean the mouth is the last thing at night to prevent sugar molecules or food particles from wreaking their havoc during sleeping hours.

How to Care for Artificial Teeth

The first false teeth were clumsy contraptions carved from ivory and held together with metal springs (George Washington's famous "falsies" were made from walrus tusks, not wood). Later experiments with celluloid proved unsuccessful because of the inflammability, as exemplified by public catastrophes in which smokers' dentures caught on fire. Whether with "partials" or full dentures, the mouths of more than half the population over 45 are now enhanced with artificial teeth, which, regardless of formulation, require daily cleansing to prevent tartar buildup and unpleasant breath. It is especially important to remove partial dentures for cleaning to avoid a collection of food fragments in the recesses around retention clips.

If the sensitive tissue around or beneath artificial teeth becomes tender, rub your gums with aloe vera gel or vitamin A (squeezed from a pierced capsule) and supplement your diet with 30 to 100 milligrams of zinc daily until the soreness disappears.

How to Deal with Discolored teeth

Depigmentation, white spots, or a mottled appearance may be the result of childhood exposure to overly flouridated water, illnesses with high fevers, prescriptive doses of tetracyline, or deficiencies of vitamins A, B, or E. Dr. Ronald T. Maitland, 1988 spokesperson for the American Dental Association, warns that abrasive pastes and polishes set up a vicious pattern of roughening and wearing away tooth enamel to make teeth more prone to staining.

Recently acquired surface discolorations from coffee, tea, acidic foods or beverages, or from smoking, that remain after normal brushing and flossing may be removed by brushing with baking soda; rubbing with a fresh strawberry; or by scrubbing with lemon peel, then thoroughly rinsing with water.

Natural Dentifrices:
FOUR NATURAL CLEANSERS FOR FIGHTING GERMS AND PLAQUE

Many dentists believe dentifrices serve only to add piquancy to the otherwise boring task of tooth cleaning. This is borne out by studies of over 50 different brands of toothpaste—none proved more effective at preventing dental caries than proper flossing and brushing with plain water[124]—and, although several flouride-containing dentifrices have acceptance as cavity fighters, *Parade Magazine* (February 7, 1988) reports that no toothpaste or gel has the American Dental Association seal for plaque removal.

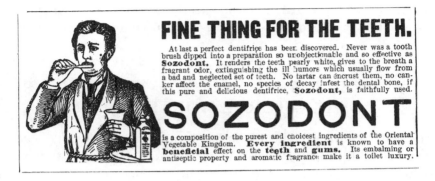

FINE THING FOR THE TEETH.

At last a perfect dentifrice has been discovered. Never was a tooth brush dipped into a preparation so unobjectionable and so effective as **Sozodont.** It renders the teeth pearly white, gives to the breath a fragrant odor, extinguishing the ill humors which usually flow from a bad and neglected set of teeth. No tartar can encrust them, no canker affect the enamel, no species of decay infest the dental bone, if this pure and delicious dentifrice, **Sozodont,** is faithfully used.

SOZODONT

is a composition of the purest and choicest ingredients of the Oriental Vegetable Kingdom. **Every ingredient** is known to have a **beneficial** effect on the **teeth** and **gums.** Its embalming or antiseptic property and aromatic fragrance make it a toilet luxury.

The recorded formula for this liquid dentifrice, marketed in 1893, shows little of benefit, or of Oriental origin: 10 ounces water, 4 ounces honey, 2 ounces alcohol, $1/2$ ounce potassium carbonate, with sufficient oil of rose and oil of wintergreen to flavor.

In 1860, borax, dissolved in water, was suggested for destroying the parasitic mites believed to exist in remnants of food fermenting between the teeth. During the 1880s, beauty-conscious ladies were advised to brush their teeth with white soap instead of harsh dentifrices, and were assured that the slightly unpleasant taste would soon pass unnoticed. In lieu of laundry products, there are other natural cleansers:

- **Apple juice or lemon juice.** Brush, then rinse with water.

- **Baking soda** has none of the silicates contained in abrasive dentifrices, and, long before modern dentists began recommending it for stain removal, soda was combined with other natural substances for cleaning teeth, killing germs, and preventing plaque.

  Mix equal amounts of soda and sea salt; mix $1/2$ cup soda, 1 tablespoon sea salt, and 1 teaspoon ground cinnamon; mix $1/2$ cup soda, $1/4$ cup dried lemon or orange peel (pulverized in an electric blender or coffee grinder), and 4 teaspoons table salt; or, make a paste with soda and a mashed strawberry or 3-percent hydrogen peroxide.

HERBAL TOOTH POWDERS

- *Black walnut* powder, brushed on the teeth, is credited with restoring tooth enamel.[154]

ᐁ **Mint leaves, Peruvian bark, and rosemary leaves,** lightly roast-
ed and ground to a powder with charcoal, cleanse and polish teeth.

25 HERBS YOU CAN USE TO MAKE YOUR OWN NATURAL MOUTH RINSES

The Federal Drug Administration has found most ingredients in commercial mouthwashes useless; many unsafe.[137] For easily prepared,
natural "mouth rinses," steep one to three ounces of any of the following herbs (singly or in combination) to make double-strength tea.
For germ-fighting benefits, soak the herbs in $2/3$ cup ethyl alcohol (or
80-proof vodka) for one week; strain and dilute with $1^1/_3$ cups distilled water.

ᐁ **Agrimony:** astringent, good for receding or bleeding gums,
promotes healing after tooth extraction

ᐁ **Angelica root:** relieves pain, promotes healing

ᐁ **Anise seeds:** aromatic flavoring, relieves pain

ᐁ **Camomile:** reduces gum inflammation and pain, aids healing

ᐁ **Cardamom:** freshens breath, used as flavoring

ᐁ **Catnip:** relieves mouth soreness

ᐁ **Cinnamon:** freshens breath

ᐁ **Cloves:** freshens breath, kills germs, reduces pain

ᐁ **Comfrey:** astringent, good for bleeding gums, relieves pain

ᐁ **Eucalyptus:** antiseptic

ᐁ **Fenugreek:** freshens breath, relieves mouth inflammation

ᐁ **Golden seal:** astringent, antiseptic (has an antibiotic action similar to tetracycline and streptomycin)

ᐁ **Horsetail:** freshens breath, strengthens tooth enamel

ᐁ **Lemon balm:** freshens breath, relieves mouth soreness

ᐁ **Myrrh:** antiseptic, astringent, aids bleeding gums and mouth
inflammation

ᐁ **Peppermint and Spearmint:** antiseptic breath fresheners promote healing

- **Plantain:** helps bleeding gums, reduces pain and mouth inflammation

- **Rosemary:** freshens breath

- **Sage:** strong astringent, reduces saliva production, folk remedy for bleeding gums

- **Sandalwood:** astringent, disinfectant

- **Shave grass:** reduces bleeding, improves healing and prevents scarring after dental surgery

- **Thyme:** scientifically proven antiseptic which gives a famous mouthwash its characteristically unpleasant flavor

- **White oak bark:** astringent, relieves canker sores, strengthens gums, helps set loose teeth

- **Winter savory:** scientifically confirmed antiseptic

- **Witch hazel bark:** relieves soreness and bleeding gums

THREE EASY ANTISEPTIC MOUTHWASH RECIPES

1. *Food flavorings (extracts).* Shake 1 to 2 tablespoons extract with a mixture of $1/2$ cup *each* ethyl alcohol (or 80-proof vodka) and distilled water. Use almond to soothe pain; lemon for bleeding gums; peppermint, spearmint, or vanilla for flavor; wintergreen for killing germs, reducing pain, and strengthening gums.

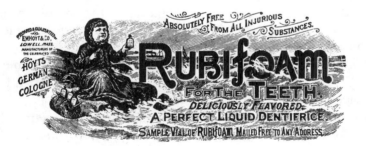

2. *Mint flavored.* Soak $1/2$ teaspoon *each* crushed cloves, myrrh, thyme, and spearmint in $3/4$ cup ethyl alcohol for 1 week, shaking the bottle daily. Strain, add 10 drops oil of peppermint and $1 1/2$ cups distilled water.

Or, combine 1 cup *each* ethyl alcohol and distilled water with 1 teaspoon *each* peppermint and wintergreen oil.

3. *Nonalcoholic.* Boil hyssop leaves in vinegar to cover, strain, and use as a rinse to relieve a sore mouth.

Or, steep $1/4$ teaspoon *each* of anise, mint, and rosemary in $3/4$ cups boiling water for 10 minutes. Strain and use as a rinse for bleeding gums or an irritated mouth.

Or, combine 2 tablespoons *each* dried eucalyptus leaves, lemon balm, peppermint, plantain, sage, and thyme. Boil 4 teaspoons of the mixture in 1 cup water for 10 minutes. Let stand, covered, for another 10 minutes. Strain and bottle for an all-purpose mouthwash.

HOW TO BANISH BAD BREATH

The most obvious cause of unpleasant mouth odor is strongly flavored food such as garlic or onion. Eating the fresh parsley or cilantro often served as a garnish with halitosis-generating meals; chewing cloves, cardamom or dill seeds, or chlorophyll-thymol tablets from health food stores are convenient away-from-home breath purifiers.

Less obvious is the fact that fragments of food lurking between the teeth may cause even the blandest of meals to create offensive mouth odors. The 98.6-degree temperature in the mouth instigates the decomposition of bits of meat, eggs, and similar foods within a few hours. When you neglect to sequester a few bites of fibrous veggies to munch on for teeth cleansing after dessert—and immediate brushing is not feasible—hie yourself to the powder room and clear the crevices with a toothpick.

Brushing your tongue each time you brush your teeth reduces mouth odor 60 percent more effectively than just brushing and flossing your teeth;[86] rinsing with mouthwash adds the finishing touch. If that combination plus these natural remedies does not resolve the problem, visit your dentist and physician to be sure decaying teeth, kidney dysfunction, or digestive problems are not responsible.

᙭ Eat acidophilus yogurt every day, or take acidophilus supplements with each meal.

- Rinse your mouth two or three times a day with equal parts of horseradish and honey diluted with water. Or, swish with triple-strength tea made from equal amounts of golden seal, myrrh, and rosemary.

- Drink a cup of fenugreek, peppermint, or rosemary tea each morning and evening. Add $1/4$ teaspoon anise, cinnamon, cloves, or mace to each cupful to increase the efficacy of the tea.

- Drink 2 cups a day of this Breath Freshening Tea:

  2 tablespoons *each* anise, camomile, lemon balm, and peppermint

  1 tablespoon *each* angelica root, cloves, echinacea, and dried parsley

  Soak 1 teaspoon of the dry mixture in 1 cup cold water for an hour, bring to a boil, cover, and steep for 5 minutes, then strain.

13

WATCHING OUT FOR YOUR EYES: HOW TO RELIEVE EYESTRAIN AND OTHER COMMON AILMENTS

When it comes to creating a first and lasting impression of beauty, the eyes have it. Romantic poets refer to them as windows of the soul; pragmatic physicians believe they mirror the state of physical health. Regardless of how others view our eyes, their well-being is essential if we are to see out of them. Sunglasses help prevent damage from ultraviolet rays; goggles guard them while we gaze at underwater wonders or work with equipment that might produce flying fragments; wearing collars with room for two fingers between fabric and neck allows an ample supply of nutrient-bearing blood to reach them. (A study at Cornell University revealed that 67 percent of the white-collared males tested were suffering from eye impairment due to restricted circulation from too-tight collars.)

HOW TO NOURISH YOUR EYES

What we ingest has a profound effect on our eyes. Thirty-five hundred years before vitamins were "discovered," Egyptian physicians successfully treated night blindness with ox liver, and in 500 B.C., Hippocrates was prescribing raw liver (2 ounces = 30,000 IUs of vitamin A) for his patients with dimming sight. Vitamin A has been acknowledged as the "eye vitamin" since World War II fighter pilots dined on carrots (26,000 IUs of vitamin A per cup) to restore their night vision. Although excess vitamin A stored in the liver can be harmful, there is little danger of toxicity from the vitamin-A precursor, beta carotene, in foods or supplements because the body converts it to vitamin A only as needed. Good vision also depends on a well-balanced diet and a constant supply of specific vitamins and

162

minerals. Many ophthalmologists recommend taking one or two tablets daily of a comprehensive "eye vitamin" supplement containing

Beta carotene (5,000 IU)

Vitamin C (60 milligrams)

Vitamin E (30 IU)

Copper (2 milligrams)

Selenium (40 micrograms)

Zinc (40 milligrams)

To help delay the development of cataracts, doctors sometimes advise much larger amounts of these nutrients.

Studies conducted by the former U.S. Department of Health, Education, and Welfare established that smoking reduces visual acuity, color perception, and night vision by decreasing the amount of oxygen delivered to the eyes by the blood vessels. Taking additional vitamin C (25 milligrams per cigarette smoked) and extra B-2 (30 to 50 milligrams plus a daily B-complex supplement) helps nullify the adverse effects of nicotine and carbon monoxide. Other recent findings link eye disorders to specific dietary overindulgences: alcohol blurs vision by interfering with the optic nerve; animal fats, refined carbohydrates and sugars, and excess salt adversely affect vision by altering the viscosity of fluid within the eye and changing the focal length of the eye's refraction. An excess of refined sugar also depletes calcium and chromium from the elastic cells in the eyes, causing the eyes to stretch out of shape and lose their normal focusing ability.[75, 100]

Drinking a glass of water containing 2 teaspoons *each* apple cider vinegar and raw honey at each meal is a folk remedy credited with maintaining good eyesight.[90] Eating raw fruit and vegetables benefits the eyes by providing enzymes necessary for vitamin and mineral assimilation, and a daily glass of any of the following mixtures is reported to improve vision in two weeks.[127, 192]

> $3/_4$ *cup carrot juice* + $1/_4$ *cup spinach juice.*
> $2/_3$ *cup carrot juice* + 1/4 *cup celery juice* +
> *1 tablespoon spinach juice.*
> $2/_3$ *cup carrot juice* + $1/_4$ *cup green lettuce juice* +
> *1 tablespoon cod liver oil.*
> $1/_2$ *cup carrot juice* + $1/_2$ *cup celery juice.*

Techniques for Reducing Eye Fatigue and Increasing Muscle Strength

Quick-start Morning Massage

Including a brief eye massage in your morning beauty routine improves circulation to distribute nourishment to the eyes, helps eliminate any puffiness, and gives you a youthfully wide-eyed start on the day.

1. Dab oil or cream on the under-eye skin. Put the first two fingers of your left hand one-half inch from the outside corner of your left eye; pull to the left to slightly tighten the skin. With your right index finger, start under the inside corner of your left eye and massage around it with gentle, circular movements. Change hands and repeat with the other eye.

2. Place your index fingers on the lower eye sockets, one-half inch from the outside corners of the eyes. Press and massage for 10 seconds.

3. Press the index finger of each hand under the center of each eyebrow. Close your eyes and rest the second finger of each hand on the eyelid. Try to open your eyes against this gentle pressure. Relax and repeat 5 times.

4. Open your eyes wide. With your fingertips, push up on your forehead just above each eyebrow for 5 seconds. Relax and repeat 5 times.

Six Simple Eye Calisthenics

Like all muscles, those controlling eyeball movement grow stronger with exercise, and tire if held in a fixed position too long. Interspersing eye calisthenics with periods of visual concentration lessens eye fatigue and increases the strength of these six pairs of orbital muscles.

- Hold your index finger about 10 inches in front of your eyes. Look at the tip of your finger, then look into the distance. Repeat 10 times.

- Look steadily at an object on the wall while slowly rolling your head in a circle. Close your eyelids and slowly roll your eyes in clockwise, then counterclockwise, circles. Repeat 5 times.

🐚 Without moving your head, look up, down, left, and right, as far as possible. Dart quick glances at the corners of the room. Close your eyes for 5 seconds, then repeat.

🐚 Blink both eyes as fast as you can 15 times. (Blinking exercises two other sets of muscles: sphincter muscles that contract when you close your eyelids, another pair that raises the lids.) Wink one eye at a time while keeping the other eye open, 10 times for each eye. Tensing the entire face on the same side as the wink helps prevent bagging or dark circles under the eyes.

🐚 Open your eyes as wide as you can. Slowly roll them in a circle to the left, then to the right. Close your eyes for 5 seconds between each of 5 repetitions.

🐚 For a complete regimen, try this variation of Yoga therapy for improving eyesight and relieving eyestrain:

1. Sit upright. Slowly nod your head 3 times toward your chest, your left shoulder, your back, and your right shoulder.

2. Slowly roll your head clockwise, then counterclockwise.

3. Inhale with your eyes tightly closed; exhale, open your eyes and blink rapidly 10 times.

4. Without moving your head, move your eyes in a slow circle to the left, then to the right. Look diagonally toward the corners of the room, then up and down.

5. Vigorously rub your hands together. Close your eyes, cover them with your palms, and take 5 slow, deep breaths.

"PALMING": THE BEST WAY TO REST YOUR EYES

"Palming," first introduced by Dr. William H. Bates,[79] is still considered the best way to relax tired eyes.

1. Sit comfortably in an armchair or at a table with your elbows supported. Close your eyes and cup your palms over them without touching the eyelids.

2. Relax and take slow, deep breaths until the restful gray you "see" with your closed eyes turns into velvety blackness.

3. Open your eyes and blink rapidly a few times.

GETTING THE RED OUT: FIVE NATURAL SOLUTIONS FOR BATHING YOUR EYES

Many strange substances have been used to cleanse and refresh eyes, get the red out, and relieve the feeling of grit behind the eyelids. Inserting drops of castor oil, milk bottled with a white poppy, or a wash made with dried hen's dung were once popular. For added sparkle, Spanish señoritas squeezed the oil from orange peel into their eyes and colonial Americans "flirted in" soapsuds; both mistreatments seemed effective because the irritation causes the eyes to form tears to wash away the discomfort.

Human tears are Mother Nature's prescription for bathing the eyes. To simulate tears, use filtered sea water (purchased in bottles at health food stores), or a saline solution made from $1/4$ teaspoon salt dissolved in $1/2$ cup water. Folk practitioners suggest dissolving 2 tablespoons of clean rock salt in 1 quart of rain water (or bottled water), then immersing the face and blinking the eyes several times to wash the eyes and clear redness; or using one of these natural eye washes and drops:

1. **Baking soda:** $1/2$ teaspoon dissolved in $1/2$ cup water.

2. **Herbal teas,** made from 1 level teaspoon of dried herb steeped in 1 cup boiling water and well strained.

    Borage helps clear redness and relieves stinging from cigarette smoke or wintry winds.

    Camomile relieves watery or inflamed eyes, and speeds healing of eye infections.

    Elderflower clears redness.

    Eyebright cleanses the eyes and improves sight.

    Fennel, prepared from powdered seeds and strained through a paper coffee filter, refreshes weary eyes, reduces inflammation or watering, and is suggested as a twice-daily eyebath for glaucoma or other ocular diseases.

    Golden seal, *lemon grass*, *red raspberry*, or *sassafras teas* may be used as either drops or washes to relieve eyestrain and refresh the eyes.

Pekoe tea, 1 teaspoon of the brew diluted with 1/4 cup water, may be used for either drops or baths to relieve eye irritation resulting from hay fever.

3. **Honey**. Stir $^1/_2$ teaspoon into $^1/_2$ cup lukewarm water.

4. **Milk**. A few drops of milk will relieve eye irritation caused by grains of salt or pepper. Equal parts of milk and water or strained sassafras tea may be used for refreshing eye drops or washes. For sore eyes, try this eighteenth-century potable eye bath: Boil 4 ounces camomile tea in 2 cups milk until reduced to 1 cup. Dissolve 2 tablespoons brown sugar in the hot liquid, stir in $^1/_2$ cup rum, strain, and bottle.

5. **Rose petal water**. Boil unsprayed, fresh rose petals in water to cover. Strain into a sterilized bottle for use as eye drops or baths to strengthen the eyes and relieve irritation caused by hay fever.

NINE SOOTHING COMPRESSES AND POULTICES FOR REFRESHING TIRED, IRRITATED EYES

When using eye compresses or packs, reclining (preferably on a slant-board) for 10 to 15 minutes enhances their benefit. Wet tea-bag compresses are one of the most effective ways to refresh tired, itchy, puffy, or watery eyes. Make-ahead pads of cotton saturated with witch hazel and stored in a jar in the refrigerator are even more convenient.

1. *Alum water*. Saturate eye pads in a solution of $^1/_8$ teaspoon alum and 1 cup water.

2. *Beets*, cooked, chilled, grated, and sandwiched between pieces of gauze, help relieve eyestrain. Direct application of raw cucumber slices is equally effective.

3. *Bread*. Toast and cool a slice of stale bread. Cut in half, soak in ice water, then wrap in cloth for eye compresses.

4. *Herbal poultices*: Borage, camomile, elderflower, eyebright, fennel, hyssop (by itself or mixed half-and-half with St. John's wort), rose hip, sassafras, slippery elm, verbena, or witch hazel bark in moistened tea bags (or compresses of wet tea leaves wrapped in cloth).

5. *Golden seal tea* brings relief to tired eyes. Steep $1/4$ teaspoon of the dried herb in $1/2$ cup boiling water. Cool, strain, then use to saturate eye pads.

6. *Milk*, warmed to room temperature and used to saturate eye pads, puts the sparkle back in weary eyes.

7. *Orange juice*, freshly squeezed and strained, then used to moisten gauze pads, is an eye refresher.

8. *Papaya-mint* or *plain papaya tea bags* soaked in hot water, then chilled, not only refresh tired eyes but also reduce under-eye bags.

9. *Potato*, hand-grated or processor-pureed, raw potato wrapped in gauze is a time-tested remedy for tired eyes and sandy eyelids.

NATURAL REMEDIES FOR SIX COMMON EYE PROBLEMS

BLACK EYES

Apply an ice pack or a cold compress (soft-pack frozen veggies are fine, but raw beef steak is no longer advised) for 15 minutes once each hour for 4 or 5 hours. Or, boil hyssop leaves, slippery elm bark, or soapwort roots until tender, wrap in gauze, and secure over the eye at bedtime. Do not remove until morning.

BLOODSHOT EYES

Capillary weakness resulting from deficiencies of vitamin C and bioflavonoids may be responsible for redness that does not clear with natural eyedrops and baths. If the problem continues after dietary supplementation of 5,000 milligrams vitamin C plus 1,000 milligrams bioflavonoids daily, consult your physician—allergies or conjunctivitis might be the cause.

DARK CIRCLES OR BAGS BENEATH THE EYES

These beauty detractors may not be due to either debauchery or illness. Under-eye tissue is so fragile that pockets can develop as repositories for fat or fluid, and is so transparent that the veins may show through as dark shadows.

- ✌ Compresses of moist camomile, pekoe, or rose hip tea (or warmed castor oil or olive oil) help remedy the problem if left in place for 15 minutes to several hours daily.

- ✌ Placing half a fresh fig or a poultice of grated raw cucumber under each eye for 15 minutes each day has been effective in some cases.

- ✌ Nighttime "fluid pooling" may be responsible for morning puffiness; try sleeping with two extra pillows tucked under your head. Or, freeze babies' teething rings, wrap in soft cloth, and place over your eyes for a few minutes.

DROOPY EYELIDS

- ✌ For immediate, temporary relief, chill 2 teaspoons in ice water and place them over your closed eyelids.

- ✌ If weakened muscles are the cause, increase your dietary protein and add supplements of vitamin C, bioflavonoids, and vitamin E. Then strengthen the miniature muscles with exercise. Several times daily, cup your palms over your eyes and stretch the eyelids upward and outward for 10 seconds. Or, squeeze your eyes tightly shut; slowly relax the squeeze and lift your eyebrows, stretching the lids upward as far as possible without opening your eyes. Relax and repeat 5 times.

- ✌ Lids swollen from fluid accumulation may respond to 50 milligrams per-day supplements of vitamin B-6 plus compresses of moist camomile or pekoe tea bags.

DRY EYES

Inadequate nutrition or lack of humidity in desert-dry air or overheated rooms may instigate itching and burning not caused by allergy or eyestrain. An improved diet with daily supplements of 300 milligrams of Omega-3, plus frequently misted house plants or a humidifier, help moisturize eyes as well as skin. More often, dry eyes result from failure to blink as often as we should to keep our eyes lubricated. To remedy the problem, take a 10-second "break" of rapid blinking while changing focus from near to far during close work, deliberately blink at the end of each line of reading material, and use natural eye drops or washes every day.

Eyelid Lumps and Inflammations

Sties (tender bumps and little abscesses that suddenly bulge out between the roots of the eyelashes) and *chalazions* (slower-growing cysts that form on the edge of an eyelid when a gland inside the lid becomes plugged) usually can be cleared with natural remedies.

- Saturate a lint-free cloth (or gauze eye pads) with hot water and hold against the sty for 10 to 15 minutes at a time, 3 or 4 times daily.

- A moistened pekoe tea bag, or a compress of warm castor oil or dampened baking soda wrapped in cloth and left in place overnight, often drives away burgeoning sties by morning.

- A persistent sty can be treated with a poultice of grated raw potato, which may bring it to a head so it will burst and dissipate.

Blepharitis, eyelid inflammation with crusting and scaling at the base of the lashes, is related to abnormally increased dandruff and often contains infectious bacteria. If natural eye drops and dandruff treatments (see Chapter 14) do not resolve the problem, professional care should be sought.

How to Cultivate Long, Luxurious Lashes

Each lash has an individual life cycle consisting of a six-month growth period followed by a resting period during which it separates from the root so a new lash can form in the follicle. A few eyelashes are dislodged daily by washing or rubbing the eyes, and the unnoticeable process continues. The massive lash-and-brow fallout sometimes engendered by severe malnutrition or lengthy illness is usually followed by regrowth after good health is regained.

Cutting off your lashes in the hope of having them grow in longer and thicker doesn't work, but there are natural means of encouragement that have proven successful:

Castor oil or olive oil. A nightly brushing with either of these oils is an old-fashioned, slow-but-sure treatment practically guaranteed to produce long, silky eyelashes.

"Huile de Ricin," an exotic sounding French formula for luxurious lashes, can be duplicated by adding a sliver of lemon peel to the small bottle of oil used for daily brushing.

Liquid protein, sold as a dietary aid, strengthens and lengthens eyelashes when brushed on nightly.

Petroleum jelly, applied each night and morning, helps correct brittle, breaking eyelashes and makes them appear longer.

Vitamin D. Each evening, snip a capsule of vitamin D and pat the contents over your lids and lashes. Fantastic results have been reported after less than three months of this treatment.[33]

How to beautify your brows

Eyebrows should compliment your face and accentuate your eyes, not attract attention to themselves. To encourage growth and thickening, rub lanolin or any of the eyelash-stimulators into the brows each evening before bed. If your eyes are close set, removing a few extra hairs from the inner edge of the brows can give you a more wide-eyed appearance; otherwise, brows should begin directly above the inner eye corners. Besides plucking the stragglers under and between your eyebrows, you may want to adjust their shape to conform to your facial structure.

Arched if your face is round.

Rounded if your face is heart shaped.

Slightly arched if your face is square or rectangular.

Straight if you have a long slender or oval face.

To eliminate tweezing discomfort when removing superfluous hairs, and to leave the vacated skin smooth and attractive:

1. Wipe your brows with an alcohol- or astringent-saturated cotton ball to remove any traces of oil.

2. Brush your brows the "wrong way" with an eyebrow brush or child's toothbrush to clear out any leftover makeup or flaky skin, then stroke them back into place.

3. For ouchless plucking: Press an ice cube over the area for a few seconds, blot with a tissue, then tweeze one hair at a time in the direction of hair growth.

4. Finish by again wiping the area with alcohol or astringent, then apply a moisturizer or a coating of honey. The honey not only softens the skin, but also acts as a natural bactericide.

Overly thick, bushy eyebrows (masculine or feminine) can be trimmed with manicure scissors or thinned with tweezers. To train your eyebrows and keep them in line: Start by brushing them straight up on your forehead, then coax them into the proper shape with the side of the eyebrow brush. Smoothing on a dab of petroleum jelly or hair-styling gel while brushing will help keep them in their place.

14

HAIR CARE:
TIPS ON CONTROLLING,
CONDITIONING, AND COLORING

Crowning glory and face framer, hair shelters our heads from heat, cold, and injury. It has held an aura of fascination since fairy-tale Rapunzel lowered hers as a ladder for her lover, Lady Godiva made her famous ride, and wasp-waisted nineteenth-century ladies piled so much of it under their hats that they had to perambulate with out-thrust bosoms and bustled buttocks.

Hair grows approximately one-half inch per month until it reaches a length of 10 to 12 inches, then growth slows to half speed. After a three-year *anagen* (growing) phase, cell production ceases for three months (the *telogen* or resting phase) while replacements are formed. The inner core of the hair receives nourishment from blood vessels in the scalp. The outer layer (the *cuticle*) is composed of overlapping scales that, when hair is well cared for, lie flat to seal in natural oils and reflect light from our shining tresses. When internal supplies are inadequate, or when external abuse roughens the outer layer, dull, lifeless-appearing hair results.

How to Nourish Your Hair

Healthy hair depends on a nutritionally sound diet. Protein deficiencies can halt the growth phase, causing hair to shed prematurely. Excessive amounts of sugar, refined carbohydrates, or alcohol can deplete the B-for-beautiful-hair vitamins. Smoking robs the body of vitamin C and constricts the supply-carrying blood vessels. In addition to iodized salt or kelp salt-substitutes to furnish iodine, suggested hair-enhancing daily supplements are 1 multivitamin-mineral, 25,000 IU vitamin A in the form of beta carotene, 1 B-complex stress tab, 1,000 milligrams vitamin C, and 15 to 30 milligrams of zinc.

Do-it-Yourself Scalp Massages That Stimulate Blood Flow

A tight scalp restricts the flow of nutrients and prematurely moves hair into the preparing-to-fall-out stage. If your hair is oily, massage gently. If it is dry, massage more vigorously to stimulate the oil glands. For a quick daily massage, use your fingertips to massage tiny circles from the nape of your neck to your forehead, then across the hairline. For a once-or-twice weekly massage:

1. Brush your hair to remove contaminants and tangles.

2. Sit comfortably. Droop your head toward your chest and rotate it slowly to the right, then to the left.

3. Still leaning forward, place the palms of your hands (fingers separated) underneath your hair. Using push-and-relax movements, work your hands upward from the nape of your neck. Raise your head and reverse the process from forehead to nape. Repeat until your scalp feels tingly and warm.

Brushing: Why Gentle Is Better

Gentle brushing encourages blood circulation, stimulates the sebum-producing glands and distributes their oils to glimmerize hair strands. It also dislodges dry scalp flakes and whisks them away along with dust or hairspray residue. Brushing upward from the nape of the neck while bending forward adds volume after you flip it back into place. Overly vigorous brushing damages hair by stripping away outer cells to expose the inner shaft, breaking brittle hair, or by dislodging not-yet-ready-to-depart hairs.

How to Dry Clean Your Hair

These rub-in, brush-out cleansers can be utilized to remove surface soil, oil, and odor during illness or for any-time waterless freshening.

☙ **Almond meal, bran, cornmeal, oatmeal, sawdust, or talc** can be sprinkled through the hair, massaged in for 5 minutes, then brushed out. Mixing a tablespoon of baking soda with any of these substances aids odor control.

☙ **Borax,** dissolved in alcohol and rubbed into well-brushed hair, then removed with a towel is a hundred-year-old solution.

☙ **Egg white,** beaten to a stiff meringue, rubbed into the hair and scalp and allowed to dry before being brushed out, is used for bedridden patients in European hospitals.

☙ **Witch hazel** or an antiseptic mouthwash, applied to the scalp and thoroughly brushed out, relieves "itchies" and removes surface contaminants. For blondes, 3-percent hydrogen peroxide will serve the same purpose and lighten hair roots.

HOW TO SHAMPOO FOR BEAUTIFUL HAIR

During the Middle Ages, shampooing bouffant coiffures was a semiannual event. A century ago, ladies' magazines declared that hair could be washed as often as once a month. For your daily or weekly shampoo:

1. Rinse your hair with warm water.

2. Pour a little shampoo into your hands, then massage it into your scalp and hair. Always use as little shampoo as possible, and, if you are using a commercial product, dilute it with water.

3. Rinse with warm water until all the shampoo has gone down the drain. If your hair doesn't feel squeaky clean, apply a second lathering and repeat the rinsing.

4. Wrap a towel around your head; press to blot excess water, then dry gently.

DO-IT-YOURSELF SHAMPOOS THAT CLEAN AND ENHANCE YOUR HAIR

Body-cleansing bar soaps are not intended for hair. They can roughen the outer layer, dry the hair and scalp, and often contain chemicals that penetrate into the bloodstream through hair follicles. Alkaline hair products destroy the protective acid mantle and leave a film that, unless removed with an acidifying rinse, dulls hair and can create dandruff. You can improve commercial shampoos by adding a few drops of lemon juice to each application, or by combining equal amounts of shampoo and triple-strength herbal tea (camomile for light hair, rosemary or sage for dark). Or, you can concoct your own shampoo.

CASTILE SHAMPOO

For shimmering blonde or silver hair, try this simple formula: Grate a 4-ounce bar of castile soap into a quart jar. Fill with water and let stand. Shake before using. Follow with a rinse of 2 tablespoons strained lemon juice in 3 cups water.

HERBAL SHAMPOOS

For a cleansing, although not very sudsy, shampoo with an acceptable pH: Simmer $1/4$ cup dried comfrey root or rosemary in 3 cups of water for 15 minutes. Strain, then add $1/2$ cup grated castile soap and 1 teaspoon olive oil. Stir to dissolve the soap. For more lather, add 2 tablespoons of commercial shampoo.

❧ HERBAL EXTRAVAGANZA ❧

> *5 cups water*
> *$1/4$ cup each birch buds and leaves, marigold petals*
> *$1/4$ cup dried orange peel from the spice shelf*
> *2 tablespoons each camomile and red clover*
> *1 tablespoon each orris root, nettle, rosemary, and sage*
> *$3/4$ cup grated castile soap*
> *2 tablespoons aloe vera gel*

Bring water and herbs to boiling in a glass or enamel pan, cover, and simmer for 15 minutes; steep for 30 minutes. Strain all but 1 cup of the liquid into a bowl with the soap, and beat until frothy. Whisk the remaining liquid with the aloe vera gel, then beat into the soapy mixture. For a sudsier shampoo, add $1/2$ cup commercial shampoo.

OIL-ENRICHED SHAMPOOS

To moisturize dry, brittle hair and add shine to normal hair, mix equal amounts of vegetable oil and your regular shampoo for the first lathering. Rinse thoroughly, then wash again with plain shampoo. For conditioning plus shine, add a few drops of jojoba or wheat germ oil or the contents of a 400-IU vitamin E capsule to enough of your regular shampoo for one lathering.

PROTEIN SHAMPOOS

Shampoos with a protein content of 40 to 50 percent increase the tensile strength of hair, boost body, help repair dry hair, and add sheen. Commercial shampoos rarely contain more than 1 percent protein; you can improve them by adding natural protein.

- Soften half a packet of unflavored gelatin in 2 tablespoons cold water. Heat by placing the cup in a pan of boiling water or in a microwave oven for a few seconds, stir to dissolve, then add 1 tablespoon of mild shampoo.

- Whir 1 whole egg in an electric blender. Add 1 packet unflavored gelatin and $1/3$ cup baby shampoo. Let stand for 5 minutes, then blend thoroughly. Or, whisk an egg with 2 tablespoons *each* water and your usual shampoo, plus 1 teaspoon *each* lemon juice and olive oil; reserve the surplus in the refrigerator. Or, whisk 1 egg yolk with the amount of shampoo you normally use.

- Separate an egg and beat the white. Mix in enough shampoo for two applications. Apply half the mixture, leave on for 5 minutes, then rinse. Massage the egg yolk into your scalp and hair; wait 5 minutes before rinsing with lukewarm water. Work in the remainder of the egg-white mixture and rinse thoroughly.

SUDSLESS SHAMPOOS

- **Alcohol and water.** Combine in the proportions of 1 part alcohol to 3 parts water.

- **Borax and sage tea or water.** Mix 2 tablespoons of borax with 1 quart of liquid.

 ❧ **Egg shampoos.** A whole egg or an egg yolk beaten with water is a soap-alternative for improving dry hair. For an "exemplary shampoo," the egg yolk can be beaten with rum.

GUIDELINES FOR CHOOSING A HAIR STYLE THAT FLATTERS YOUR FACE

Upswept sides counterbalance gravity's sags, a double chin, or a short neck. A narrow jaw or receding chin can be modified by curls brought forward below the ears. A side part with soft curls framing the upper part of the face minimizes a prominent chin or a wide jaw-line. An oval face is compatible with all styles; hair-styling basics for other face shapes are

Diamond: bangs with volume at forehead, sleek sides, fullness at lower portion of face.

Heart: center or side part with wave across forehead, fullness at lower portion of face.

Long: bangs, width at sides, fluffed around the ears.

Round: sleek at sides with hair piled atop the head.

Square or rectangular: off-center part, bangs that sweep across forehead, sides drawn upward from ears to feathery curls on top.

HOW TO STYLE AS YOU DRY

Hair expands and loses its elasticity when wet. Vigorous rubbing with a towel, or stretching with a brush or a fine-toothed comb, can break or dislodge waterlogged hair strands. Many hairstyles require only finger arranging and air drying; setting lotions coat each strand with a protective film for added body and style-holding.

NATURAL SETTING LOTIONS, MOUSSES, AND GELS

 ❧ **Beer,** allowed to stand until the carbonation dissipates, helps hold a set and control flyaway hair. Mix the beer half-and-half with water as a final rinse, or pour it into a spray bottle and mist your damp hair. Or, add 1 tablespoon lemon juice to $1/3$ cup beer and comb it through your hair.

❧ **Egg white,** stiffly beaten, can be used as a protein-enriching styling mousse.

❧ **Flaxseed or quince seed.** Simmer 1 tablespoon of seeds in $1/2$ cup water until slightly thickened. Strain before using.

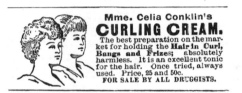

❧ **Gelatin.** Soften $1/2$ packet unflavored gelatin in 2 tablespoons cold water. Add $1/3$ cup boiling water, stir until dissolved, then blend in $1/2$ teaspoon *each* lemon juice and cologne.

❧ **Lemon juice,** misted from a spray bottle and combed in, adds resiliency, body, and highlights to light hair.

❧ **Milk**—whole, for dry or normal hair; skim for oily hair—is an excellent wave set. For a gentle set, blend 1 teaspoon instant nonfat dry milk with $1/3$ cup water.

❧ **Rosemary tea,** brewed double strength, is a damp-weather curl preserver for dark hair.

Curling Cues

Always leave a bit of leeway between curlers and your scalp, and remove them as soon as your hair is dry. Thermostatically controlled hot rollers are considered safe, as are clips or plastic-tipped bobby pins. Heat from curling irons, crimpers, or hair dryers can be damaging if not carefully controlled. Back-combing or teasing is an unnatural way to style hair; the "body" it produces by roughing the cuticle can strip away the protective outer layer and lead to hair breakage.

NATURALLY-NURTURING HAIR TREATMENTS

EIGHT PRESHAMPOO CONDITIONERS THAT ARE WORTH WAITING FOR

Massage these natural conditioners into dry hair, cover with a shower cap and allow to permeate for 30 minutes to an hour before shampooing. To speed the penetration, wrap hot, moist towels around your head.

1. *Avocado* provides protein and oil for restoring rebellious hair to glossy manageability. Simply massage a mashed avocado into your scalp and hair, or give your hair a super treat by blending the mashed avocado with a beaten egg and 2 tablespoons wheat germ oil.

2. *Egg yolk* can be used as is, or, for dry hair, mixed with 2 teaspoons castor oil and 1 teaspoon rum. For an all-purpose conditioner: Combine 1 egg yolk with $1/4$ cup yogurt, 1 teaspoon grated lemon rind, and $1/2$ teaspoon powdered kelp.

3. *Honey*. Light honey, all by its sticky self, does lovely things for light hair. For every shade of hair: Mix $1/4$ cup honey, 2 tablespoons vegetable oil, and 1 teaspoon lemon juice.

4. *Hydrolyzed protein* (predigested liquid protein marketed as a diet supplement) is a quickly absorbed substance for resurrecting lifeless hair.

5. *Mayonnaise*, store bought or prepared from the recipe in the Glossary, is a mild conditioner. For additional body and glimmer, beat 1 egg yolk and 1 teaspoon *each* vinegar and powdered kelp into each application.

6. *Milk*. Mix instant nonfat dry milk and water to a paste for a body-building pack.

7. *Molasses* (light for light hair, dark for dark hair) is an old-fashioned favorite for rejuvenating weary hair. Soften 1 packet unflavored gelatin in 2 tablespoons molasses. Stir in 1 tablespoon *each* flat beer and sweetened condensed milk.

8. *Oils.* Polyunsaturated oils combat dryness and revitalize drab, brittle hair. Warm the oil to room temperature if it has been refrigerated; shampoo twice for total removal. For extra shine and easier removal, mix 2 tablespoons oil with 1 tablespoon lemon juice and 1 teaspoon cognac. Castor oil strengthens hair weakened by overprocessing or overexposure to sun and water. Linseed oil (from a health food outlet, not a paint store) softens stiff, unmanageable hair.

AFTER-SHAMPOO QUICKER-ACTING CONDITIONERS

Conditioners such as these should be applied only to the hair, not the scalp. To use: Pour the conditioner into your hands, rub into your freshly shampooed hair, comb through for even distribution, then rinse out with tepid water after the suggested length of time. To add sheen, blend 1 tablespoon citric acid crystals with any of these conditioners. For extra body plus shine, follow any of them with a 3-minute application of mayonnaise.

- **Eggs.** Beat 1 or 2 egg yolks with 1 or 2 tablespoons of water (depending on hair length), rinse after 15 minutes. To increase the benefits, blend 2 tablespoon yogurt with each egg yolk. A whole egg can be whisked with lemon juice for a 15-minute conditioning shiner-upper, or gussied up for other head-mending nourishers.

  Combine 1 beaten egg with 1 tablespoon *each* glycerin and wheat germ oil. Or, dissolve 1 tablespoon citric acid crystals in 2 tablespoons water, then beat in 1 egg and 1 tablespoon sweetened condensed milk.

- **Fruit salad.** In an electric blender, whir $1/2$ a banana, $1/4$ of an avocado, $1/6$ of a cantaloupe, and 1 tablespoon *each* wheat germ oil and yogurt. Leave on for 10 minutes to regenerate summer-abused hair.

- **Half-and-Half** gives hair extra body when left on for 5 minutes.

CONDITIONING WITH RINSES

Adding a tablespoon of lemon juice (for light hair) or cider vinegar (for dark hair) to a quart of water for the final rinse removes dulling film and restores the pH balance. (Strain the juice through a sieve. If you rely on the juicer strainer you may think you've developed a terminal scalp disease when fragments of lemon pulp appear in your hair.)

- **Baking soda**, mixed with water in the proportions of 1 tablespoon soda to $^3/_4$ cup water, will remove hairspray residue and discourage unpleasant odor. Work the liquid through your hair, then rinse out.

- **Herbal teas** (camomile for blondes, rosemary or sage for brunettes), brewed regular strength and used for a final rinse, tone the hair and restore the acid mantle.

- **Vinegar**. Combine 2 tablespoons *each* vinegar and double-strength peppermint tea with 1 quart of water as a final rinse. To liven drab hair, mix $^1/_4$ cup vinegar with $1^1/_4$ cups water; dispel the odor by adding a few drops of oil of cloves to a pint of water and rinsing again.

Cosmetic vinegars have a more pleasing aroma plus increased conditioning benefits. Two tablespoons of any of the cosmetic vinegars in Chapter 3 may be added to your final rinse, or you can brew your own customized rinse. Each combination should be brought to a boil in an enamel or glass pan and simmered, uncovered, for 15 minutes, then covered and allowed to steep for 30 minutes before straining.

All-purpose Sparkler

1 cup each *white vinegar and distilled water*
$^1/_4$ cup each *dried nettle, red clover, and rosemary*

Light-haired Vinegar Rinse

1 cup each *white vinegar and distilled water*
3 camomile tea bags
2 tablespoons lemon juice

Dark-haired Sage Rinse

1 cup each *red wine vinegar and distilled water*
2 tablespoons dried sage

Conditioning with Tonics and Dressings

Tonics may be applied between shampoos or immediately after shampooing to condition, control, and add shine. You can substitute 80-proof vodka for the ethyl alcohol in any of these preparations.

- **Castor oil**, totally soluble in alcohol, has an advantage over other oils for hair dressings. For an instant tonic, shake $1/4$ cup water with 2 tablespoons ethyl alcohol and 2 teaspoons *each* castor oil, ammonia, and glycerin.

  Antiseptic tonics. Steep 2 tablespoons *each* nettle and sage in $1^1/_2$ cups ethyl alcohol for a week. Strain out the herbs, pour the liquid into a pint bottle, add $1/_3$ cup castor oil, and shake well. Or, steep $1/_4$ cup sage, 2 tablespoons rosemary, and 1 tablespoon nettle in $1^1/_2$ cups ethyl alcohol for 10 days. Strain; then add $1/_4$ cup distilled water and $1/_4$ cup castor oil. Shake to combine.

- **Perfumed tonic.** This exotic blend originated in Arab harems and is said to stimulate hair growth as well as furnish fragrance and shine. Add 2 tablespoons lavender water and $1/_2$ teaspoon *each* lavender oil and sweet basil oil to 1 pint ethyl alcohol. Let stand for a month, shaking every few days.

- **Rose water and glycerin**. Mix half-and-half or in a ratio of 3 parts rose water to 1 part glycerin.

How to Enliven Your Hair Color with Natural Colorants

Hair pigmentation is not necessarily permanent. Tow-headed children often become brunette adults, carrot-tops may turn into auburn-haired sirens or sires, and we all eventually grow gray. If your present hair color is less than exciting, natural substances can add pizazz. Vegetable hair dyes date back to antiquity; walnut hulls and henna are two naturally conditioning colorants currently available.

Black Walnut. The hulls of black walnuts (sold in health food stores) can be pressed to produce a juice that dyes hair dark brown. It also stains skin; wear rubber gloves when handling the hulls, and apply dye carefully. For a rich walnut hue: Combine $1/4$ cup walnut juice, 1 tablespoon ethyl alcohol, and $1/4$ teaspoon *each* ground cinnamon and cloves in a screw-top jar. Let stand for a week, shaking daily, then strain through a cloth-lined sieve and add $1/8$ teaspoon salt.

Henna. Today's henna is more sophisticated than the stewed henna-bush leaves used thousands of years ago by Persian and Egyptian beauties to color their hair and nails. Dried and powdered, henna is marketed in neutral, black, and brown, as well as red shades. It coats the hair to add body and color, then gradually fades away without leaving an obvious root line. Intensity varies with the length of application and henna is not recommended if your hair is more than 15 percent gray, if it has been bleached or colored with a metallic dye, or if you plan to have a perm in the immediate future.

HOW TO BRIGHTEN DARK HAIR

Camomile tea, brewed regular-strength, brightens dark hair without bleaching it. Rosemary and sage teas (individually or combined and steeped double strength) darken while they add glimmer. Leave the tea on your hair for half an hour, then rinse with warm water.

HOW TO LIVEN LIGHT HAIR

- **Camomile** brightens blonde hair, minimizes dark streaks, adds highlights, and abolishes the spongy stickiness that can occur with bleached hair. As a final rinse, pour regular or double-strength camomile tea through your hair several times. For additional glimmer, add 1 teaspoon lemon juice. For more bleaching action, brew triple-strength camomile tea with white wine instead of water.

- **Green pekoe tea**, brewed regular strength and used as a final rinse, adds a reddish shimmer to blonde or light brown hair.

  Cindy's strawberry-blonde hair had gradually faded to such a non-descript shade that she threatened to have it tinted before leaving for college. As an alternative, Cindy's grandmother suggested she try tea. "Worked wonders for me," she said. "My hair used to be reddish-gold, and when I was 19, my aunt accused me of coloring it. I told her honestly, 'All I do is wash and rinse it.' I just didn't mention that the rinse was green pekoe!" The tea's magic was as effective as it had been 50 years earlier; red glints illuminated Cindy's bright "untinted" hair as she boarded the plane for school.

• **Lemon** brings sunny glints to light hair. Combine $1/2$ cup water with $1/3$ cup strained lemon juice. Work through the hair, then let dry before rinsing.

> *Lemon-lime shampoo.* Combine 1 tablespoon *each* lemon juice, lime juice, and a mild shampoo. Work through your dry hair with fingers or a wide-toothed comb. Dry with a blow dryer or sit in the sun for 20 minutes. Wash out and follow with a rinse of 1 tablespoon lemon juice per pint of water. Repeat daily until the desired shade is achieved.

> *Lemon hairspray.* To combine brightening with style holding, mist with lemon juice. For more holding power, simmer a cut-up lemon in water to cover. When the lemon is tender, pour the mixture into an electric blender. Whir until smooth, then strain through a fine sieve.

• **Peroxide** brightens murky looking light hair, but is not recommended for tinted or bleached hair. Combine 2 tablespoons peroxide with 1 tablespoon mild shampoo and $1/8$ teaspoon ammonia. Work through wet hair and leave on for 4 minutes. Rinse out, then rewash with plain shampoo and follow with a lemon-water rinse. For a more pronounced effect, use 20-volume peroxide instead of 10-volume.

• **Natural frosting.** Fresh lemon juice, camomile oil, peroxide, or the lemon-lime shampoo described above, can be used to frost light brown or dark blonde hair. Use a small brush to "paint" random strands; or don a "frosting cap" (or a punctured bathing cap), pull the strands through with a crochet hook and saturate with a cotton ball. Sit in the sun a few minutes before shampooing.

How to Postpone and Rejuvenate Gray Hair

Illness may cause alternating bands of gray on each hair as pigment-forming capability fluctuates with the severity of the disease. Normal graying commences around the age of forty; premature graying is linked to heredity, stress, and nutritional deficiencies. Stress management and dietary upgrading often forestall and sometimes regress the silvering; color is not restored to already-white hairs but their replacements grow out in the original shade. Nutritionists report astounding successes with several months of a high-protein diet plus two tablespoons each of brewers yeast and vegetable oil daily, and these anti-gray-hair vitamins: 1 B-complex stress tab, 30 to 300 milligrams B-5, 2,000 milligrams choline, 400 to 800 micrograms folic acid, and 100 to 300 milligrams PABA. Nineteenth-century suggestions include these gray-hair preventives and restoratives:

- Blend 2 tablespoons castor oil and 1 tablespoon ethyl alcohol. Rub into hair roots once each week.

- Combine 2 tablespoons *each* glycerin and rose water or cologne with 1 tablespoon cider vinegar. Each morning and evening, brush your hair until your scalp tingles, then apply the liquid to the hair roots with a cotton ball.

- Drink a cup of sage tea daily and rub a bit of the brew onto the hair roots. Or, simmer 1 tablespoon *each* black pekoe tea and dried sage in 1 cup water in a covered pan for 20 minutes. Steep several hours before straining. Massage the liquid into your hair and scalp each day until hair is the desired shade, then reduce applications to twice weekly.

How to Correct Seven Specific Hair and Scalp Problems

1. Dandruff and Itchy Scalp

That little itch and the snow descending upon your shoulders may be only dry flakes from hairspray residue or shampoo buildup. Daily brushing plus frequent shampooing preceded by an oil-based conditioner and followed with an acidic rinse may be all that is required. Dandruff that persists may be the real thing, *seborrheic dermatitis*, which can develop when the sebaceous glands are overactive as a result of emotional tension or faulty diet, or can appear as a byproduct of allergy, hormonal imbalance, or infection. Studies show that many cases of dandruff are related to poor metabolization of refined carbohydrates and the resulting deficiency of B vitamins. Improving your diet and taking antioxidants (30 to 400 IU vitamin E plus 50 to 200 micrograms selenium daily) may help correct the cause. Immediate control often can be achieved with these natural precautions and remedies:

- Massage your scalp daily with castor oil or olive oil; castor oil mixed half-and-half with vinegar; vinegar or lemon juice diluted with an equal amount of water or mint tea; any of the cosmetic vinegars from Chapter 3; a mixture of 1 tablespoon glycerin and 1 teaspoon cider vinegar, or 1 teaspoon *each* glycerin and borax blended with ¼ cup distilled water; double-strength mint tea or rosemary-sage tea with 1 teaspoon borax dissolved in each cup; rubbing alcohol or witch hazel.

- Between shampoos, work cornmeal or miller's bran through your hair and brush out.

- Before shampooing, rub petroleum jelly or olive oil into your scalp and cover with a hot, moist towel for 30 minutes. Or, massage a lightly beaten egg (with or without a tablespoon of sea salt) into your dry hair and scalp. Let it permeate for 5 minutes before rinsing and shampooing. If your hair is dry, use egg yolks instead of a whole egg. If your hair is oily but your scalp is dry, substitute egg white beaten with the juice of a lemon.

- Follow each shampoo with a final rinse of strong tea: catnip, celery-seed, rosemary-mint, or wintergreen; add 1 tablespoon vinegar to increase the benefits. After the rinse, massage your scalp with a mixture of ¼ cup apple cider vinegar, 1 tablespoon witch hazel, and 2 crushed aspirins.

- Always dry your hair with fresh towels, and always use your own combs and hairbrushes; infectious bacteria is transferable.

2. DRY HAIR

The amount of sebum produced by the sebaceous glands diminishes with age and is responsible for gradually drying hair. Adding 2 tablespoons of vegetable oil plus vitamin E and cod liver oil supplements to the daily diet, brushing nightly, having occasional preshampoo oil treatments, and shampooing no more often than twice a week usually corrects this type of dryness.

Suddenly dry, lifeless, brittle hair can occur during periods of stress, pregnancy, or illness; or can be brought about by overprocessing or overexposure to extreme temperatures. Vitamin-C deficiency inhibits the oil-producing glands and may cause hair to split or break. To revitalize your forlorn tresses, pamper them with natural nurturing.

- Brush your hair gently to avoid breakage while distributing the natural oils.

- Use a preshampoo protein/oil conditioner each time you wash your hair. Extend the length of conditioner contact time or drape a heating pad set on "low" over your conditioning hair for 30 minutes.

- Enrich your shampoo with oil or protein, and use a mildly acidic solution such as 1 teaspoon lemon juice or vinegar per pint of water for the final rinse.

3. OILY HAIR

Reducing dietary fats and experimenting with these natural remedies should bring liveliness to your lank locks.

- Work a strip of gauze through your hairbrush bristles to absorb excess oil during your daily brushing.

- Before you shampoo, apply stiffly beaten egg white to your hair and scalp, then brush out after it dries. Or, dissolve 1 tablespoon salt in skim milk and rub it into your scalp. Shampoo after 30 minutes.

- Follow each shampoo with a rinse of 1 tablespoon lemon juice or vinegar per pint of water.

- Before styling your hair, rub witch hazel on your scalp.

4. SPLIT ENDS

Split ends are often a corollary of dry hair; especially when it has been overpermed, set with brush rollers, or teased while styling. Singeing split ends is not recommended (it can harm the hair shafts); trimming them off prevents the separation of cell layers from extending throughout the length of the hair. Dry-hair care, plus refraining from further hair-wrecking practices, should avoid recurrence of the problem.

5. FALLOUT AND THINNING HAIR

The diameter of each hair and their total number varies with hair color; blondes have more but skinnier hair than brunettes or redheads. As metabolic processes slow, Father Time gradually makes fat hair thin, thick hair sparse. Females are less prone to baldness than males, but our equalization of rights is rapidly equalizing hair fallout as well as pay scales because of the accompanying stress that constricts follicle openings and nourishment-carrying blood vessels. Anything that disrupts our internal system contributes to hair loss: malnutrition, pregnancy, severe illness, an underactive thyroid, certain medications, chemical or X-ray therapy.

Nutritional deficiencies or an excess of carbohydrates and animal fats can cause falling hair. Increasing protein intake by 14 grams a day (the amount in 2 eggs or $1^1/_2$ cups skim milk) increases the diameter of each hair by 14 percent;[86] B-vitamin-containing foods (see Vitamin and Mineral Chart) stimulate hair growth. To augment the daily diet, nutritionists suggest 1 multivitamin-mineral, 1 B-complex stress tab, 1,000 milligrams *each* choline and inositol, and 1,000 milligrams of vitamin C.

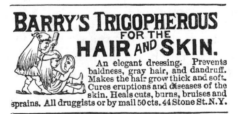

External care is also important. About 85 percent of our hair is normally in its growing phase; the hairs that fall are those that have loosened in the follicles to make way for their replacements. Overly enthusiastic brushing or toweling can prematurely dislodge these hairs, or break them off in the follicles to prevent or slow the emergence of new hair. Accumulations of dead cells, dirt, or shampoo residue can hamper regrowth by clogging the tiny openings. Consistently gentle cleanliness and these natural growth encouragers often resolve the problem.

    ❯ Two or three times a day, massage a small amount of one of these old-fashioned ointments into your scalp: a blend of 2 tablespoons *each* castor oil and lard with $^1/_4$ teaspoon rosemary oil.

Or, $^1/_4$ cup almond oil or olive oil with $^1/_2$ teaspoon rosemary oil and 3 drops lemon-grass oil.

☙ Twice daily, massage your scalp and hairline in small circular motions with your fingertips or an electric vibrator, preferably while relaxing on a slantboard with your head 18 inches lower than your feet.

Or, stimulate circulation with this 1850s cure for falling hair. Immerse your head in cold water containing 1 tablespoon salt per quart. Dry your hair, then brush until your scalp feels warm.

☙ At bedtime, try one of these natural remedies: massage your scalp with aloe vera gel, sliced raw garlic, jojoba oil, lard, or fresh onion juice. Shampoo out in the morning. To augment the benefits, rub petroleum jelly into your freshly scrubbed scalp and wipe it off with cotton saturated in a mixture of $^1/_4$ cup water and 1 teaspoon alcohol.

☙ Once each week, apply a preshampoo protein or oil conditioner, or a 2-hour preshampoo scalp-stimulator of 2 tablespoons vodka mixed with 1 tablespoon honey. Then use a protein-enriched, body-building shampoo.

☙ Use rosemary tea as an after-shampoo rinse. Or, cook $^1/_4$ pound of unpeeled chopped chestnuts in 1 quart of boiling water for 10 minutes. Cover and let stand for 15 minutes. Strain and add 1 teaspoon wine vinegar. Pour 1 cupful through your hair as a final rinse.

6. LOCALIZED LOSS

Any of the falling-hair instigators may be responsible for a receding hairline or patchy bald spots, but hair styling is the customary culprit. Men are burdened with MPB (male pattern baldness) genes; women denude their own scalps. *Alopecia areata or traction alopecia* is the technical term for what happens when we roll our hair too tightly or try to sleep on brush rollers, pull it back into a sleek chignon style, plait it into cornrows, or strangle it with rubber bands for a pony tail. Although prolonged tension can cause permanent hair loss,[159] hair usually regrows when the abusive practices are discontinued.

7. SWIMMER'S HAIR

Ocean salt, lake minerals, or the algicides and chlorine in swimming pools strip away the hair's protective covering and oils, and can turn blonde, gray, or bleached hair an eerie shade of green. To avoid these misfortunes: wear a bathing cap lined around the hairline with a 2-inch strip of chamois. Immediately after emerging, rinse your hair with fresh water or spray it with bottled water, club soda, or a solution of baking soda and water; then shampoo as soon as possible.

Judy didn't think she needed to wear a bathing cap while swimming her daily laps because she kept her head out of the water. After a few weeks, however, the sides and back of her bright golden hair acquired the greenish cast of aging copper. When shampooing failed to remove the discoloration, Judy sought professional help. "Tomato juice works better than anything else" said the salon manager. "If that doesn't get rid of the green, come in for a hot-oil pack and chemical treatment." Judy applied an oil treatment at home, left the tomato juice on her hair for 5 minutes after shampooing, and was rewarded with a return to her standard gold. To prevent future greening, Judy rinses her hair with tomato juice whenever the edges of her hair feel damp after swimming.

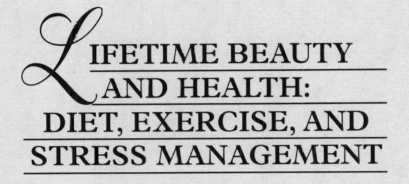

LIFETIME BEAUTY AND HEALTH: DIET, EXERCISE, AND STRESS MANAGEMENT

Ꭷ*15*Ꭷ

HOW TO EAT YOUR WAY
TO BEAUTY AND HEALTH:
THE BASICS OF BALANCING
YOUR DIET

Your glowing complexion, strong nails, sparkling eyes, shining hair, and vibrantly healthy body reflect the nourishment they receive from the foods you eat. Balancing a nutritious diet can be as simple as selecting servings from the five main food groups categorized in the U.S. Department of Agriculture's nutritional guidelines. In 1992, The Food Guide Pyramid in Figure 15-1 replaced the long-standing four-food-group pie chart that had been used to teach nutrition since the 1950s. The pie chart had outlined four food groups—meats, dairy, vegetables/fruits, and grains—but it didn't clarify how to prioritize these building blocks in relationship to daily eating habits. The new pyramid advocates a diet heavy in grains, fruits, and vegetables—with decreasing amounts of milk, yogurt, cheese, meats, nuts, fats, and sweets.

NUTRITIONAL CHOICES FROM THE FOOD PYRAMID

1. BREADS, CEREALS, AND OTHER GRAINS

The largest of the five groups in the pyramid is the bread, cereal, rice, and pasta group. These grains are our principal source of fiber (see Table 15-2). They also furnish a wealth of vitamins and minerals, and when combined with legumes or milk, provide complete protein with less fat than meat. Official guidelines recommend that you eat 6 to 11 servings from this group each day. Serving examples include:

The Food Pyramid

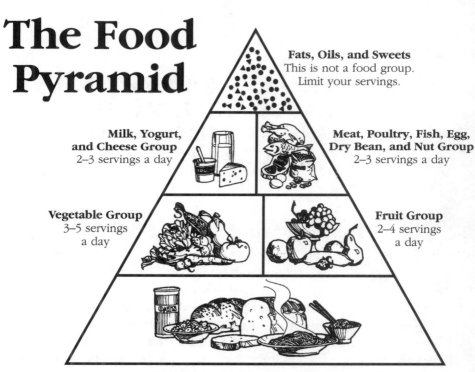

Fats, Oils, and Sweets
This is not a food group.
Limit your servings.

Milk, Yogurt, and Cheese Group
2–3 servings a day

Meat, Poultry, Fish, Egg, Dry Bean, and Nut Group
2–3 servings a day

Vegetable Group
3–5 servings
a day

Fruit Group
2–4 servings
a day

Bread, Cereal, Rice, and Pasta Group
6–11 servings a day

1 slice of bread or 1 muffin, roll, or tortilla

$^1/_2$ to $^3/_4$ cup cooked cereal, pasta, or rice

$^1/_2$ to 1 cup (depending on density) ready-to-eat cereal

2. VEGETABLES

Eating a variety of vegetables provides vitamins, minerals, fiber, complex carbohydrates, as well as enzymes and antioxidants. The Food Pyramid recommends that you eat 3 to 5 servings from the vegetable group each day. A serving size is

$^3/_4$ cup vegetable juice

$^1/_2$ cup chopped raw or cooked vegetable

1 medium-sized potato

1 small salad

TABLE 15-2:
FOOD COMPOSITION OF GRAIN PRODUCTS*

Per serving	Carbohydrate (grams)	Protein (grams)	Fat (grams)	Fiber (grams)	Calories
Breads—1 slice					
Cornbread	14	3.7	3.6	1.9	104
Pumpernickel	17	3.0	.4	1.5	79
White	12	2.0	.7	.7	62
Whole wheat	11	3.0	.6	1.3	55
Cereals					
Cornflakes (1 cup)	21	2.0	.1	4.1	95
Oats, cooked (³/₄ cup)	18	4.8	1.7	3.6	103
Shredded wheat (1 large biscuit)	20	2.0	1.0	3.3	90
Crackers					
Graham (2)	10	1.0	1.0	1.4	55
Saltines (4)	8	1.0	1.0	.1	50
Rice—¹/₂ cup					
Brown, cooked	17	1.9	.4	1.8	89
White, cooked	18	1.5	.1	.6	80

*Compiled from: *Eat Better, Live Better,*[65] *Nutrition Almanac,*[92] and *U.S.D.A. Handbook No. 8.*

To preserve their maximum benefits, subject vegetables to a minimum of preparation. When possible and desirable, eat them raw. Never soak them in water or add baking soda to enhance the color while cooking. Steam vegetables rather than boiling them. If you must boil, use as little water as possible (unless the liquid is to be consumed in soups).

3. FRUITS

Be sure to eat 2 to 4 servings of fruits each day. Servings include:

1 whole fruit, such as an apple, banana, or orange

¹/₂ cantaloupe or grapefruit

¹/₂ cup sliced raw or cooked fruit or berries

Store all leftovers tightly covered to maintain nutritional value; orange juice, for instance, loses 15 percent of its vitamin C if refrigerated for a day in an open pitcher.

Dietary fiber is the indigestible portion of plant foods. The presence of fiber in grains, fruits, and vegetables is one of the reasons they form the base of the Food Pyramid. Their fiber is divided into two categories:

- **Soluble fiber** (pectins and gums from fruits, nuts, oats, seeds, vegetables) helps the body metabolize carbohydrates and reduce cholesterol.

- **Insoluble fiber** (cellulose, lignin, and hemicellulose from whole grains) helps prevent constipation, diverticulosis, and colon cancer.

The National Cancer Institute recommends a daily mixture of 25 to 30 grams of "soluble" and "insoluble"; both categories are charted under the single heading "Fiber" in Tables 15-2 and 15-3.

TABLE 15-3:
FRUIT AND VEGETABLE FOOD COMPOSITION*

Per serving	*Vit. A (IU)*	*Vit. C (mg)*	*Fiber (grams)*	*Carbohydrate (grams)*	*Calories*
Apple, fresh	117	5	2.4	17	76
Asparagus, cut, cooked	866	25	1.7	3	20
Banana, raw	285	15	2.7	30	128
Broccoli, fresh, cut	2,580	108	3.9	5	30
Cabbage, raw, shredded	60	25	3.4	3	12
Carrots, raw, grated	11,000	8	3.3	10	42
Corn, vacuum canned	320	5	4.0	33	105
Orange, fresh	360	90	2.0	20	88
Peach, fresh	1,516	8	2.3	10	43
Peas, frozen, cooked	480	11	3.2	10	55
Potato, baked, white	—	20	1.0	21	93
Strawberries, sliced	60	60	1.8	9	40
Tomato, raw	1,100	28	1.4	6	25

*Varies with growth and preparation methods. Figures compiled from *Eat Better, Live Better*,[65] *Nutrition Almanac*,[92] and *U.S.D.A. Handbook No. 8.*

4. MILK, MILK PRODUCTS, MEAT, FISH, POULTRY, NUTS, LEGUMES

The third level of the pyramid combines the milk, yogurt, and cheese group with the meat, poultry, fish, beans, eggs, and nuts group. The new guidelines recommend that you consume only 2 to 3 servings daily from each of these two groups.

Our body looks to milk and milk products for much of its calcium needs. When the body is deprived of an adequate supply of calcium, it draws this mineral from our bony structure to maintain the soft tissues and nervous system, leaving us with porous bones and loose teeth. As reported by Jean Anderson and Barbara Deskins in *The Nutrition Bible* (William Morrow, 1995), RDAs for calcium were increased at the 1994 NIH Consensus Conference. The former RDA of 800 milligrams per day for men is raised to 1,000 milligrams through age 65. For men over age 65, and for women over age 50 who are not taking estrogen, the new RDA is 1,500 milligrams. Two cups of milk (or its equivalent in milk products) provides over half of the RDA for calcium—approximately a fourth of our daily protein—plus carbohydrates for energy (see Table 15-4). Skim and fat-free milk products furnish the benefits without the saturated fat of whole milk. You can select your quota from these serving-size guidelines:

1 cup fluid milk, reconstituted dry milk, or plain yogurt

$1/2$ cup cottage cheese (this equals the calcium in $1/4$ cup milk)

$1/2$ cup ice cream (this equals the calcium in $1/3$ cup milk)

1-inch-cube Cheddar or Swiss cheese (this equals the calcium in $3/4$ cup milk)

2 tablespoons processed cheese spread (this equals the calcium in $1/2$ cup milk)

Meat, fish, poultry, eggs, legumes, and nuts give us the protein we need to maintain beautiful externals, such as hair and nails, and vital internals, such as muscles and organs. Meat and dairy products are complete-protein foods. (Plant foods, with the exception of soybeans, must have their missing amino acids supplied by combining them with other protein sources.) Proteins are an important part of any diet, but be careful in measuring out your daily servings; the serving

TABLE 15-4:
FOOD COMPOSITION OF MILK AND MILK PRODUCTS*

Per serving	Calcium	Protein (grams)	Fat (grams)	Carbohydrate (grams)	Calories
Milk (1 cup)					
whole	291	8.0	8.1	11.0	150
2 percent	297	8.0	5.0	12.0	120
skim	302	8.0	trace	12.0	85
buttermilk	285	8.0	2.0	12.0	100
Evaporated milk ($^1/_2$ cup)	328	8.5	9.5	12.5	170
Cream, whipped (2 tablespoons)	10	trace	6.0	trace	80
Sour cream (2 tablespoons)	28	trace	2.0	2.0	50
Ice cream ($^1/_2$ cup)	88	2.5	7.0	16.0	135
Ice milk ($^1/_2$ cup)	88	2.5	3.0	14.0	92
Yogurt					
1 cup whole milk	274	8.0	7.0	11.0	140
nonfat plus added milk solids	452	13.0	trace	17.0	125
Cottage cheese					
$^1/_2$ cup large curd, creamed	68	14.0	5.0	3.0	117
low-fat, 2 percent	78	15.5	2.0	4.0	102
Cheddar cheese (1-inch cube)	204	7.0	9.0	trace	115
Swiss cheese (1-inch cube)	272	8.0	8.0	1.0	105
Parmesan cheese, grated (2 tablespoons)	69	2.0	2.0	trace	25

*Compiled from *Eat Better, Live Better*,[65] *Nutrition Almanac*,[92] and *U.S.D.A. Handbook No. 8.*

sizes are surprisingly small, as shown in Table 15-5. The protein equivalents for 1 ounce of cooked meat are

> 1 egg
>
> $^1/_2$ to $^3/_4$ cup cooked legumes
>
> $^1/_4$ to $^1/_2$ cup nuts or seeds
>
> 2 tablespoons peanut butter

TABLE 15-5:
FOOD COMPOSITION OF MEAT, FISH, POULTRY, EGGS, LEGUMES, AND NUTS*

Per serving (meats measured after cooking)	Protein (grams)	Fat (grams)	Carbohydrate (grams)	Calories
Beef—lean				
steak, broiled	18	4	0	115
($2 \times 4 \times 1/2$ inch)				
ground, broiled	23	10	0	185
($3^1/_2$-inch patty)				
Fish				
nonoily, baked (3 ounces)	22	4	0	135
tuna, oil pack, drained				
(3 ounces)	24	7	0	170
Chicken, $1/2$ breast, fried in oil	26	5	1	160
Turkey—roasted				
dark meat (3 ounces)	26	7	0	175
light meat (3 ounces)	28	3	0	150
Egg, 1 large, boiled	6	6	trace	80
Legumes—dry, cooked, drained ($1/2$ cup)				
black-eyed peas	6	trace	17	80
lima	8	trace	25	130
red or white	8	trace	21	115
soybeans (complete protein)	11	6	11	130
Nuts—$1/4$ cup				
Cashews	6	16	10	199
Pecans, broken	3	17	4	160
Walnuts, chopped	4	16	4	161
Peanut butter (2 tablespoons)	8	16	6	180
Sunflower seeds, hulled ($1/4$ cup)	9	15	7	178

*Compiled from *Eat Better, Live Better*,[65] *Nutrition Almanac*,[92] and *U.S.D.A. Handbook No. 8.*

    Calcium and protein are two important nutrients found abundantly in this Pyramid level, but sometimes they work against each other. To maintain a full supply of calcium and prevent osteoporosis, many women have increased their intake of milk and milk products (as well as calcium-fortified antacid tablets) beyond the recommended allowances. One way to increase your calcium supply is to decrease the intake of foods high in animal proteins. Research reported in the *American Journal of Clinical Nutrition*[104] reveals that high-protein diets can cause a negative calcium balance, even in the presence of more than adequate dietary calcium. This happens because sulfur-rich proteins make extra acid in the body; as acids wash through the bones, they dissolve calcium, which is then eliminated through the urine. *The American Medical Association Family Medical Guide* (Random House, 1994) advises a daily total of 5 or 6 ounces from the Meat group for sedentary and moderately active adults; a total of 7 ounces for active men and very active women.

5. FATS, OILS, SWEETS

At the very top of the pyramid are fats, oils, and sweets. This is not a recommended food group. They occupy the smallest section of the whole pyramid because they are items that should be consumed sparingly.

HOW TO EAT BY THE NUMBERS

For a more exactingly balanced diet you can divide foods into three categories (carbohydrates, fats, proteins) and work with percentages. The National Institutes of Health recommends that the diet for a moderately active adult consist of 55 to 60 percent carbohydrate, 25 to 30 percent fat, and no more than 15 percent protein.[182] Being precise requires an elaborate set of charts, but you can approximate with the food-composition information in this chapter.

- One gram equals $1/28$ of an ounce; 100 grams ($3^{1}/_{2}$ ounces) equal approximately $1/2$ cup of juices and foods such as cooked vegetables. One milligram equals $1/1000$ of a gram; a microgram is $1/1000$ of a milligram.

- A calorie is a measure of the amount of energy produced when a food is "burned" by the body. Excess calories are stored as body fat. Caloric needs can be estimated by multiplying your ideal weight by 15. For instance, if you weigh 125 pounds, 1,875 calories a day should maintain your weight.

  Carbohydrates, at 57 percent of the 1,875 calories, equal 1069 calories or 267 grams.

Conversion Formula		
Carbohydrates	4 calories per gram	112 calories per ounce
Fats	9 calories per gram	252 calories per ounce
Proteins	4 calories per gram	112 calories per ounce

Fat's 30-percent proportion equals 562 calories or 62 grams.

Protein, computed at 13 percent, equals 243 calories or 61 grams for a 125-pound individual.

CARBOHYDRATES

Complex carbohydrates from the starches and fibers of plant foods are the hi-octane fuel that furnishes energy most efficiently. Simple carbohydrates include the glucose and fructose from fruits and vegetables, lactose from milk, and sucrose from cane sugar. Fructose is gradually assimilated because of the accompanying fiber. Candy or sugary desserts, especially when eaten alone, immediately raise the blood sugar level, provide a brief spurt of energy, then leave us with the wearies because the insulin released to cope with the sudden surge of glucose also disposes of sugar that was already in the blood. Molasses, honey, and brown sugar contain minuscule amounts of vitamins and minerals, but from a nutritional standpoint, sweets are unnecessary; the body readily converts complex carbohydrates into glucose for our energy needs. As long as most of your carbohydrate quota is supplied by vegetables, fruits, grains, and legumes (and you are neither diabetic nor hypoglycemic), occasionally indulging a chocaholic craving or a yen for lemon meringue should not unduly upset your dietary balance.

Table 15-6 shows the caloric breakdown of bakery products and desserts.

FATS AND OILS

Without at least one tablespoon of fat every day, fat-soluble nutrients are not assimilated, hair is lackluster, skin flakes, and joints creak. The fatty acids from unsaturated fats are termed "essential" because they cannot be produced from other fats within the body. Fats from plant products (except for coconut or palm oil) are unsaturated and remain liquid at

TABLE 15-6:
FOOD COMPOSITION OF BAKERY PRODUCTS AND DESSERTS*

Per serving	Carbohydrate (grams)	Protein (grams)	Fat (grams)	Calories
Cake				
Angel food	24.0	2.8	.1	108
Devil's food cupcake with chocolate frosting	28.0	2.1	8.2	184
White, 2-layer with white frosting	94.2	5.0	19.3	562
Candy				
Chocolate fudge (1-inch piece)	34.0	1.2	5.5	180
Marshmallow (2 large)	9.4	.2	trace	38
Cookies—1 average				
Brownie with nuts	25.0	3.3	16.0	243
Chocolate chip	6.0	.5	3.0	52
Fig bar	11.5	.6	.9	55
Danish pastry, without nuts	30.0	4.8	15.2	274
Doughnuts—1 average	17.0	1.5	6.1	129
raised, jelly filled	30.0	3.4	8.8	226
Pie—$^1/_6$ of 9-inch pie				
Apple	59.9	3.5	17.4	402
Lemon meringue	52.7	5.2	14.3	356
Pecan	70.5	7.0	31.5	574
Pumpkin	37.1	6.0	17.0	319

*Compiled from *The Dieter's Companion*,[69] *Nutrition Almanac*,[92] and *U.S.D.A. Handbook No. 8.*

room temperature; animal fats are saturated, contain cholesterol, and harden at room temperature. Hydrogenated vegetable fats have been converted to a solid form that, according to reports in *Prevention* (June 1988), may be more harmful than naturally saturated fats. Michael E. DeBakey[53] has found that cholesterol levels are not affected by an occasional steak or a few eggs each week. (See Table 15-7.)

PROTEINS

For complete proteins, combine foods such as cereal and milk, bread and peanut butter or cheese, or beans and rice; or utilize the already complete proteins from animal products. All foods (except fats and

TABLE 15-7: FOOD COMPOSITION OF FATS AND OILS*

per tablespoon	Total Fat (grams)	Fatty Acids Saturated (grams)	Unsaturated Oleic/Linoleic (grams)	Cholesterol (mg)	Calories
Butter	11.8	7.2	3.2	30	100
Margarine					
regular	11.8	2.1	8.4	0	100
whipped	8.0	1.4	5.7	0	70
Lard	12.8	5.1	6.4	12	116
Vegetable shortening	12.0	3.2	8.8	0	110
Oils					
corn	13.6	1.7	11.1	0	120
olive	13.5	1.9	10.8	0	119
peanut	13.5	2.3	10.4	0	119
safflower	13.6	1.0	11.6	0	120
Mayonnaise	11.0	2.0	8.0	5	100
Salad dressing					
French	6.0	1.1	4.5	0	65
Italian	9.0	1.6	6.6	0	70

*Varies among different brands. Compiled from *The Dieter's Companion*,[69] *Eat Better, Live Better*,[65] and *Jane Brody's Nutrition Book*.[29]

sugars) contain some protein. A pint of milk provides 16 grams of protein, two slices of wheat bread furnish 6 grams; filling out the 61-gram quota (267 calories) for a 125-pound person presents no problem. The trick lies in keeping fat and cholesterol within sensible limits.

Only about 15 percent of our cholesterol is acquired from foods; the remainder is manufactured by the body to help produce new cells and to keep the brain and nervous system functioning. There are two kinds of cholesterol: the damaging, low-density lipoproteins (LDL) which cling to arterial walls; and the protective, high-density lipoproteins (HDL) which help the body eliminate excess cholesterol.

Eggs, the most perfect protein, have their yolks loaded with cholesterol, yet contain lecithin (a phospholipid that helps regulate cholesterol), and, according to a report in *Nutrition Action Health Letter* (July/August 1989), each egg now contains 22 percent less cholesterol than the "official" measurement of 274 milligrams shown in Table 15-8. Shellfish are so low in saturated fat that their cholesterol content is not considered nearly so health-threatening as the lesser amounts from highly saturated sources such as red meat, whose fat and cholesterol is also being reduced by dietary improvements.

CONDIMENTS AND SEASONINGS

Apparently insignificant extras can wreak havoc with a perfectly balanced diet. (See Table 15-9.)

SALT/SODIUM

Whether provided by Mother Nature or added to foods as table salt, salt is vital for physical and mental health. No human system can function without it. The sodium in it controls the body's moisture content and thus the amount of blood within it. It regulates what goes in and out of every body cell. But too much salt contributes to a number of health problems that can be prevented by limiting our intake.

Increases in blood pressure are the most frequently reported changes caused by too much salt. When the body has too much sodium, blood pressure increases to force out the excess through urine or sweating. This additional strain on the arteries makes them more susceptible to blood clots and rupture or stroke. The risk increases with age because blood vessels become less flexible, contributing to consistently higher blood pressure. High blood pressure also causes the heart to work harder, until it wears down and fails to pump efficiently, making hypertension a major contributor to heart attacks.

An article in the *Nutrition Action Health Letter* (March 1994) [102] noted that systolic blood pressure rises an average of 15 points between the ages of 25 and 55. If lifetime salt intake were lower by about one teaspoon a day (that's 2,300 mg of sodium), blood pressure would still rise with age, but the increase would be 6, not 15 points. That would mean a 16-percent drop in coronary heart disease deaths and 23-percent fewer stroke deaths at age 55.

High blood pressure is not the only danger posed by excess salt. Other health problems include:

> ❧ *Osteoporosis.* Most people rightly think of too little calcium as the cause of osteoporosis, but too much sodium is another culprit. The reason is simple: The more sodium you excrete, the

TABLE 15-8:
FOOD COMPOSITION OF PROTEINS*

| Protein Source | Protein (grams) | Fatty Acids | | Cholesterol (mg) | Calories |
		Saturated (grams)	Unsaturated Oleic/Linoleic (grams)		
Beef, lean, cooked, 3 ounces	26	2.7	2.7	80	172
Cheese—1-inch cube					
Cheddar	7	6.1	2.3	30	115
Mozzarella	8	4.4	1.7	25	90
Cream cheese, 1 ounce	2	6.2	2.6	30	100
Chicken, broiled, 3 ounces	21	1.1	1.9	60	120
Egg—1 large					
Whole, boiled	6	1.7	2.6	274	80
White only	3	0	0	0	15
Yolk only	3	1.7	2.6	274	65
Fish—3 ounces					
Haddock, breaded, fried	17	1.4	3.3	60	140
Shrimp, canned, drained	21	.1	.2	113	100
Tuna, water pack, drained	24	1.5	2.2	48	105
Frankfurter, 1, 2 ounces	7	5.6	7.7	35	170
Milk—1 cup					
Whole	8	5.1	2.3	35	150
1 percent	8	1.6	.8	8	100
Yogurt, low-fat, 1 cup	13	.3	.1	12	125

*Varies with product and preparation. Compiled from *The Dieter's Companion*,[69] *Eat Better, Live Better*,[65] and *Jane Brody's Nutrition Book*.[29]

more calcium you lose. Excess sodium is as important a calcium-waster as excess protein.

ॐ *Stomach cancer.* Excess salt irritates the stomach lining, causing cells to reproduce more often. That alone could increase the risk of cancer. In animal experiments, it has been found that salt makes cancer-causing chemicals more potent.

To reduce your intake of excess salt, you can throw away your salt shaker. Use herbs or a squirt of lemon juice instead. But that's only a start, because a mere 10 percent of the sodium the average American consumes comes from the shaker. The other 90 percent comes from the foods we eat—by far, the most comes from processed foods. Watch

**TABLE 15-9: FOOD COMPOSITION OF CONDIMENTS
AND SEASONINGS***

Per amount shown	Sodium (mg)	Fat (grams)	Carbohydrate (grams)	Calories
Salt—1 teaspoon				
Garlic or seasoned	1,850	.1	.7	4
Table, iodized	2,300	0	0	0
Sugar, granulated, 1 teaspoon	trace	0	4.0	16
Jam or preserves, 1 tablespoon	2	trace	14.0	54
Jelly, 1 tablespoon	3	trace	12.7	49
Sauces—1 tablespoon				
Barbecue	130	1.7	1.2	15
Catsup	177	.1	4.3	19
Mustard, brown	352	1.7	1.4	25
Mustard, yellow	337	1.2	1.7	20
Soy	1,209	.2	1.5	8
Tartar	99	8.1	.6	74
Olives—canned, 2 large				
Green	61	1.0	.2	10
Black	38	.9	.1	9
Pickles				
Dill, 1 (4 × 1³/₄ inches)	1,924	.3	3.0	15
Sweet, 1 gherkin (1¹/₂ ounces)	128	.2	18.0	73
Sweet relish (1 tablespoon)	107	trace	5.1	21

*Varies according to brand. Compiled from *The Dieter's Companion*,[69] *Nutrition Almanac*,[92] and *Tufts University Diet and Nutrition Letter* (December 1985).

out for most brands of frozen dinners or pizza, processed meats (like hot dogs or bacon), processed cheese, canned or dried soup, salad dressing, canned meats, beans, or vegetables, tomato sauce, and fast foods.

Beverages to be Sipped with Discretion

Alcoholic libations, coffee, tea, and caffeine-containing soft drinks have a mild diuretic action, so do little to replenish fluids lost through excretion and perspiration. Soft drinks contain sugar or artificial sweeteners of questionable virtue, plus phosphorus that can reduce the body's absorption of calcium unless quaffed in moderation.

Alcohol. For those who enjoy imbibing a bit of the bubbly, there are encouraging words: A study reported in the *Tufts University Diet and Nutrition Letter* (August 1995) reported that some 40 studies have consistently linked the consumption of all kinds of alcohol to a reduced risk of heart disease.

   ❧ Alcohol protects against heart disease by thinning the blood. It appears to render cells in the blood called platelets less sticky and therefore less likely to aggregate and form a clot that could block the flow of blood to the heart. Alcohol's greatest benefit to cardiac health appears to be that it raises HDL-cholesterol from 10 to 20 percent (HDL cholesterol is the "good" kind that clears cholesterol from the blood rather than causing the buildup of debris along the artery walls).

If you're a woman, don't pop the cork just yet; there's also a down side to this news. Consider that in a Harvard study of almost 90,000 women, three to nine drinks a week reduced the risk of heart disease by 40 percent (that's the goods news). But in these same women, alcohol consumption raised the risk of breast cancer by 30 percent (that's the bad news). When making decisions about alcohol consumption, doctors advise women to consider their personal health profile. You might want to abstain or at least drink on a very infrequent basis if you have one or more risk factors for breast cancer: A mother or sister who has developed the disease, onset of menstruation before age 12, first pregnancy after

30, never having children, menopause later than 55. On the other hand, if you do not have any particular risk factors for breast cancer yet have developed some heart disease risks—high blood pressure, diabetes, or high blood cholesterol—you might choose to continue moderate drinking if that is already your habit.

Moderate drinking for women means one drink a day. This is less than the recommended maximum of two drinks a day for men for several reasons: Women have proportionately more fat and less water than men, so alcohol does not get diluted so well in their bodies. Also, women have less of an enzyme called alcohol dehydrogenase, which breaks down alcohol before it reaches the bloodstream, so alcohol is more likely to go to their heads.

"Moderate" drinking for older people is also no more than one drink a day. Researchers at the Centers for Disease Control and Prevention have found that although older drinkers metabolize alcohol as efficiently as younger ones, an identical dose of alcohol produces a higher blood alcohol concentration in an older drinker because total body water content decreases with age.

Drinking while taking medications is a dangerous idea; many medications don't interact well with alcohol. Heart drugs like Nitrostat, for instance, can combine with alcohol to make blood pressure drop precipitously. Drinking also increases the risk of gastrointestinal bleeding in people who regularly take aspirin (like some arthritis sufferers). And medications like anticonvulsants have a sedative effect that might work with alcohol to heighten a sleepy or fatigued effect. Anyone who takes a particular drug on a regular basis should speak to a physician about its interaction with alcohol before mixing the two.

Drinking beyond moderation has direct adverse effects on the heart and causes one's risk of death from other illnesses to go up sharply. Specifically, excessive drinkers have a greater chance of dying from several different types of cancer, including cancer of the esophagus and stomach and perhaps cancer of the colon and rectum as well. They are also more likely to die of a stroke, cirrhosis of the liver, falls, and automobile accidents as well. Researchers agree that no one should take up drinking for the express purpose of staving off heart disease. The potential for alcohol abuse is too strong, and there are much safer and generally more healthful ways to protect the cardiovascular system:

following a low-fat diet, eating more vegetables and fruits, exercising more, and losing weight.

The calories in alcoholic beverages need to be considered too. Alcohol offers nonnutritious calories that can be converted to energy by the liver, but if those calories are not immediately used for that purpose, they are stored as fat. Most alcoholic drinks contain at least 100 calories each. At a drink a day, this can easily add more than 10 pounds to your total body weight in less than a year.

1 jigger ($1^1/_2$ ounces) distilled liquor = 100 calories

1 can (12 ounces) regular beer = 150 calories

1 can (12 ounces) light beer = 70 to 120 calories

4 ounces champagne = 84 calories

4 ounces dry wine = 102 calories

4 ounces sweet wine = 165 calories

Coffee and Caffeine. Caffeine, a central nervous system stimulant, is the most widely used psychoactive drug in the world. Fifty percent of the American population drinks at least two cups a day—enough to increase mental alertness and lessen fatigue.

On the up side, caffeine (also found in tea, colas, chocolate, and headache medicines) has been absolved of earlier charges associating it with birth defects, cancer, and fibrocystic breast lumps (*Health*, November 1987). And researchers at Harvard have found that women who drink six or more cups of coffee a day are no more likely to have heart attacks than women who don't drink coffee at all (*Tufts University Diet and Nutrition Letter*, April 1996)[187].

Too much caffeine, however, constricts blood vessels, depletes calcium supplies, speeds up respiratory and heart action, causes irregular heartbeat, and instigates irritability, twitching muscles, and insomnia. Author James J. Gormley (*Better Nutrition*, May 1996)[72], warns:

- Caffeine significantly increases blood pressure and, consequently, the risk of stroke.

- Much of the coffee we drink comes from countries which use U.S.-made pesticides that are banned here but are allowed to be exported to these other coffee-producing countries.

ॐ Caffeine causes small blood vessels in the eyes to constrict, which reduces the vessels' ability to transport nutrients to the eyes and to remove waste products and toxins.

ॐ Coffee drinking contributes to iron loss (since tannin, found in coffee, binds to iron, preventing its absorption) and to zinc loss (affecting eyesight, immunity, and sex drive).

ॐ Because coffee is a diuretic, calcium, potassium, magnesium, and sodium are excreted before they can be utilized.

ॐ Babies whose mothers drink coffee during pregnancy can become addicted to caffeine before birth. Mothers who did not drink coffee during pregnancy, but did before and after, set their babies up for colic, excessive fussiness, and sleeplessness.

Decaffeinated Coffee. Removing the caffeine dispenses with most of coffee's suspected or acknowledged dangers, but both regular and decaf increase the secretion of stomach acid which can initiate indigestion or aggravate ulcers.

CAFFEINE CONTENT OF BEVERAGES*

Per serving	Milligrams of Caffeine
Coffee—6-ounce cup	
drip	130–180
perked	120–140
instant	70–100
Tea—6-ounce cup	
steeped 2 to 5 minutes	20–100
instant	40–60
Colas and caffeine-containing soft drinks, 12-ounce can	30–70
Hot cocoa, 6-ounce cup	5–35

*Varies with strength and brand. Compiled from *Earl Mindell's Shaping Up With Vitamins*,[116] *Eat Better, Live Better*[65] and *Managing Your Mind and Mood Through Food*.[197]

Tea. Steeping time regulates potency as well as flavor; shortening the brewing time to one minute can reduce the caffeine to 10 milligrams per cup. Besides caffeine, pekoe contains tannin (an astringent that can irritate an empty stomach).

Herbal Teas. Some herbal teas should be imbibed judiciously. Fox-glove is the equivalent of digitalis; Indian hemp is the original name for marijuana; ginseng is a more potent stimulant than caffeine; carcinogens have been detected in sassafras; the alkaloids in comfrey root have been linked to liver cancer; and cathartic herbs (aloe, buckthorn, dock root, senna leaves) can cause diarrhea.

Most herbal teas are beneficial. There are antioxidant herbs (rosemary is more effective than BHA and BHT); beautifying herbs (see Sections 1 and 2); soothing, sleep-inducing herbs (camomile, catnip, dandelion, hops, lobelia, valerian); and energizing teas brewed from blackberry or raspberry leaves, cardamom, ginger, ginseng, goldenseal, lemon balm, rosemary, sage, or yerba mate. See Chapter 19 for details on brewing herbal teas.

How to tailor your own "look beautiful, feel great" diet

Nowhere is it graven in stone that we must eat three meals a day with specific foods at each one. Although *when* you consume *which* portion of your daily quota of nutrients doesn't affect their beautifying properties, it does affect your mental acuity and energy level. With either home-prepared or commercially produced natural foods, you can tailor your own "look beautiful, feel great" diet to provide peak energy when you need it, keep your blood sugar and disposition on an even keel, and summon the sandman at day's end.

- **Protein foods** increase alertness by stimulating the brain's production of mentally energizing chemicals from the amino acid tyrosine.

- **Complex carbohydrates** from fruits, vegetables, and whole grains are the most efficient energy source.

- **Simple carbohydrates** from sugar and refined flours give a "quick fix" injection of energy, then trigger the "wearies" by releasing insulin and serotonin.

- **Fats** slow digestion, thus creating mental lethargy by diverting blood away from the brain to the stomach.

- **Excess calories** do more than produce bulges. Ingesting over 600 of them at one sitting lulls both body and soul—witness the living-room loungers after a family Thanksgiving dinner.

WHY YOU SHOULD ADD PHYTOCHEMICALS TO YOUR DIET

The new buzzword when discussing nutrition and health is "phytochemicals." Phytochemicals are elements of chemistry within natural foods that have been proven to retard cancer development and growth. One such substance is sulforaphane, which researchers from Johns Hopkins University School of Medicine extracted from broccoli and gave to rats treated with a carcinogen that causes mammary tumors. The substance significantly reduced the size and number of the tumors and delayed their development. The researchers say the substances enhance the performance of enzymes that protect against cancer-causing agents.

Actually, phytochemicals work at several steps in the process of cancer development. "At almost every one of the steps along the pathway leading to cancer," says epidemiologist John Potter of the University of Minnesota, "there are one or more compounds in vegetables or fruit that will slow up or reverse the process." Take a look at the sampling below.

SEVEN FOODS THAT WARD OFF CANCER

- **Tomatoes** are rich in *p-coumaric acid* and *chlorogenic acid*, which block the formation of nitrosamine compounds, strongly linked to stomach, liver, and bladder cancer. Strawberries, pineapples, and peppers are also rich in these acids.

- **Broccoli** also contains *phenethyl isothiocyanate*, which prevents carcinogens from binding to DNA, and *indole-3-carbinol*, which causes estrogen to break down into a harmless metabolite rather than the form linked to breast cancer.

❧ **Cabbage** harbors a high concentration of *indole-3-carbinol* along with *oltipraz*, which increases enzymes that protect against a wide range of cancers, and *brassinin*, shown to protect against mammary and skin tumors.

❧ **Garlic** and **onions** contain *allylic sulfides*, which work by waking up enzymes inside that which detoxify cancer-causing chemicals.

❧ **Hot chili peppers** have heatwaves of *capsaicin*, which keeps toxic molecules (especially those in cigarette smoke) from attaching to DNA—the spot where sparks ignite into lung and other cancers.

❧ **Citrus fruits** and **berries** are storehouses of *flavenoids*, which keep cancer-causing hormones from latching onto a cell.

❧ **Soybeans** contain *genistein*, which seems to keep tiny tumors from connecting to capillaries that carry oxygen and nutrition. This may explain why Japanese men who relocate to the West and adapt to a low-soy diet have a significantly increased rate of prostate cancer.

The research into phytochemicals has been spearheaded by a recent conference in Washington, D.C., with doctors, college professors, and researchers from around the world attending and lecturing. The National Cancer Institute is so excited it has launched a multi-million-dollar project to find, isolate, and study phytochemicals. The National Cancer Institute, the American Cancer Society, and many other authorities now agree that fresh fruits and vegetables are important in maintaining good health.

How TO ADAPT YOUR DIET TO YOUR LIFESTYLE

Cramming all your food-group servings into one meal a day would be impossible and unhealthful; eating several times during the day bolsters biological rhythms. Eating between meals is no longer frowned upon, and some health experts recommend a "grazing diet" consisting of nutritious snacks spaced throughout the day like an ongoing progressive meal.

The generally accepted pattern calls for eating approximately one fourth of the day's allotment within three hours of awakening. Unless a siesta is on your agenda, a high-protein 300-calorie lunch is advisable. For normal evenings, fill in any missing food-group servings or category percentages, and let your bathroom scale be your guide. If you need to remain dynamic for several more hours, dine on modest portions of high-protein, complex-carbohydrate foods and save the soporifics for a bedtime snack, or until you are ready to relax.

How to Supplement Your Diet with Vitamins and Minerals

Eating a sensible diet should, and often does, fulfill all our nutritional needs. However, soil depletion or production and preparation methods may decrease the nutrient content of foods, and circumstances frequently interfere with best of dietary intentions. As precautionary insurance, most health care professionals advise taking a daily supplement containing 100 percent of the RDAs. If you are pregnant, ill, or taking medications, you should not take more than the RDA of any supplement without the approval of your doctor.

Originally established as the minimum daily requirement (MDR) for nutrients to prevent deficiency diseases, the guidelines were expanded to the recommended daily dietary allowances (RDAs) believed adequate for the nutritional needs of healthy individuals. For the 1990s there are new terms of identification. RDAs (recommended daily allowances) developed by the Food and Drug Administration as USRDAs are now RDIs (reference daily intakes) and are one of the sources for DVs (daily values) shown on food and supplement labels. Currently, the numerical values of RDIs are almost identical to the RDAs (recommended dietary allowances) prepared by the Food and Nutrition Board of the National Research Council, but changes are anticipated. Already being implemented is the replacement of IU (international unit) with RE (retinol equivalent) as the unit of measure for vitamin A and beta carotene (which the body can convert to vitamin A).

The external and internal benefits of specific vitamins and minerals, as well as their RDAs, are shown on the Vitamin and Mineral Chart, and the amounts suggested for enhancing beauty are given in Sections 1 and 2.

Researchers are finding that antioxidant vitamins, minerals, and other substances can prevent or at least postpone many of the degenerative ailments associated with aging. Chemical particles called free radicals are formed by oxidation within the body and acquired from external contaminants in foods, water, and the air. Unless neutralized by antioxidants, free radicals damage cells, weaken the immune system, can contribute to the development of maladies such as arthritis and cataracts, and are suspect in cancer and heart disease. To assist the body's own free-radical fighting system, Jean Carper, author of *Stop Aging Now* (Harper-Collins, 1995), and *Earl Mindell's Anti-Aging Bible* (Simon & Schuster, Fireside, 1996) suggest the following daily supplements of antioxidants.

Beta carotene (10 to 25 IU)

Vitamin C (500 to 1,000 milligrams—in divided doses)

Vitamin E (100 to 400 IU—up to 800 IU of
D-alpha-tocopheryl succinate)

Selenium (50 to 200 micrograms)

Coenzyme Q-10 (30 milligrams)

These primary antioxidants work individually against specific kinds of free radicals and, in many instances, are synergistic so that taking them together is more effective than taking larger amounts of just one or two would be. Other antioxidant substances include garlic, the herb ginkgo biloba, the amino acid glutathamine, the enzyme superoxide dismutase (sold as SOD), and zinc.

❧ *16* ❧

BEAUTIFUL MOVES:
HOW TO HAVE FUN
WHILE YOU EXERCISE

Amid 1890's advertisements for constricting corsets and smelling salts to ward off fainting spells, ladies' magazines warned their gentle readers that perfect health could not be attained through enervating indolence. Now that the feminine ideal of languorous fragility has been replaced by one of radiant vitality, achieving a combination of beauty and health calls for more than external pampering and internal nourishing—it requires the movement of 696 muscles. The body keeps 200 of them in tone by cardiovascular and digestive functions; moving the rest is up to us. And not all the beautiful moves can be classed as "exercise."

BREATHING TECHNIQUES THAT BEAUTIFY AND REVITALIZE

To experience our full potential, most of us need more oxygen. With "normal" shallow breathing, only the upper portion of the lungs is utilized and less than a sixth of the air in our lungs is changed with each breath. Consciously controlled deep breathing promotes oxygenation of the blood and elimination of waste carbon monoxide. Just a few deep breaths each hour can have a beautifying, revitalizing effect. To evaluate your present lung capacity:

> ❧ Exhale and measure the circumference of your chest at the level of the breastbone. Inhale deeply and remeasure. Physical fitness expert Nicholas Kounovsky[95] says the expansion increase should be $2^1/_2$ inches for women, $3^1/_2$ inches for men.

🍃 Watch a second hand while taking a deep breath and holding it as long as possible (55 seconds is average). Exhale and wait as long as you can before taking another breath (15 seconds is average).

Complete breathing requires slow inhalation of air into the lower lobes of the lungs by expanding the stomach area, then slow exhalation to expel stale air by tightening the diaphragm. Hatha yoga breathing calls for inhaling for a count of 8, holding your breath for a count of 4, then exhaling for a count of 8. A variation, called "healing breath," consists of breathing in for a count of 3, holding your breath for a count of 12, then breathing out for a count of 6. To strengthen your breathing muscles and acquire more oxygen:

🍃 Whenever convenient, count as you breathe. Inhale normally and exhale twice as long as you inhaled.

🍃 While walking, inhale for 3 or 4 steps and exhale for 6 or 8 steps. After a few weeks you can deepen your breathing by inhaling for 5 or 6 steps, exhaling for 10 or 12.

LOOKING GOOD: THE RIGHT WAY TO STAND UP

Actresses employ a stoop-shouldered, head-thrust-forward, abdomen-protruding stance to portray elderly crones. "Standing tall" with head erect, back straight, and stomach pulled in reverses the effect. Besides being unattractive, poor posture is unhealthful for men as well as women. When shoulders hunch and the spine curls, the body's scrunched-up organs cannot function properly and waistlines thicken.

Uncomfortable rigidity, however, isn't necessary. Imagining yourself as a manikin manipulated by a puppeteer can ease the strain of maintaining young-looking posture. For effortless erectness, think string plus balloon. From the moment you arise, imagine that a helium-filled balloon is attached to the middle of your skull, supporting your weight. Let your arms and shoulders relax comfortably while your stomach flattens and your chin lifts. When walking with your weight-carrying balloon in place, swinging your legs from the hip joints rather than from the knees will present the smoothly elegant stride of native water-bearers or models who practice with books balanced on their heads.

Howto sit tall

In our world of *homo sedentarius*, sitting is what we do most, but not necessarily best. It takes millenniums for evolutionary alterations to become operative, and chairs were introduced just 5,000 years ago as status symbols for kings and priests. So far, the only adaptation is derrier spread—each seat at the La Scala in Milan was recently widened 5 inches! Studies indicate that maximum comfort is achieved when body weight is shared between the feet and the hips, or when legs and feet are elevated.

- A back support and your imaginary helium-filled balloon can relieve the discomfort of "sitting up straight." Elevating your feet, or one foot at a time, on a 6-inch footstool concealed beneath your desk helps prevent the back strain that can result from hours of nonphysical labor.

- A chair with adjustable seat-height can be helpful. Hunching over a desk not only encourages the development of a double chin, it creates internal imbalances in the neck, back, and hips.

- Crossing your legs is neither injurious nor varicose-vein producing if you restrict the crossing to ankle level or raise them to a "high crossing" (when suitably attired) of one ankle resting on the knee of the other leg.

- Pumping a rocking chair back and forth is excellent therapy for an aching back, ups blood circulation in your feet, and stimulates muscles in the lower leg.

Howto make little moves for big benefits

A balanced diet provides the wherewithal for beauty, health and energy, but our sedentary lifestyles create a vicious cycle; poor circulation which deprives skin, hair, and nails of needed nutrients; muscle deterioration; sluggish metabolism that piles on the pounds; and listless lethargy that overwhelms natural buoyancy. Muscle movement is an investment in energy that pays dividends of increased mental alertness and physical well-being, and offers a bonus benefit. It burns calories. The more calories we burn, the more nutritious food we can ingest without gaining weight; and the more vibrantly beautiful we become.

Internal metabolic processes require approximately 50 calories per hour while we are sleeping, sitting, or standing. Every little move increases caloric consumption and potential energy; avoiding movement can have the opposite effect. A systems analyst gained 6 pounds during the first six months following a promotion that entitled her to a garage parking space next to the elevator instead of one on the outskirts of the lot. She analyzed and remedied the problem by getting off the elevator two floors below her office and stair-climbing the rest of the way every morning and noon.

According to a report in *American Health* (May 1987), exercising enough to burn 2,000 calories a week improves fitness and extends life. To use up 100 calories you can swim one-third of a mile, walk one mile, bicycle four miles, or simply make the most of each daily activity. You don't have to participate in marathons or work out with sophisticated health-club equipment to be physically fit. Ordinary, everyday moves can be parlayed into an amazing amount of calorie-consumption; studies show that consistent, moderate exercise increases longevity more than rigorous athletic training.[100]

- Climbing stairs for 5 minutes burns 73 calories; descending stairs, 28.

- Typing on an electric typewriter or computer keyboard uses 105 calories per hour.

- "Light" housework uses 180 calories per hour; washing windows or scrubbing floors, 225. (As a result of extensive studies, Russian gerontologists arrived at an unsurprising conclusion: women live longer than men because they rarely retire from active work.[124])

Without counting either minutes or caloric expenditures, there are countless ways to extend your use of personal energy and keep your muscles supple.

 ❧ Use footpower instead of horsepower: get off the bus at the stop before your destination, walk up one or two flights of stairs instead of taking the elevator or escalator, park at the far end of the shopping mall rather than in front of the store.

 ❧ Use hand power instead of electric power: resurrect your potato masher and rotary egg beater, hand-chop the soup or salad vegetables, wash and dry those few dishes without waiting to fill the dishwasher.

 ❧ Move your legs while you stand and wait or work: wherever you are, rise up on your toes and rock down on your heels. At the ironing board or kitchen sink, alternate side leg lifts and back kicks with marching in place.

 ❧ Make the most of every move: bend and stretch from the waist when making beds or retrieving small objects from the floor. Place frequently used supplies on high shelves so you stretch to reach them. Racewalk or jog from room to room. Bend one knee at a time and lunge like a fencer while vacuuming.

THREE QUICK EXERCISES YOU CAN DO AT HOME OR IN THE OFFICE

Muscles tire from lack of movement as well as from exertion. Exercising for a few seconds relaxes and invigorates a chair-weary body:

 ❧ Stand tall, lift your arms above your head, and lightly clasp your hands. With your head centered between your arms, bend to the right, swing across to the left, then return to the starting position. Repeat in the opposite direction.

 ❧ While standing, slowly lift one knee toward your chest; clasp both hands around the knee to pull it up and in as far as possible without strain. Deep breathe in and out. Release your hands and lower your knee. Repeat twice with each leg.

 ❧ Lean against a wall with your arms straight out in front, your back flat against the wall, and your heels as close to it as is comfortable. Lift your arms to touch the wall above your head, then swing them down to your sides as if making angels in the snow. Repeat three times.

SECRET MANEUVERS: HOW TO EXERCISE WHILE SITTING

When standing isn't feasible, exercise while sitting down. If no one is watching, do a slow neck roll or extend both arms and flap your hands. If you have an audience, perform out-of-sight moves so that only your muscles will know and benefit.

- 🕭 Rotate your ankles, then rock from heels to toes.

- 🕭 Sit tall and tighten your stomach muscles. Place your palms on the desktop and slowly lift one leg at a time for a count of 5; relax for 5 seconds, then press both feet on the floor with as much force as possible for 5 seconds.

- 🕭 Tense your left buttock for 5 seconds; relax for 5 seconds. Repeat with the right side, then tense both at the same time.

- 🕭 Press your hands into your thighs for 5 seconds, relax for a count of 5; then pull up on your thighs for 5 seconds without raising your hands.

STAY-IN-BED STRETCHES

Shortly after the turn of the century, Sanford Bennett published *Exercise in Bed* (Hilton, 1907) containing an hour-long series of movements to tone and rejuvenate the entire body. In October 1987, Tara Bennett-Goldman reported in *American Health* and *Good Housekeeping* that in-bed exercises help readjust the circulatory system and muscles from horizontal relaxation to vertical activity. Moving like a sleek cat for three reps of each exercise in the following three-minute morning motivator can get you going before you get out of bed. Just throw back the covers, lie flat on your back, and begin.

1. Slowly stretch your arms above your head, your toes to the foot of the bed.

2. Stretch both arms toward the ceiling, spread your fingers, tense and curl them like a cat's claws; then fling your arms out and bring them back so your palms press together.

3. Clasp your hands behind your head and bend your knees to place your feet flat, 10 inches apart. Pull your pubic bone toward your navel while pressing with your feet and raising your hips. Slowly lower your hips and straighten your knees.

4. Raise your right knee to your chest, clasp it with both hands and pull it toward your chin. Slowly lower your knee against the pressure of your hands. Repeat with the left leg. Then draw both knees to your chest and hold them with your arms. Tense your stomach muscles and gently rock your knees from side to side.

5. Bend your left knee to place the heel on your right thigh. Grasp your left ankle with your right hand and gently pull the heel up your thigh until moderate tension develops. Hold for 20 seconds. Repeat with the opposite leg.

THE SIX-MINUTE SHAPE-UP GUIDE FOR TONING AND LIMBERING

A lithe body with firm, resilient muscles is our prerogative regardless of age. There is no biological reason for body fat to increase while muscle and bone tissue decrease at the current rate of 1 percent each two years. Hippocrates' observation, "That which is used develops, that which is not used wastes away," is particularly applicable to joints and muscles. If not exercised, joints stiffen, muscles weaken, and flab develops. As little as six minutes a day of proper exercise can reverse this process, shape up the body, and restore youthful bounce and glow. The "shaping up" is automatic. A pound of fat occupies 20 percent more space than a pound of muscle, yet requires fewer calories for maintenance. By exercising, you can exchange bulges for sleek sinew and wear a smaller size without losing any weight. If you are dieting to lose pounds, exercise not only speeds fat loss by burning extra calories, it also prevents muscle loss and saggy skin.

How to Move Safely

Recent fitness enthusiasm has led to reevaluation of the therapeutic benefits and the possible pitfalls of exercise. New-and-improved exercises have been developed to replace strenuous calisthenics that can be hazardous to joints and muscles.

- **Deep-knee bends and duck walking** are no longer recommended because they put too much strain on the knees.

- **Bent-knee hang downs,** performed slowly, without force or jerky bouncing (which can cause microscopic tears in muscles) replace the locked-knee toe touches that overstress back, knees, and hamstring muscles.

- **Bent-leg raise-ups,** with the lower back pressed into the floor, arms crossed over the chest or behind the head and shoulders raised only high enough to clear the floor, replace straight-leg sit-ups that place excessive stress on the lower back and hip flexor muscles.

- **Single leg lifts,** with one knee bent and foot flat on the floor, are safer than double leg lifts that overstress the lower back.

- **Rear thigh lifts,** while on all fours, with the thigh slowly brought up parallel to the torso and the knee bent to form a right angle, safely work buttock muscles without the back strain or neck and shoulder contortions of the old "donkey kicks," which called for rapidly lifting one leg as high as possible.

Before embarking on any exercise program it is wise to have a medical checkup. If your arteries have hardened you may need to exercise in a horizontal position because blood vessels expand naturally when you are on a level plane; when you exercise in a standing position, your heart must pump blood uphill through forcibly expanded blood vessels over 70 times every minute.[120]

- **Start slowly.** Begin your regimen by performing each exercise only twice, then gradually work up to the desired total. Starting each session with slow moves allows your muscles to warm up. A warm shower increases muscle flexibility by as much as 20 percent. Exercising in front of an air conditioner or in 65-degree air can reduce the range of motion by 10 to 20 percent.

- **Let your digestive organs do their job** before drawing their needed blood away to move other muscles. Twenty minutes is considered essential to avoid possible indigestion or cramping, an hour is better. Exercising before a meal is ideal because it may decrease your appetite and improve your digestion.

- **Use an exercise mat or a carpeted surface** for all seated or prone-position exercises. (Beds do not offer sufficient support for exercises other than the stay-in-bed stretches.)

- **Breathe while you move.** Inhale with the easy move; exhale with the difficult one; holding your breath strains the cardiovascular system.

- **Move at your own pace.** Professionals may move faster than you should; slow and sinuous movement is best for improving flexibility, smooth and rhythmic for muscle toning.

- **Individualize your full-body program** by selecting several exercises from both of the following categories. Build up to the number of repetitions needed to reach your goal: 6 reps of each for a total of 6 minutes a day to maintain flexibility and muscle tone; 10 reps of each for a total of 12 minutes to stretch and strengthen muscles.

  If you have a sturdy door with a firmly anchored doorknob, you can add this allover conditioner: grasp one side of the knob with each hand, keep your tummy tucked in, your back and arms straight while you slowly squat until your hips touch your heels, then slowly pull yourself up to a standing position.

- **Exercise with a partner** to add the pleasure of companionship and to maintain a consistent regimen. Melanie and Carl are a case in point. Although she hadn't gained weight, time and gravity were increasing the circumference of Melanie's waist. She had been exercising sporadically, but her busy schedule and waning enthusiasm always provided excellent excuses for putting her after-work firming-up program on hold. When she dissolved in tears because Carl had to help zip her into the snug-fitting dress that had "shrunk" while hanging in the closet, he came up with the solution. "Let's set the alarm fifteen minutes earlier in the morning and shape up together. My belts are getting a little tight, too." Clothes now fit the way they should, and neither Carl nor Melanie is tempted to forsake their slightly competitive few minutes of before-breakfast camaraderie.

Upper Body Exercises

- Stand with your feet wide apart. Fold your arms in front of your waist and cup each elbow with the hand of the other arm. Slowly raise your folded arms over your head as far back as possible without discomfort, then slowly lower them to the starting position.

❧ Stand with your arms straight out in front, palms down. Bend your elbows down to raise your hands, palms up, directly above your shoulders. Slowly raise both palms straight up as though you were lifting a heavy box. Hold the imaginary box steady for a few seconds before slowly lowering it and returning to the starting position.

❧ Stand with hands loosely clasped behind your back. Keep your arms straight while slowly bringing your elbows as close together as possible without strain.

❧ Lie face down with your knees bent, ankles crossed, and your feet raised several inches. Bend your elbows and place your palms flat on the floor under your shoulders, fingers pointed inward. Keep your head and torso in a straight line while slowly pushing up until your arms are fully extended to share the weight with your knees. Slowly lower your body almost to the floor and push back up again.

MIDDLE AND LOWER BODY EXERCISES

For maximum benefit, complete the repetitions for each separate exercise before going on to the next one in a group of complementary exercises such as this first one.

❧ Stand tall with feet 24 inches apart, arms outstretched at shoulder level. Twist at the waist to reach forward, then backward with each arm.

Lower your left arm and slide it down to your knee as you bend to the left and raise your right arm. Reverse to bend to the right.

Leave your feet in position, bend forward from the waist (without locking knees) and let your arms swing loosely between your legs for 10 seconds—with fingers curled if your hands touch the floor.

❧ Sit with knees bent, feet flat on the floor, and arms folded in front of your chest. Keep your spine straight while you lean back until you feel the abdominal muscles tighten. Hold for 5 seconds before returning to the starting position.

Straighten your arms and place your hands flat on the floor behind you. Straighten and raise your right leg, then bend the right knee and slip the right foot under your left knee without touching the floor. Straighten the right leg, return to the starting position. Relax and repeat with the opposite legs.

ᕦ Lie on your back with hands under your head. With knees bent, toes pointed, and both feet clear of the floor, raise your head and alternate legs while twisting to touch the right knee with the left elbow, left knee with right elbow.

ᕦ Lie on your back with knees up, feet flat on the floor, and arms crossed over your chest with the fingertips at shoulder level. Press down with your lower back while slowly raising your head and shoulders toward your knees until your shoulder blades are clear of the floor, then lower to the starting position.

As an alternative: Lie on the floor with your hips close to the legs of a straight chair, your feet and calves resting on the chair seat. Grasp the bottom of the chair legs with your hands and slowly pull yourself up until your shoulders are raised. Keep your lower back in contact with the floor while returning to the starting position.

ᕦ Lie on your back with knees bent, arms at your sides, palms down. Slowly raise your legs and pelvis off the floor until your knees are almost over your face. Return to the starting position.

Leave your hands at your sides. Lift and straighten your legs over your hips. Slowly separate your legs as wide as possible without strain, then bring them back together.

ᕦ With knees slightly flexed, bend over and place your palms on the floor. Without raising your head, walk on all fours as if you were a primordial creature.

Drop to your knees, leave your arms extended, and round your back up for a count of 5. Rock back so your hips are over your heels, slide your arms out in front of you, and rest your forehead on the floor for 5 seconds.

Heartfelt Moves: 13 Benefits of Aerobic Exercise

Stop-and-go sports and exercises such as those in the preceding sections improve flexibility and help you keep trim. EMS (Electronic

Muscle Stimulators) help rehabilitate muscles damaged by severe accident or disease but, as explained in the February 1989 issue of *Mayo Clinic Nutrition Letter*, they will not make you either beautiful or fit. A regular program of continuously sustained aerobic activities (walking, swimming, rowing, etc.) maintain vibrant beauty and health by strengthening the cardiovascular system and deepening breathing to provide more oxygen, and they offer an extensive array of potential rewards.

1. **Alleviated tension and elevated mood.** Sustained movement at target heart rate causes your body to produce greater amounts of the beta-endorphins, which counter stress and depression, increase tolerance to pain, and account for the euphoric "runner's high." In a study of 300 people, Dr. Robert Thayer of California State University at Long Beach found that moderate aerobic exercise was the best way to alleviate a bad mood and become more alert.

2. **Aroused alertness.** A 30-minute bout of aerobic exercise has been shown to improve short-term memory and increase mental performance by 25 percent.[99]

3. **Better regulated blood-sugar levels**. Physical activity improves glucose tolerance and reduces insulin resistance. If you have diabetes, however, be sure to check with your doctor before beginning an aerobic regimen; it might trigger hemorrhaging if you suffer from retinopathy.

4. **Extended lifespan.** A 17,000-person study being conducted by Stanford Medical School indicates that each hour of aerobic activity increases anticipated longevity; by 1.95 hours if you are 40 years old; by 2.61 hours if you are 60.

5. **Improved skin tone.** Regular exercise slows cell degeneration and collagen breakdown (the prime instigators of wrinkling) and keeps your skin glowingly healthy because of the extra oxygen and nutrients provided through stimulated blood circulation.

6. **Increased energy.** As explained in *Mayo Clinic Nutrition Newsletter* (October 1988), energy levels increase as the body adapts to exercise, muscles become better able to utilize oxygen, the heart's pumping capacity improves, and the resting

pulse slows. The average resting heart rate is 78 per minute, with a variance of 10 considered normal. By conditioning your heart through exercise, you can reduce the resting rate to 70 or less, which allows your heart to pump the same amount of blood with fewer beats.

7. **Lowered cholesterol.** Habitual aerobic exercise has been shown to bring about a dramatic drop in elevated cholesterol levels, along with an increase of the blood substance that dissolves heart-attack-instigating clots.[33,124] A report in the March 1988 issue of *American Health* states that the proportion of "good" HDL cholesterol is raised when you walk or run 12 miles each week at any pace; achieving your target heart rate is not essential to this benefit.

8. **Lowered blood pressure.** A study in *Medicine and Science in Sports and Exercise*, reported by *Prevention* (April 1994) states that three to five days a week of aerobic exercise done for 20 minutes to an hour can subtract up to 10 millimeters of mercury from both the top and bottom numbers of your blood-pressure readings. That means that someone with high-normal pressure (say, 139 over 85) may be able to jump back into the normal category (less than 130 over 85) with a simple, almost-daily routine.

9. **Reduced weight and girth.** In addition to immediately decreasing appetite, eight to twelve minutes of aerobic activity contributes to weight loss by burning between 80 and 200 calories, boosts the metabolic rate so that you continue to burn calories at a higher rate for up to two days, and builds lean tissue which occupies less space than the replaced fat, thus reducing your inches.

10. **Relieved PMS.** Regular exercise has an effect on female hormones that may prevent or abate premenstrual tension and water retention.

11. **Stimulated immune system.** According to worldwide tests reported in *Prevention* (February 1988), the amount of virus- and cancer-fighting lymphocytes in the blood are more than doubled by an hour of bicycle riding or other moderate aerobic activity. Overly intensive training, however, can hamper

immunity; with the exception of daily walks, you should adhere to the classic recommendation of three to four 30-minute aerobic sessions per week.

12. **Stronger bones.** Studies conducted at the University of Oregon indicate that a program of regular exercise increases bone density to offset the decline in bone mass which normally commences after the age of 40. Developing peak bone mass through exercise and adequate calcium consumption before the age of 35 protects against osteoporosis later in life; consistent postmenopausal exercise plus calcium can replace lost bone density.

13. **Disease prevention.** In *The Brown University Long-Term Care Quality Letter*[177], Dr. Bess Marcus reports that recent research indicates that even light and moderate exercise can have a significantly positive impact on many chronic health problems that affect older adults, including coronary heart disease, hypertension, colon cancer, osteoporosis, and psychological distress.

How to Target Your Heart Rate

The heart's ability to speed up with exercise diminishes so predictably that "maximum heart rate" has been established as 220 minus a person's age. Numerous studies show that the "normal" decline in cardiac capacity can be combated by any activity that brings the heart rate into the target zone of 60 to 80 percent of its maximum and maintains it from 5 to 20 minutes. The least complex method of targeting your heart-rate goal is to subtract your age from 220, then multiply that total by the desired percentage. For instance: if you are 40 years old, your target heart rate would be 126 (220 minus 40 = 180 multiplied by .70); the acceptable "low" would be 108, the "high," 144.

If you don't have an electronic pulse monitor, you can check your heart rate by pausing while exercising, placing your left middle fingers next to your windpipe or over the pulse on your right wrist, counting it for 6 seconds, then multiplying by 10. (The medical practice of counting for 15 seconds and multiplying by 4 is impractical during exercise because the heartbeat slows rapidly when physical activity is discontinued.)

EIGHT WAYS TO AVOID AEROBIC ADVERSITIES

Before embarking on any fitness program, it is wise to obtain your physician's approval, then:

1. ***Schedule your aerobic sessions several hours after eating so your digestive system is not disrupted.*** "Carbohydrate loading" an hour before exercising is no longer advocated even for competitive athletes.[99]

2. ***Warm up first.*** When your body is at rest, approximately 85 percent of your blood supply is in your chest and abdomen. As activity begins, blood moves to the working muscles which then "heat up" to such an extent that they could boil a quart of water in an hour. If your muscles are abruptly required to stretch and squeeze to their limit, ligaments may tighten around joints and, in extreme cases, muscles can tear. Studies reveal that 60 percent of sports injuries are traceable to improper warm-up techniques.[75]

   The length of your warm-up and the movements involved depend on your starting condition and the type of exercise. If you have been up and moving, going for a walk will entail no warm-up. If you plan to leap out of bed and onto your bike for a 15-minute spin, play fair with your muscles by performing some limbering exercises. Then begin your aerobic activity at low intensity; walk before you run, swim a slow lap instead of diving in and breast-stroking at top speed.

3. ***Cool down.*** Allowing your muscles a cooling off period is as crucial as warming them up. Abruptly stopping a workout can cause a sudden drop in blood pressure that may produce dizziness plus blood pooling and an aftermath of painfully tight muscles. Gradually slowing your activity for the final 5 minutes (or performing mild stretching and bending exercises after a bout of rope jumping or other activity that does not lend itself to low intensity) permits a return to normalcy without danger.

   If you have been perspiring heavily, wait for your temperature to drop before showering. A cool shower will shock your system; a hot one can draw so much blood to the skin that there might not be enough left to supply your internal organs. If you've overexercised, a tub-bath herbal soak of juniper or lemon balm often relieves the worst of the muscle pain.

4. ***Approach your aerobic goals sensibly.*** Consistency is the key to muscle conditioning; strengthening occurs during the 48 hours following vigorous exercise. If the activity is not repeated within 72 hours, muscles begin to shrink and lose their new-found flexibility at the rate of about 1 percent per day.

The standard regimen calls for three or four weekly sessions of approximately 30 minutes each (5 to 10 minutes for warm up, 12 to 20 minutes at target heart rate, 5 to 10 minutes to cool down). Research reported in *University of California, Berkeley Wellness Letter* (November 1988) indicates that "interval training" of 3 to 5 minutes at target heart rate, 3 minutes of slowed-down activity (60-percent heart rate), then another 3 to 5 minutes at high intensity produces 10 percent greater gains in aerobic capacity than steady-speed sessions. Lower intensity, longer-duration activity forces the body to break down stored fat for energy.

5. ***Put your program on hold if you have a fever or virus.*** Elevating your temperature even higher by exercising can aggravate your illness, and viruses make muscle fibers more susceptible to tears and injuries.

6. ***"Think" yourself into a successful regimen.*** By remembering that you are working with Mother Nature to help your body—not striving to punish it or yourself—you can turn what might be a disagreeably boring workout into a pleasurable experience. Experiment until you discover which of these options works best for you: Mentally envision the eventual results of your efforts. Concentrate on your muscular movements while visualizing your body reshaping itself into more glamorous contours. Or, evolve a meditation-type mantra such as whispering "down" every time one foot hits the ground. Or, imagine an applauding audience admiring the grace and aplomb with which you whip through your exercise session. Or, disassociate yourself from the entire process by wearing a radio or tape-playing headset if outdoors, or by watching television while pedaling, rowing, skiing, or walking with indoor exercise equipment.

7. ***Dress in comfortable clothing with properly fitted shoes designed for your chosen activity.*** For outdoor activities in cold weather, wear gloves and a hat to hold heat in your body. In the summer, a white or light-colored hat will reflect the sun's rays. Leg warmers help avoid cramping by keeping your muscles warm, but rubber or plastic "conditioning suits" can cause dehydration and deprive your skin of oxygen. (The pounds of liquid lost reappear as soon as you drink a few glasses of water; the harm to your system lingers.)

8. ***Replenish fluids and nutrients.*** Thirst is not always a reliable guide to Mother Nature's needs. Fluid losses from perspiration during strenuous activity can deplete your water-soluble vitamins and minerals as well as liquids. Sports medicine specialists advise drinking a glass of cool water 20 minutes before, at 20-minute intervals during, and immediately after exercising.[71] Nutritionists suggest a daily multivitamin-mineral supplement as insurance, extra vitamin E to protect cell membranes from destruction by oxidation from the increased oxygen intake,[174] and a diet rich in potassium-containing foods (see the Vitamin and Mineral Chart) to prevent leg cramps. Taking a 500-milligram vitamin-C-plus-bioflavonoids tablet before and after exercising is a muscle-stiffness preventive.

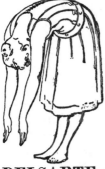

Clothing should be even less confining than this whaleboned waist advertised in 1892.

NINE AEROBIC EXERCISES THAT STRENGTHEN THE CARDIOVASCULAR SYSTEM

Customizing your beautifying, cardiovascular-improving program can be as simple as getting up earlier and walking to work. If you prefer to move in the company of others, sign up for a class, join a club, or exercise with a friend. You can opt for a single activity or, with your muscles kept in shape by daily toning exercises, vary your program to avoid monotony. Aerobic dancing, cross-country skiing, cycling, jogging or running, rope jumping, rowing, swimming, walking—whatever works for you is "right" for your body as long as your doctor approves and you always warm up and cool down.

1. AEROBIC DANCING

Whether you participate in a class or work out in privacy with a video tape, aerobic dancing is a fun way to keep fit. Low Impact Aerobics (LIA or soft aerobics) have replaced the ballistic, bouncy routines that resulted in high injury rates. Wearing aerobic shoes with rearfoot and lateral support further lessens the possibility of shin splints or foot problems.

Calories burned: 60 to 90 each 10 minutes, depending on the intensity of activity.

2. CROSS-COUNTRY SKIING

The movements required for cross-country skiing utilize muscles in the arms, legs, and trunk in equal measure, and are virtually free of injury-initiating stresses. Easily stored "ski machines" allow you to benefit from this aerobic exercise in the comfort of your own home, without waiting for the snow to fall.

Calories burned: 70 to 200 each 10 minutes, depending on tempo.

3. CYCLING

Enthusiasm for this activity began in 1891 when the "safety bicycle" replaced prior models with their huge, unmanageable front wheels. If you live in an area where outdoor biking is feasible, our twentieth-century models offer designs for city, mountain, or all-terrain cycling. To alternate outdoor riding with indoor pedaling, you can put your bike up on rollers in your living room. If back-to-nature biking is impractical or undesirable (half an hour amid city traffic fills your lungs with as much carbon monoxide as ten cigarettes[137]), invest in a stationary exercycle which offers similar cardiovascular, upper-leg, and buttock-toning benefits.

Calories burned: 65 for each 10 minutes of pedaling at 10 mph with a heart rate of 130.

4. JOGGING AND RUNNING

Jogging is usually classified as running when the speed exceeds six miles an hour. Either activity is great for your heart, and for weight reduction, but both are so joint-jarring and injury-ridden they should be undertaken only with medical approval. Begin your program by alternating five minutes of brisk walking with five minutes of slow jogging, then gradually increase the jogging segments. Jog or run for your set period of time, not for distance or speed. The ideal pace is one that keeps your heart rate within the target zone while leaving you with enough breath to carry on a conversation. According to Dr. Thomas McMahon (*Prevention*, December 1987), bending your knees just ten extra degrees and taking "scurrying" steps emphasizes the role of thigh and buttock muscles, reduces the amount of shock transmitted through the body by 80 percent, and uses up 25 percent more calories than the customary gait.

Calories burned: 80 for 10 minutes of jogging at 5 miles per hour; 130 when running at 10 miles per hour.

5. JUMPING ROPE

If you want to improve your cardiovascular system with the least expenditure of time, and you have your physician's approval, this is the ideal aerobic activity. The President's Council on Physical Fitness and Sports found five minutes of rope jumping the equal of fifteen minutes of jogging. Although it seems too good to be true, utilizing your six minutes of daily exercise as a warm-up; jumping for five minutes, five times a week; then doing walk-around household chores for two minutes while you cool down can take care of your fitness regimen.

Both *Joy of Jumping*[31] and *The Hop, Skip and Jump Way to Health*[118] recommend building up to 500 continuous jumps by beginning with 10 jumps per session several times a day. To ease into the program, jump one foot at a time; to increase the benefits, jump with both feet and jump higher than the suggested one inch off the floor. If your ceiling is too low, or if you don't have a rope, you can simulate by assuming the position (upper arms near the ribs, forearms at a 45 degree angle) and rotating your wrists while jumping.

Calories burned: 63 for each 5 minutes at 120 to 140 turns per minute.

6. ROWING

Whether stroking across the water in a shell or rowing a machine while watching television, this is a superb, full-body exercise. The popularity of home exercise equipment has led to multi-action combinations such as rower-cycles and rower-skiers that cost no more than membership in a fitness club. Rowing is an effective back-strengthener often prescribed for those with lower back and disk problems, but it is not suitable for certain physical conditions. Check with your doctor before experimenting.

Calories burned: 60 to 325 each 10 minutes, depending on intensity of activity.

7. SWIMMING

The buoyancy of water so reduces stress on joints and ligaments that swimming is a perfect exercise for the elderly or for anyone with physical problems, yet its muscle toning and aerobic benefits equal those of land-based activities. Body beautifying as well as cardiovascular-conditioning, swimming also bolsters bones. In *Clinical Research* (January 1987), Dr. Eric Orwoll cites tests showing that swimming is as efficient as weight-bearing exercise in building bone mass to retard osteoporosis.

Maximum heart rate for swimming is slower than for other activities because water absorbs body heat and the horizontal position eases blood circulation. To compute your 12- to 20-minute target zone:

subtract your age from 205, then multiply by the desired percentage between 60 and 80. (For our 40-year-old, 125-pound example, this would be 115 at 70 percent of maximum heart rate.)

Calories burned: 50 to 115 each 10 minutes, depending on the vigor of exertion.

8. WALKING

Although it may not seem like exercise, walking provides the same benefits as other aerobic activities, and can be practical as well as healthily beautifying. You can substitute your walks for riding (as in walking to work) or combine them with necessary errands. Carrying heavy objects or wearing ankle weights is not advisable because of the possibility of straining the body's joints by upsetting nature's balance between arms and legs; but hand weights of one to three pounds, designed for walkers or joggers, can safely be used to increase the effort.

Begin by "strolling" on alternate days, gradually increase your pace to raise your heart rate into its target zone for at least 12 minutes with a cadence of 90 to 120 steps per minute. For precise monitoring (and for fascinating diversion), splurge on a wristwatch-pulse counter and a pedometer. To avoid becoming overheated as your muscles warm up, dress for a temperature 10 to 20 degrees warmer than it actually is, then walk *with* the wind as you start out; *against* it as you return. Walking in a light drizzle or amid drifting snowflakes is delightful, but, if the weather outside is frightful or if your neighborhood is rife with potential danger from mortals or motor fumes, walk in the comfortable safety of a shopping mall or purchase a treadmill.

- **Strolling** (1–2 mph): burns approximately 30 calories each 10 minutes, seldom achieves target heart rate but lowers cholesterol and may be utilized as warm up and cool down for fitness walking.

- **Brisk walking** (3–3$^1/_2$ mph, 50 calories per 10 minutes)

- **Striding** (3$^1/_2$–5$^1/_2$ mph, 50–75 calories per 10 minutes): long, swift strides expend almost as much energy as jogging, without the sometimes-injurious jarring impact.

- **Racewalking** (4–6 mph, 65–120 calories per 10 minutes): This full-body exercise uses the same number of muscles as swimming, and has become so popular with celebrities that its exaggerated hip-swing is regarded as sexy. Racewalking requires a warm-up and cool-down of limbering exercises, plus mastery of its unique moves.

1. Keep your feet close to the ground, reaching forward with one heel while pushing off with the toe of the other foot. Straighten the knee of the advancing leg as the pushing-off toe maintains ground contact until the reaching heel touches down so there is a split-second of double support.

2. Rotate your pelvis to direct your movement in a straight line so your feet land directly in front of one another.

3. Keep your hands in loose fists, your arms bent at right angles, and swing your elbows high—left arm and right leg forward, right arm and left leg back. Your shoulders should lift and lower with each stride; your head glide smoothly, parallel with the ground.

9. ORIENTAL MOVES

For over six thousand years, Ch'i Kung, Dao Yin, T'ai Chi Ch'uan, Yeng Shu, Yoga, and similar disciplines have been practiced by Far Eastern peoples. All adhere to the Taoist principle of mind-body unification and control to prevent and correct ailments, improve bodily functions, and reverse the aging process. The physical portions of two of these disciplines, T'ai Chi Ch'uan and Hatha Yoga, have been adopted by the Western world. Yoga is not sufficiently vigorous to accelerate the pulse into its target heart-rate zone, but both are excellent fitness exercises that benefit the cardiovascular system.

T'ai Chi Ch'uan: Originating in Tibet and perfected in China during the Sung Dynasty (960–1278 A.D.), T'ai Chi Ch'uan is now practiced daily by millions of Orientals who perform the 128 stylized, dancelike postures each dawn and dusk in a twenty-minute ritual of constant motion designed to allow the free flow of energies throughout the body. Usually referred to as T'ai Chi, it can be learned from illustrated texts such as *Knocking at the Gate of Life*[35] and *The Chinese Way to a Long and Healthy Life*[134] or by attending classes at health clubs, YMCAs, and community centers. Condensed versions of

T'ai Chi include fewer postures; at Rancho La Peurta in Mexico, the slow, smooth motions are completed in ten minutes to the accompaniment of Latin music.

The broad range of curative powers claimed by its adherents may be questioned by skeptics, but, although performed with deliberation, target heart rate can be achieved after only one minute of the exercise.[57] Pennsylvania's Swathmore College has incorporated T'ai Chi into its football team's training schedule, and an international lecturer testifies to its fitness and stamina building. On a tour of the Orient this 70-year-old became so intrigued by the early-morning sight of young and old Chinese performing T'ai Chi that she studied and regularly practiced the movements. The following year, she impressed herself and the men she hired to cut down one of her trees. For four hours, while they sawed the tree into logs for her fireplace, she picked up the wood, trundled it 30 yards in a wheelbarrow, unloaded and stacked it—and suffered no painful after-effects the next day.

Hatha Yoga: Even more ancient than T'ai Chi Ch'uan, Yoga has two distinct aspects. The spiritual side, concerned with knowledge and meditation, must be pursued under the guidance of a guru. The physical, Hatha Yoga, which emphasizes deep breathing and sinuous poses to foster flexibility and extend life, has achieved international acclaim. After the *asanas* (poses) have been mastered under the tutelage of an instructor, it can be practiced at home. (Because Hatha Yoga affects every part of the body, it is wise to check with your physician before attempting any of the advanced poses.)

In India, where it is regarded as a cure for everything from gout and wrinkles to sexual impotence and the common cold, each of the 25 Yoga centers in Delhi has a daily attendance of 1,500. In America, where Hatha Yoga classes are taught in health clubs, Y's, and senior centers, it is credited with almost as many bodily benefits; including increased stamina, relieved stress and tension, reduced bronchial difficulty, and improved musculature to alleviate lower back pain.[100]

TAKE THE PLUNGE INTO WATER WORKOUTS

Everyone can get a good physical workout in water—from beginning exercisers to professional athletes and from senior citizens to pregnant women. Water exercising is great for overall body health because it works on seven aspects of fitness: flexibility, aerobic and anaerobic capacity, musculoskeletal resiliency, strength, power, and speed. Water workouts are very different from "swimming." To enjoy the benefits of water exercise, you don't have to be able to swim. You don't have to be in great physical shape. You don't even have to get your hair wet. Water workouts really are for everyone. Even if you have not exercised in months or years, you can enter the water and begin immediately.

THE MAGIC OF WATER

The magic of a water workout lies in water's support for the body (buoyancy), water's resistance to body movement, and the wonderful feeling of invigoration that only water exercise can give.

Buoyancy: Water buoyancy lets you run, walk, leap, stretch, and pivot without the jolts that can cause injuries when you do them on land. Water acts as a cushion for your weight-bearing joints, preventing injury, strain, and reinjury common in other exercise programs.

Resistance: Because water is denser than air, your muscles work harder in water than if you were simply moving your arms and legs through air on land. Water is a natural weight-training machine that is instantly adjustable: The harder you push and pull and kick in the water, the more resistance you meet from it.

AEROBIC EXERCISE

As explained earlier, in order to experience an aerobic training effect, you must achieve a working heart rate that is continuously elevated to your target heart rate zone for 20 to 30 minutes, three to five times a week. You can reach this goal in water much more easily than on land because the water keeps you cool, your body buoyancy takes the strain off your muscles and joints, and your heart will pump harder without taking your breath away. On land, continuous aerobic exercise can make your muscles feel heavy. An hour of running, aerobics, power walking, mountain biking, or rope jumping jolts the skeletal system. In water, however, aerobic work is achieved effortlessly. Although you feel a sense of great strength against resistance, you finish the workout feeling fresh.

MENTAL STRENGTH

What an amazing change in attitude you will experience as soon as you enter the water! Stress washes away. Anger, disappointment, and aggravation go with it. The moment you become immersed in water, you have entered a new environment of sensation and perception. You can learn to use this quality of water to diffuse built-up negative emotions and to enjoy life while getting physically fit.

REHABILITATION

Many people turn to water for rehabilitation. Whatever the injury or disability, water workouts soothe the body and mind. Water offers freedom of movement and security to injured patients as no other exercise medium can. The moment you slide into the water for an emergency water workout, you feel significantly better. Pain is reduced; mobility is regained. In water you can move, stretch, walk, and even run when all that seemed impossible on land.

Water exercise is a perfect activity for anyone who has enjoyed daily exercise but now has a traumatic or chronic injury. If you know you shouldn't bicycle today because of a sore knee, train in the water instead. If your elbow hurts and you can't play tennis, train in the water. Therapists even use water to help patients who have fallen off ladders, tripped on the sidewalk, tried to lift heavy boxes, suffered whiplash, pain in the back or neck, sprained ankles, knee and hip replacements. All sorts of people with all sorts of ailments have found they can begin an active program of stretching and conditioning right away instead of lying in bed for a week and having their muscles atrophy. Many therapists believe that water workouts can cut recovery time by up to half.

Water workouts are also good for anyone with arthritis. The Arthritis Foundation promotes water exercise because workouts in warm pools can decrease pain and stiffness. The Foundation and the YMCA have developed a widely offered aquatic program. This involves gentle exercises in 83- to 88-degree water under a trained instructor's supervision. You don't have to know how to swim to participate. For details, call the Arthritis Foundation at 1-800-283-7800.

Water workouts are also being recommended to some patients recovering from cancer surgery. Once they receive medical clearance, breast cancer patients who have had surgery may enroll in the YWCA's Encore program. This national support program's meetings include group discussion, as well as land and water exercise. Water workouts can help with the painful swelling that can occur when surgeons remove lymph nodes in the armpit to see if the cancer has spread. Also, gentle movement increases the range of motion of joints in areas where scar tissue forms following cancer surgery.

CROSS TRAINING

Although many athletes and exercisers turn to water workouts during a crisis, increasing numbers are using water as a training tool and as a preventative measure as well. When a land exercise causes pain in a joint or muscle, smart exercisers immediately go to the water and take a day off without really taking a day off. Instead of pounding the pavement twice a day, seven days a week, distance runners often do several of their long runs in deep water. Instead of sprinting on the synthetic track five days in a row, Olympic hopefuls often substitute one of their weekly workouts with sprints in water. Professional football, soccer, tennis, and basketball players have recently begun water training programs. Like professional and Olympic athletes, you can avoid strain and injury while moving closer to your fitness goals by letting water work its magic for you.

TIPS FOR SAFE AND ENJOYABLE WATERPOWER WORKOUTS*

&. If you are alone in a pool, make sure someone is nearby in case of emergency. Always use the "buddy system" whenever you exercise in open water—river, bay, ocean, or lake. If you can't find a friend to join you, have someone watch from shore. If you aren't familiar with the water's currents, surface, texture of the bottom, or possible underwater obstacles, ask a local resident or lifeguard about possible dangers before you enter the water. If you wish, you can modify some of the exercises, working against currents or waves to make them more difficult. In rocky areas, wear a pair of water-training shoes.

&. Don't drink alcohol before a water workout. Alcohol impairs your balance, coordination, and judgment, and it alters your body's physiological response to exercise.

---

*Reprinted with permission from *The Complete Waterpower Workout Book* by Lynda Huey and Robert Forster (Random House, 1993).

🍃 Wait at least two to three hours after a big meal before starting a hard workout. If your workout is gentle, you can decrease the waiting time to one hour.

🍃 Most pools are cool, so as soon as you slide into the water, begin jogging or bouncing for a warm-up. Bouncing is a rhythmic up-and-down movement in which your knees bend, then straighten, then bend again.

🍃 When you bounce or jump, inhale at the height of the jump and exhale at the lowest point near the water. This prevents you from accidentally swallowing water.

🍃 Move to a spot in the pool where you can stand in chest-deep water and extend your arms fully without hitting any obstacle, a swimmer, or another water exerciser.

🍃 To avoid blisters on your toes or on the balls of your feet, find a pool with a friendly bottom surface or buy some water-training shoes.

🍃 Begin the exercises slowly. If your body feels strong and energetic, increase the pace of the movements as well as the height of the jumps. If you feel tired, move more slowly and sit lower in the water. Don't be surprised if your body changes the way it feels midway through the workout. Obey it.

🍃 If you are a nonswimmer, consider joining a class to learn to swim. You will feel safer each time you enter the water.

How to Get Going

If you join an organized exercise group, the instructor will lead the way through the vast variety of exercises you can comfortably do in the water. If you're on your own, create an exercise routine for yourself, as you would on land. Begin with a 5-minute warm-up of running and bouncing across the shallow end of the pool. If you have a sore ankle, foot, shin, knee, hip, or back, put on a flotation belt. Wearing it throughout your workout reduces impact on your weight-bearing joints. Work for cardiac fitness by running, jumping, jogging, and so on. Work for muscle strength by moving your legs and/or arms through the water with ever-increasing speed and power. Work for flexibility by stretching out your legs, arms, and back to a point that is comfortable, holding for a few seconds, and then resting. You can adjust the intensity of your workout by changing the speed of your movements or by moving into slightly deeper or slightly shallower water.

Think of all the land exercises you'd like to do but avoid because you don't have the muscle power or stamina; try them in the water and you'll be in for a wonderful surprise. Without the sweat and strain of land exercises, you'll be able to perform beyond your most daring expectations.

TRY WEIGHT LIFTING FOR STRENGTH TRAINING

The adage "use it or lose it" is, unfortunately, especially true regarding the body and its muscular strength, endurance, and flexibility. The body's efficiency improves with use and it deteriorates with disuse. Strength-training exercises are designed to keep your muscles strong and healthy.

Strength training (sometimes called weight training) exercises specific muscles by relying on the resistance of barbells, dumbbells, machines, rubber cords, a partner, or even your own body weight. Its goal is the improvement of fitness levels and personal appearance.

IT'S FOR EVERYBODY

Weight lifting, once the domain of biceps-popping body builders, has gone mainstream and is now a big hit in all age categories and with exercisers of all different ability levels. Health clubs are filled with strength-training enthusiasts, and high schools, colleges, and universities are offering strength-training courses to thousands of students. In addition, strength-training programs are also gaining in popularity among older populations, including individuals with osteoporosis and patients in cardiac rehabilitation programs.

Strength training is especially popular among women. These exercises offer women the opportunity to make noticeable changes in body composition, appearance, and health. Improvements involve increases in strength and tone (with minimal muscle enlargement), decreases in subcutaneous fat, and a reshaping process that results in a more attractive appearance. Most interesting is the news about strength training and osteoporosis. Studies are consistently finding that strength training helps women preserve bone density while improving muscle mass and strength, thus offering prevention against osteoporosis. Even frail, elderly women have boosted bone density and muscle strength and functioning after working out with weights. Not only does strength training have a very potent effect on bones, but it can improve balance, muscle strength, and activity levels as well. Even your posture will improve as your upper body grows strong enough to keep your trunk from curving into a tired stoop.

A LIST OF BENEFITS

The major benefits of strength training are

- Increased muscular strength.
- Increased local muscular endurance.
- Increased bone density.
- Prevention of injury during sports and recreational activities.
- Improved performance capacity in sports and recreational activities.
- Positive influence on body composition.
- Improved strength balance around joints.
- Improved total body strength.

A SAMPLING OF EXERCISES

A fitness instructor at your local health club, Y, or fitness center can tailor a strength-training program to your specific needs. Here are a few examples, just to get you going and give you an idea of how easy it is to build up muscular strength.

To strengthen bones and muscles, experts suggest that you perform eight to ten strength-training exercises involving the body's major muscle groups two to three times a week. Choose a weight (which can be a dumbbell, a rubber cord, or even partner resistance) that you can use at least eight but no more than ten times before muscle fatigue sets in.

PARTNER EXERCISES

To strengthen the shoulders: With a partner standing behind you, raise your arms out from your body until they are parallel to the floor. At the same time, have your partner gently push down on your arms to offer resistance so that the move takes about 6 seconds. After three or four repetitions, switch roles by having your partner try to lift your arms from your sides while you push down to resist.

To strengthen the hamstrings group located on the back of the upper leg: Lie on the floor on your stomach with your knees bent at about a 45-degree angle. Have your partner kneel facing the soles of your feet and grasp your lower leg just below your heels. Bend your knees until your heels touch your buttocks. Have your partner apply pressure to resist the movement, but allowing completion of the movement in about 6 seconds. Repeat three to four times.

CORD EXERCISES

You can purchase the thick rubber cord used in these exercises from most sporting good stores.

To strengthen arm biceps and some muscles located on the front of the forearm: Grasp the handles of the cord and stand on the center of the cord, keeping your back straight and holding your head upright. Moving only your forearms, pull the handles upward until the elbows are completely bent. Then return the arms to the starting position. Repeat until you feel your muscles begin to tire.

EXERCISING BY YOURSELF

To strengthen the lower back: Lie on the floor on your stomach. Place your arms out in front of your body. Slowly raise your head, shoulders, chest, and legs off the ground at the same time. (You'll look like you're flying.) Then slowly resume the starting position. Repeat three or four times.

To strengthen shoulder rotator cuff (needed for virtually all throwing activities, tennis strokes, and swimming):

1. Lie on the floor on your back. Grasp a light dumbbell (about 1½ pounds) in one hand. Keeping your upper arm at your side with

the back of the forearm down on the floor, bend your elbow to a 90-degree angle. Raise the dumbbell until the forearm is pointing directly at the ceiling (with upper arm still at your side). Then lower the dumbbell back to the starting position. Repeat 10 to 15 times with each arm.

2. Stand erect holding a light dumbbell in one hand with palm facing the body. Slowly raise the dumbbell directly out to the side until the arm is parallel to the floor. Then slowly return the arm to the starting position. The elbows should remain straight, but not locked, throughout the entire movement. Repeat 10 to 15 times with each arm.

Strength training offers a variety of health benefits to exercisers of all ages and abilities. However, if you have high blood pressure, heart disease, arthritis, diabetes, osteoporosis, or are over 50 and have been totally sedentary, you should talk to your doctor before you begin lifting weights.

❧ *17* ❧

MAKING THE LEAST
OF STRESS

Stress is Beauty Enemy Number 1. External appearance mirrors internal health—emotional as well as physical—and reflects stress reactions. Linked to the brain by thousands of nerve endings, skin not only blushes when we are embarrassed and pales when we are frightened, it can react to too much stress by drying out and itching or wrinkling; becoming too oily and erupting with blemishes; or by developing eczema, hives, or psoriasis.

How stress and illness interact

The Physical Connection

In the 1960s, Doctors Holmes and Rahe devised a "Stressful Events Rating Chart" as an indicator of illness potential. On a scale of 1 to 100, the chart depicts receiving a traffic ticket (11 points) at the bottom; getting married, buying a house, being fired, or retiring (approximately 50 points each) in the middle; divorce (73 points) or the death of a spouse (100 points) at the top. If your total score for a 12-month period falls between 150 and 300, your chance of suffering serious illness is 53 percent; if your points exceed 300, the probability is 80 percent.

Further studies reveal that an accumulation of minor stresses can be equally hazardous—responsible for a myriad of apparently unrelated disorders such as arthritis, chronic fatigue, colitis, dandruff, dental caries, depression, hair loss, headaches, high blood pressure, indigestion, peeling fingernails, sexual dysfunction, tinnitus, and ulcers. Evolution's pokiness is at the root of these stress-induced misfortunes. Our bodies have not yet developed the ability to discriminate between a traffic snarl and the growl of a saber-tooth tiger entering the cave; they still react to stress with the "fight-or-flight" response.

1. Stress hormones—adrenaline, noradrenaline (epenephrine, norepinephrine), cortisol—are released to prepare the body for action.

2. Breathing becomes shallow and rapid; heartbeat, blood sugar, and cholesterol levels rise; digestive processes slow and practically come to a halt.

3. If the stress continues, or is not released after a brief period, the body resumes its most vital functions but remains on "red alert" (free-floating anxiety).

4. If unrelieved stresses occur frequently, the body becomes exhausted: accident prone, mentally inefficient and depressed, physically vulnerable to illness, and aesthetically unattractive.

THE MENTAL CONNECTION

Stress has almost as many definitions as it does causes and effects. In the health sciences, stress is defined as something that is (or is believed to be) a threat to the continuance of existing lifestyle. Any change, positive or negative, can trigger the stress response. Frustration is stress that comes when things don't turn out the way we want them to, when we feel thwarted, or when we lose control of our lives. (Studies reported in the August 1988 issue of *University of California, Berkeley Wellness Letter* reveal that lower echelon workers are more prone to stress-related problems than upper echelon decision makers.)

Our safe, civilized society abounds with stressors: long lines at check-out counters, ringing telephones and busy signals, computer glitches, the constant pressures of multi-faceted career and homemaker roles . . . Mental reaction to stress is a matter of individual perception. A stepped-up deadline may be a creative challenge to one person, a traumatic catastrophe to a co-worker. By identifying personal stress-triggers, avoiding or modifying as many as possible, and learning to demobilize physical reactions to stresses that cannot be altered, we can maintain an inner serenity that preserves our health and radiates vibrant beauty.

THE NUTRITIONAL CONNECTION

Diet augments relaxation and exercise. Poor nutrition is in itself a stress, low blood sugar initiates the stress response, and physical or mental stress depletes essential nutrients—another vicious cycle in the making. By providing your body with a well-balanced diet (see Chapter 15) you can protect yourself against many of the harmful effects of stress and the fatigue of its aftermath. Nutritionists and holistic physicians advise taking extra vitamin C (up to 1,000 milligrams per hour during extreme stress) and one to three B-complex tablets each day.

Natural Tranquilizers: "Eat something; you'll feel better," is a folk-remedy truism with a factual nucleus. A bite or two of anything temporarily alleviates stress by providing a few moments of pleasurable self-gratification. Chewing or sipping substances that offset stress can give longer-lasting relief.

- Eating an ounce of gumdrops, jelly beans, or dry cereal without milk, can foil the fluttering butterflies in your midsection. Sweet, starchy carbohydrates (without fat, fiber, or protein to slow their assimilation) immediately prompt the body to secrete opiate-like endorphins as well as the serotonin that eases anxiety and tension. Ration them carefully—doubling the amount might put you to sleep.

- Drinking a cup of any of the herbal teas listed for encouraging sleep will help calm daytime nervousness. Herbalists suggest brewing up a mixture of equal parts of balm leaves, hops, lavender flowers, and primrose; and as reported in *Prevention* (September 1988), tests at Rutgers University show valerian to be an efficient tranquilizer with no side effects.

- Sipping half a cup of this "super milk" every few hours will calm your nerves, keep your blood sugar on an even keel, and help replenish the protein and potassium used up by stress reactions. Combine in an electric blender and whir until smooth:

    > *2 cups fluid lowfat milk*
    > *¹/₂ cup instant nonfat dry milk*
    > *1 sliced banana*
    > *1 tablespoon brewer's yeast*

- Optional additions for increased benefits: 1 tablespoon lecithin granules, miller's bran, peanut butter, protein powder, or wheat germ.
- Taking dolomite or other calcium-magnesium tablets provides quick-acting, between-meals nerve-soothing.

The Mind/Body Connection

There is definitely a connection between the way we feel mentally and the way we feel physically. Just as a negative state of mind has the ability to cause illness, a positive state of mind seems to have the power to ward off illness. Since the thirteenth century, the sick and infirm have made pilgrimages to France hoping for a "miracle" at the fountain of Our Lady of Lourdes. More than 6,000 persons have claimed cures since 1858. Is it divine intervention or spontaneous remission generated by high hopes that returns physical health to these people? No one knows for sure, but researchers are beginning to see for a fact that optimistic and positive thoughts can strengthen the immune system and restore good health. Daily, they gather evidence that the mind plays an essential role in the physical processes that accompany remission from serious illnesses.

Recently the Institute of Noetic Sciences collected more than 3,500 accounts of spontaneous remissions from 830 medical journals in more than 20 languages. Excerpts of these true and astonishing reports were published in 1993 by the Institute in *Spontaneous Remission—An Annotated Bibliography*. Each story tells a similar tale: firm belief in the possibility of a cure accompanies most "miracle" recoveries. If a positive mental state can overcome terminal disease, imagine what it can do for general, day-to-day health!

Six Ways to Dodge or Diminish Stressful Situations

An astounding amount of stress is self-instigated, or self-perpetuated, and, therefore, subject to self-destruction.

- Re-evaluating goals and establishing priorities often relieves the stress of trying too hard to achieve or acquire more than is needed or really wanted—and makes it easier to say "no." Saying "yes" to the best of friends or the worthiest of causes is foolish and stressful when it deprives you of high-priority family or private time.

&. Guilt trips can be canceled when you accept the fact that no one is expected to be 100 percent perfect 100 percent of the time; make appropriate amends or apologies; and regard each gaffe or goof-up as a learning experience.

&. Anger, disappointment, and frustration are seldom self-made, but their damaging effects can be limited by following the advice of ancient philosophers and modern psychologists: keep your head, perspective, and sense of humor; move on to something positive; and dissipate physical reactions through relaxation and exercise. Losing your "cool," devoting sleepless nights to ruminating over what you "shudda said," plotting revenge, or wallowing in your woes merely creates more stress.

&. Worry can be either a stressor or a stress reliever. Utilizing "worrying time" to formulate a series of "just in case" alternatives eliminates debilitating "stewing" and leaves you confidently in control. If the disaster should occur, you are prepared; if plan A fails, you have plans B and C to fall back on.

&. Martyrdom was saintly for Joan of Arc and the heroines in Victorian novels; in our culture it is a stressor you're better off without. Instead of being overwhelmed by the constant care of infants or invalids, arrange for an occasional surrogate. If sitters or nurses are neither available nor financially feasible, try for a trade-off. One housebound mother of five retains her equilibrium by working two half-days each week in a bookstore while the owner revels in taking over as part-time grandma.

Rather than suffering in silence while stressing yourself out with an unfair workload, admit you aren't Superwoman and ask for assistance. If no one rallies 'round, help yourself—even if it entails requesting a job transfer or foregoing a luxury to pay a weekly cleaning service.

&. Hassles (ordinary occurrences that burgeon into stressors) can be manipulated into manageability if tackled on their own turf. For instance: if you're frazzled out before your day's work commences, the cause could be the early-morning hassle of getting your family off to school and work. Having everyone's clothing and accouterment laid out the night before and making bunches of lunches on the weekend (frozen sandwiches self-defrost by lunchtime) avoids the stressful confusion of sewing on a shirt button and searching for a misplaced paper while spreading peanut butter.

An additional hassle might be your daily commute. (The September 1988 *University of California, Berkeley Wellness Letter* reports that each year hundreds of drivers get angry enough to assault offending motorists with deadly weapons—California freeways accounted for 70 such cases in 1987.) Try changing your route or your mode of transportation: form a carpool or withdraw from one; take a bus, ride your bike, walk . . . do whatever it takes to make the least of your stress and the most of your life. Your good looks and good health are worth it.

HOW TO RELAX

Consciously breathing deeply is the opening gambit for all types of deliberate relaxation because it reverses the stress-instigated shallow, rapid respiration that changes blood chemistry. Inhaling for 6 seconds, holding your breath for a count of 3, then exhaling for 6 seconds is a complete-unto-itself stress-reliever when repeated for 2 minutes.

PROGRESSIVE RELAXATION

Relaxing on cue requires practice, but once mastered, the stress-relieving relaxation response can be achieved with a few deep breaths. "Progressive Relaxation," based on a 5,000-year-old Yoga tranquility exercise and well publicized by Dr. Herbert Benson,[14, 15, 16] can be varied according to environmental circumstances and personal preferences.

1. Sit or lie in a comfortable position with your eyes closed.
2. Breathe deeply.
3. Tense, then relax each muscle group. Begin with your feet, move up through your legs, torso, arms, neck and face, and concentrate on the feeling of tension sliding away. Some experts recommend

starting at the top and working down to your feet, others suggest talking to the different parts of your body, telling them to relax.

4. Remain relaxed while breathing naturally for 5 to 30 minutes. Slowly counting down from 10 to 1 can increase the depth of relaxation. Imagining yourself slowly descending on an escalator past placards bearing numbers from 10 to 1, and telling yourself, "Ten, I am growing more relaxed. Nine, I am growing . . ." may help achieve relaxation.

5. At the end of your session, saying, "When I count from 1 to 5 I will open my eyes and feel refreshed and energetic," helps produce the desired effects. Before resuming normal activities, blink your eyes, yawn, and stretch.

USING A MANTRA

There is nothing mystic about a mantra. It need not be a secret incantation assigned by a guru, it can be any sound or word you select as an adjunct to deep breathing and relaxation. Inhale through your nostrils, exhale through your mouth; concentrate on and softly hum the word of your choice.

MEDITATING

Absence of thought, not profound rumination, is the goal of this form of meditation which reduces the activity of the nervous system. Focusing on a mantra or the words of a brief phrase or prayer helps exclude interference from external distractions. If other thoughts intrude, push them out of your mind and return to your passive repetition.

VISUALIZING

Imagining yourself in a peacefully pleasant situation can enhance physical and mental relaxation. For the greatest benefit, make your mental imagery detailed and vivid. If you visualize yourself lying on a beach, "see" the blue sky and swaying palm trees, "hear" the cry of a gull and the soothing sound of waves lapping at the shore, "feel" the warmth of the sun and the grittiness of the sand, "smell" the tangy salt air. For a two-minute stress reliever:

1. Lie down, sit comfortably, or stand and lean against a wall. Close your eyes.

2. Tense all your muscles while you inhale deeply for 6 seconds. Let your body go limp while you exhale. Take a few normal breaths, then repeat the sequence.

3. Visualize the word "calm" or imagine a calm, happy scene for about a minute, then open your eyes, yawn and stretch.

PROGRAMMING YOUR SUBCONSCIOUS

Sequestered within every sub-subconscious is an eager-to-please, primordial genie with awesome powers. Aside from attending to autonomic (involuntary) physical functions, it docily waits to be summoned. When, through relaxation, the confining "stopper" is removed, the genie can be instructed to relieve stress, influence reactions and future behavior, and improve everything from your appearance to your tennis serve. The potential is practically unlimited, but, like man-made computers, Mother Nature's genie must be programmed by conscious thought in terms it can understand. It has been corked up during our eons of mental development, so orders must be issued as simple statements of facts to be accomplished, and illustrated with visualizations of the desired results. However they're labeled (Autogenic Training, Guided Meditation, Psycho-Cybernetics, Psychosynthesis, Scientology, Mind Control, Transcendental Meditation, etc.), here are the basic guidelines for conscious-subconscious communication:

- Use positive statements and images. If you want to stop biting your fingernails, say, "My nails are growing longer and more lovely," while imagining yourself admiring your attractively long-nailed fingers. *Don't* say, "I'm not going to bite my nails any more," and *don't* visualize your raggedy fingertips.

- Concentrate on only one situation per session. For instance: if you have prepared a speech but are uptight over delivering it, table your nail-growing or whatever improvement you have been working on. "Walk" yourself through the presentation at each of several relaxation sessions to establish a "memory" of success that will relieve stressful feelings and make your speech a foregone smash. "See" yourself walking onstage and smiling confidently at the audience, "feel" the lectern as you arrange your notes, "hear" the responsive laughter when you pause after your comic line, and "enjoy" the applause as you return to your seat.

Learn to Relax with Biofeedback

Biofeedback gives you concrete evidence of the mind's influence on the body's functions. In a healthy person, the workings of the body are performed and regulated by the brain and central nervous system. The mind, however, often interferes when under stress, which produces tension in the body. Biofeedback can teach you how to restore a relaxed mind/body balance.

With biofeedback, physical signs of stress are measured with equipment that records nerve and brain waves, heart rate, skin temperature, blood pressure, muscle tension, and states of arousal, excitement, or nervousness. When hooked up to this equipment, you are alerted by signals such as alarms and flashing lights when your body is responding to stress. You then learn how to turn off the alarms and lights by changing your body's physical reaction. You learn how to use things like relaxation and autosuggestion exercises, visual imagery, and meditation and prayer to relax and slow your heartbeat or your muscle tension and so on. For example, if the equipment signals that your heart rate is increasing, you can slow the heart beat by imagining a calm, peaceful place where you feel relaxed and safe.

The goal of biofeedback training is to teach you how to recognize the physical signs of stress and how to relax and stop them. Most people need about six weeks of lessons with a psychologist trained in biofeedback to reach this goal. When you gain awareness of the relationship between your physical state and your mental state, you no longer need the biofeedback equipment because you have learned how to use natural relaxation strategies as an effective remedy to combat stress.

How Exercise Helps to Control Stress

Relaxation is the ideal prophylactic for stress; exercise, the perfect antidote. The body is designed to release tension through physical activity, which instigates the production of tranquilizing endorphins and burns up the superfluous chemicals, sugars, and fats produced during stress. Chronic stress contracts muscles and deprives them of oxygen, causing them to become tense and painful. Taking a brief "exercise break" can de-stress your muscles and dissipate accumulating stress. Dr. Robert Thayer, of California State University at Long Beach, has found that a brisk ten-minute walk decreases tension and elevates the mood of his subjects for an hour. When you are at work and an outdoor walk isn't feasible, try striding up and down the hall, climbing stairs to the next floor, or executing a few "jumping jacks" in the powder room.

Several studies have shown that people who follow a regular program of aerobic exercise have fewer stress hormones circulating through their systems and have better stress tolerance than their sedentary counterparts. Combining aerobics with relaxation and guided imagery relieves existing stress and provides a defense against future stresses.

1. Perform any aerobic activity to bring your heart rate into its target zone for 1 to 2 minutes.

2. Relax limply and visualize a peaceful scene for 1 to 3 minutes.

3. Repeat the 5-minute cycles of alternating movement and relaxation 6 to 10 times.

NINE NATURAL AIDS FOR COMBATING STRESS

Swings or hammocks were once prescribed as therapeutic "passive exercise." Rocking in a chair relieves muscular tension and lulls adults as well as infants. Listening to music—peacefully melodic sounds, not toe-tapping rhythms—soothes body and mind. Here are some other natural aids for combating stress.

1. *Approach it positively.* Regarding a partially filled glass as half empty or half full has less to do with stress tolerance than the pessimistic refusal to refill it lest the liquid evaporate or be spilled. Optimists are sometimes proven wrong, but they live longer and enjoy life more.

2. *Call time-out.* The amount and type of personal "down" time required varies with each individual, but we all need some of it. Whether it is an evening to devote to a beautifying facial and bath or an uninterrupted half day to read or pursue a hobby, we must do something for ourselves on frequent occasions. This

was the prescription a wise doctor gave one of his patients whose sudden rise in blood pressure was accompanied by an assortment of minor ailments. When queried about what she had been doing, her prideful statement that career and family duties occupied all her waking hours elicited no praise, merely the terse comment, "That could be the problem. Take some time out for yourself and come back in a month. You may not need any medication." She didn't. By delegating a few of her supposedly indispensable chores she "found" time for personal pleasures and was rewarded with a clean bill of health at her next medical checkup.

3. *Care for a pet.* Many studies show that interaction with an animal brings about a decrease in stress reactions. Even aquarium-watching is soothing—witness the proliferation of tension-dispelling fish tanks in doctors' and dentists' offices.

4. *Cry it out.* Emotional tears, not those engendered by dicing onions, carry off harmful stress chemicals.

5. *Laugh it off.* Norman Cousins' book, *Anatomy of an Illness*, established the value of humor in healing. Laughter also relieves tension. Laughing at professional comic routines is great therapy; chuckling at the funny side of our own discomfortures helps keep them in perspective.

6. *Put it into words.* Translating your innermost thoughts into conscious words can blow off steam, reduce worry, and increase stress tolerance. If you are being beset by stressors, write out a description of each one, along with a list of things you can do to modify or abolish it. If you are furious at your boss, compose a letter containing all the caustic comments you've been squelching. Read it over, then tear it up. If you would rather verbalize than put words on paper, turn on your tape recorder, shout out your fury or describe your woes to an imaginary therapist. Play it back, then erase the tape.

7. *Sleep it off.* Sleep is an antidote to stress. It reverses stress-instigated physical changes and helps replenish depleted neurochemicals. How much sleep we need is genetically determined, can vary from 3 to 11 hours out of each 24, decreases as we grow older, and increases when we are under stress. However, wakefulness in times of stress is part of the fight-or-flight sur-

vival mechanism and, unless controlled, stress and sleeplessness can create a viciously self-perpetuating cycle that leaves us looking and feeling drained. Sleep experts offer the following tips for encouraging a good night's rest.

ᐳᎶ Avoid caffeine-containing beverages for 4 hours before bedtime.

ᐳᎶ Cut down on smoking before bedtime. Nicotine is a central nervous system stimulant that produces almost the same effects on the body as caffeine. Nicotine causes an increase in blood pressure, an increase in heart rate, and stimulation of brain wave activity, all of which can affect sleep.

ᐳᎶ Avoid the alcoholic nightcap. Alcohol has an initial sedative effect that leads to quick sleep, but this is followed by disturbed, lower-quality sleep later in the night.

ᐳᎶ Check out the side effects of your medications. Difficulty falling asleep, frequent interruptions during sleep, and early morning awakenings all can be a result of the medications you take.

ᐳᎶ Unwind by doing something unstressful (read, watch television, take a bath) before preparing for bed.

ᐳᎶ Eat a *light* snack: crackers and cheese, a small bowl of cereal and milk, or a scoop of ice cream.

ᐳᎶ Drink a cup of warm milk with a spoonful of honey or blackstrap molasses. Or try a soporific herbal tea (blackberry, camomile, catnip, dandelion, hops, lavender flowers, lemon balm, peppermint, red clover, sage, skullcap, St. Johnswort, valerian). For a potent nightcap: mix 2 tablespoons valerian root with 1 tablespoon *each* lavender flowers, lemon balm, and passion flowers. Steep 1 teaspoon of the herbal mixture in 1 cup hot water for 10 minutes.

ᐳᎶ Take a multivitamin-mineral supplement every day—low levels of magnesium, iron, or copper can interfere with sleep. For occasional wakefulness, try melatonin. Available in synthetic form in tablets or capsules, melatonin is a hormone that helps regulate sleep-wake cycles. If you are taking prescribed medications, consult your physician before trying melatonin; if you have an autoimmune disorder or are pregnant, do not take melatonin. For healthy adults, one or two capsules (totaling no more than 5 milligrams) are believed to be a safe sleep-aid that compensates for the gradually decreasing amounts of melatonin produced internally.

- Perform a few gentle bending and stretching exercises.

- Vigorous exercise performed in the late afternoon or the early evening will force the body temperature to dip much lower during sleep. This lower temperature brings deeper sleep with fewer awakenings. (But be careful: experts say that if vigorous exercise is performed too close to bedtime, an elevated body temperature may make it difficult to fall asleep.)

- Practice your progressive relaxation technique after you are in bed. Visualize yourself sleeping peacefully. Implant the suggestion that you are going to drift off into sound sleep, then awaken refreshed at the sound of the alarm.

8. *Soak it away.* Before being supplanted by drugs, baths were used to quiet violent patients in mental hospitals. Dr. Richard S. Gubner, medical director of Safety Harbor Fitness Center in Florida, recommends 15-minute hot (102 degree) baths. Dr. Jens Henriksen, medical director of the Chattanooga Pain Center in Tennessee, says body-temperature bathwater is more relaxing. Herbalists suggest adding herbs to increase the benefits (see Chapter 8).

Personal preferences for body-soul pampering are the best guides. One busy career woman combines relaxation and meditation with her morning bath. She fills the tub with very hot water, relaxes and shuts out all thoughts by concentrating on the velvety blackness she visualizes with closed eyes. By the time the cooling water rouses her in 15 to 20 minutes, she is ready to meet the day—stress-free and confident that she can handle whatever happens.

9. *Utilize available assistance.* Sharing stresses with discreet clergy, family members, or friends can resolve many stressful difficulties. If you need help in mastering relaxation and coping techniques, there are classes and seminars on everything from Arica and Biofeedback to Zen Buddhism, and professionally prepared tapes covering all areas of stress control.

Stimulating Stressors That Help Fight Boredom

Stress management entails more than coping with our fight-or-flight response; it includes creating stimulating stressors. This apparent incongruity is explained by the fact that *stress underload* (the psychologists' term for boredom) is itself a negative stress than can lead to the same disorders as stress overload. As we mature, our minds gain the capacity to process ever-increasing amounts of information. If no new challenges are provided, the brain may damage the body just to relieve the monotony, or combat its boredom by egging us on to neglect our jobs, overeat, take drugs, or pick fights with our friends.

Stress-underload remedies are remarkably similar to those for controlling stress overload. Changing routes or modes of transportation provides a positive, challenging stress while diminishing commuting frustrations. Learning to care for the pet you acquired to help you relax is exciting. Joining an aerobics class, establishing exercise routines, perfecting progressive relaxation techniques—all help feed the brain's demands for stimulation.

The "time out for yourself" prescription offers unlimited, ongoing opportunities for adding zest to your life. You can take a class or teach a class, attend a concert, paint a picture, plant a garden, study a foreign language, write a book, join a club or start one. The activity needn't be self-centered—organizing a rummage sale for your favorite charity, reading and writing letters for the visually handicapped, or taking your kids to the zoo are other options. "Success" lies in the fun and fascination of learning and doing; "change" is the name of the game. You may enjoy experimenting with different experiences every few weeks, or you may discover latent talents that lead to a second career or after-retirement income.

Life and its beautifully healthful potential are gifts from Mother Nature. By making the most of what we have been given, we not only improve our outward attractiveness, we also add zestfully happy, productive years to our lives.

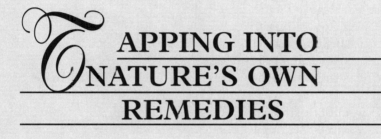

TAPPING INTO NATURE'S OWN REMEDIES

18

THE SIMPLE, FUN, AND POWERFUL
LURE OF AROMATHERAPY

Aromatherapy is a healing treatment that utilizes the aromatic essential oils of both cultivated and wild plants. Essential oils are found in the petals (lavender), leaves (basil), wood (cedarwood), fruit (orange), seeds (sesame), roots (ginger), gum (myrrh), and resin (pine). In many cases, the oils are located in more than one part of the plant. An orange, for example, has essential oils in the white flowers, the rind, and the leaves.

Used medicinally over the centuries, essential oils are now finding their way back into the family medicine cabinet as a trusted alternative natural therapy. These oils can assist in the treatment of almost every type of ache and pain, as well as soothe away stress and emotional strain.

WHERE TO FIND ESSENTIAL OILS

The use of aromatherapy to treat common illnesses may sound to some like old-wives' tales, but, in fact, the use of essential oils as medical therapy is already a well-established part of your health regimen. Peppermint, for example, is used in toothpaste, mouthwash, and soaps for its clean, fresh scent and its antiseptic properties that kill bacteria. Eucalyptus, with its antiseptic and mentholated action, is in cough drops and inhalation remedies because of its decongestant and antibacterial action. The antiseptic properties of pine are used in bathroom cleaners, and the aphrodisiac powers of sandalwood and jasmine are often in perfumes and colognes. These uses of essential oils are just the beginning—there are so many other ways they can be used in your daily health and beauty regimen.

You can purchase essential oils for the "recipes" below in health food stores, in herbal shops, and in bath and beauty shops. Once you're on the lookout, you'll be surprised how many stores sell these truly "essential" oils.

Choosing an Oil to Fit Your Needs and Your Moods

There are hundreds of essential oils on the market today. The following collection represents a good cross section of diversity. Some oils are calming; others are invigorating. Some are used to treat skin ailments; others are known as nasal decongestants or laxatives. Each selection also recommends the best way to use the oil: either by inhalation, water therapy, or massage. The details about these three ways to use aromatherapy are explained later in the chapter. The following group of essential oils, gathered from Carole McGilvery and Jimi Reed's *Essential Aromatherapy* (Smithmark, 1994) and Lynn Parentini's *The Joy of Healthy Skin* (Prentice Hall, 1996) will give you a good start in your selection adventure.

Bergamot

Bergamot has an uplifting, clean citrus scent (familiar to some as a flavoring in Earl Grey tea). It has powerful antiseptic and cooling properties. As an antiseptic, it has proved effective in the treatment of mouth and skin infections, and sore throats. It can lower fever and help with bronchitis and indigestion. It is excellent for inflamed, irritated, and even blemished skin.

Uses: Inhalation, water therapy, and massage. Diluted in water it can be used as a mouth rinse or gargle. Use as a compress over skin infections.

Caution: Keep in mind that bergamot can cause photosensitivity, so avoid the sun and tanning salons while using this oil.

Chamomile

Chamomile is a familiar herb often used as a tea to aid digestion, calm nervousness, and induce a peaceful night's sleep. The essential oil from this plant is particularly noted for its anti-inflammatory, analgesic, and sedative properties. It is used to soothe the discomforts of burns, dermatitis, diarrhea, fever, indigestion, insomnia, and menstrual problems.

Uses: Water therapy.

Caution: If you are allergic to ragweed, asters, or chrysanthemums, be careful with this oil; use a weak solution and test it on your arm a few hours before bathing.

CYPRESS

Coming from the evergreen family, cypress essential oil has a woody and slightly spicy aroma reminiscent of pine needles. It is most noted for its astringent and antispasmodic qualities. Use cypress to find relief from colds, coughs, flu, hemorrhoids, and menstrual and menopausal problems. It also acts as a sedative to soothe nervous tension.

Uses: Inhalation, water therapy, and massage. Its astringent properties make it suitable for use in cleansers for oily skin.

Caution: Not to be used by anyone suffering high blood pressure.

EUCALYPTUS

Eucalyptus has a cool, camphorous smell. It is used worldwide as an inhalant for colds and the flu. It not only helps to open the nasal passages, but it acts as an antibacterial and antiviral agent, helping to stop the spread of germs. This essential oil's antiseptic and bactericidal properties make it an excellent oil for treating skin sores, infections, burns, or inflammations. Its ability to open air passages makes it a favorite in the treatment of asthma, sinusitis, and bronchitis.

Uses: Inhalation, water therapy, and massage. Dab on a handkerchief to clear congested sinuses.

FENNEL

Fennel has a fresh, clean licorice aroma. Popular for its use as a diuretic and a mild laxative, fennel essential oil has been found effective for constipation, digestive problems, kidney stones, menopausal problems, and nausea. It is also often helpful for increasing milk supply during breastfeeding.

Uses: Massage. Can be infused in teas.

GERANIUM

Geranium has a sweet, floral essence and blends well with other essential oils. With both sedative and uplifting properties, it is often used to treat nervous tension and depression. Its stimulating action is good for the skin.

Uses: Inhalation, water therapy, and massage.

LAVENDER

Lavender has a clean, light, floral aroma with a woody overtone. It has both sedative and antiseptic properties. It is extremely comforting and soothing to one's state of mind; it is excellent for treating migraines. It also will kill bacteria on the skin and soothe inflammation.

Uses: Inhalation, water therapy, and massage. Use as a cold compress or place a few drops in boiling water and inhale for headaches and migraines. A warm towel wrap will soothe nervous exhaustion. A late-night lavender bath will help combat insomnia.

NEROLI

Neroli has a floral fragrance similar to lilies. It is a sedative and antidepressant. Neroli oil counters anxiety, hysteria, and combats insomnia. It also revitalizes dry and mature skin.

Uses: Inhalation, water therapy, and massage.

PEPPERMINT

With its strong refreshing fragrance, peppermint essential oil is excellent for digestion, as a decongestant, and for skin disorders. It is used to treat the discomforts of colds, flu, flatulence, headaches, indigestion, nausea, toothache, and sunburn.

Uses: Inhalation, water therapy, and massage. A few drops of the oil on a handkerchief can be inhaled to relieve headaches and symptoms of motion sickness. Used in a footbath, it relieves tired, sweaty feet. Used as a compress it can relieve hot flashes.

Caution: For skin treatment, do not use a concentration greater than 1 percent because it can cause irritation.

SANDALWOOD

Sandalwood has a lingering woody, sweet, exotic fragrance. This versatile oil can soothe nerves and smooth and soften dry, mature, or sun-damaged skin. Its antiseptic qualities help kill bacteria on the skin and its soothing action helps relieve inflammation. It is also used as an expectorant and antispasmodic to treat bronchitis and coughs. Sandalwood is regarded as an aphrodisiac.

Uses: Inhalation and massage. Or apply in a warm compress to treat the skin.

THREE WAYS TO USE ESSENTIAL OILS

Essential oils enter the body in three ways: (1) They can be inhaled when the oil droplets are dispersed into the air; (2) they can soak into the skin when mixed with water in baths, compresses, and the like; and (3) they can be absorbed directly into the skin through massage.

Whether in mist or liquid form, essential oils are able to penetrate easily through the skin due to their small molecules. This sounds surprising because usually oils have large molecules that sit on the surface of the skin. But essential oils do not have an oily texture. Actually, they are the complete opposite of oils because they are not heavy or greasy. These oils are called "volatile" liquids because they evaporate when exposed to the air. They feel as light to the touch as water or alcohol. They disappear almost instantly when applied to the skin.

Try inhalation, water therapy, and massage according to the following instructions. You'll soon wonder how you ever got along without these wonders of nature.

INHALATION

Breathing in droplets of an essential oil brings its healing and soothing powers directly into your body. There are a number of ways to mist the air:

- **Steam:** Add 6 to 12 drops of the selected oil to a bowl of steaming hot water. Place a towel over your head and breathe deeply. This is an excellent way to treat respiratory problems as well as to give your face a deep cleansing.

&❧ **Fragrancers:** These attractive pots are easy to use. Fill the top bowl with water and add 3 to 6 drops of the essential oil on the surface. The candle in the pot underneath heats the water, slowly releasing the natural fragrance of the oil into the room.

&❧ **Diffuser:** You can buy an electrical diffuser that gently mists the essential oil into the air.

&❧ **Humidifier:** You can add an essential oil to the water of a humidifier to mist the air. Or you can simply add a few drops of oil to a small bowl of water and place it on top of a radiator.

&❧ **Light bulb:** You can disperse an essential oil into the air by placing a few drops of the oil on a light bulb. Place 2 or 3 drops on the bulb while it is still cold. (Never place it on a hot light bulb.) As the bulb heats up, it will speed up the evaporation process and fill the room with fragrance.

&❧ **Handkerchief:** Add 3 or 4 drops of an essential oil to a handkerchief. Place the handkerchief to your nose and inhale. This is especially useful on the go to help calm nerves or clear congestion.

WATER THERAPY

Bath: Taking a bath mixed with an essential oil is a wonderful way to combine skin penetration and inhalation—and it makes you feel great! Don't run an extremely hot bath. Lukewarm water is the best temperature for therapeutic value; because the water is close to your body's temperature, it produces a relaxing and soothing action.

Add 5 to 10 drops of the essential oil to the bath while the water is running. Before you enter the tub, swish the water around so the essential oils mix well with the water. (Essential oils can mark plastic baths if they are not dispersed thoroughly.)

If you have dry or sensitive skin, mix the essential oils with 1 ounce of a carrier oil such as sweet almond oil, wheat-germ oil, or macadamia nut oil. Then add this mixture to the bath and swish to mix.

Now lie back in the water and breathe in deeply to inhale the oil droplets rising and evaporating from the bath water. At the same time, relax and let your body absorb the oil directly.

Shower: You can use essential oils in your shower, too. After washing and rinsing your body, dip a wet sponge in an oil mix of your choice and squeeze and rub this over your whole body while under a warm shower spray.

Foot Bath: Add a few drops of your favorite oil to a bowl of hot water and soak your feet. You might choose peppermint to refresh or lavender to soothe.

Sauna: Add 2 drops of an essential oil to a half pint of water. Throw the water over the coals to evaporate.

MASSAGE

As a therapy in its own right, massage is a great natural way to beat stress, promote relaxation, relieve muscle tension and stiffness, and encourage better circulation. On a mental level, massage can promote a calm state of mind, increase alertness, and reduce mental stress. (See Chapter 20 for all the details of the use of massage as a natural remedy.) When you add aromatherapy to this art of natural care, your mind and body will also respond to the therapeutic action of the oil.

Of course you'll need a partner to massage those hard-to-reach places, but even without a partner, you can massage essential oils into your skin for their soothing and medicinal properties.

A FEW MASSAGE TIPS

- Do not apply an essential oil directly to the skin (unless directed by an experienced aromatherapist) because it could cause an irritation.

- Mix and dilute essential oils with what is called a carrier or base oil. Some excellent oils for this purpose are almond oil, macadamia nut oil, and apricot kernel oil.

- Choose the massage oil that best fits your needs and moods at the moment. See the list beginning on page 266 to select the oil you need for calming nerves, restoring vitality, or soothing the discomforts of physical ailments.

- Before applying the oil, warm it in your hands so that it is slightly warm when applied to the skin.

- Avoid showering for up to three to four hours after an essential oil massage, because you don't want to rinse away the therapeutic value of the oils.

ENJOY AND BE SAFE

Natural organic aromatic essences are extremely safe when used properly. They have an advantage over drugs because they are excreted, leaving no toxic residues behind. Side effects are virtually nonexistent. But you do have to be careful; aromatherapy is not something to use without guidance. There are hundreds of essential oils, each with various health-promoting qualities, but if combined incorrectly or used in the wrong dosage, some can become quite toxic. When treating serious diseases or skin disorders, it's wise to use aromatherapy under the supervision of someone trained in their use, like a professional skin-care specialist employed by many spas.

♔ *19* ♔

A MEDICINE GARDEN: HOW TO USE HERBS TO TREAT COMMON SYMPTOMS

Healing herb plants are our earliest medicines—their curative powers date back to the beginning of recorded history. Today many are being rediscovered and reappreciated. Even pharmaceutical companies are responding to the public's demand for chemical-free, all-natural products, so you'll often find that many of the symptom-easing preparations lining the aisles of drugstores are actually modified or synthetic versions of herbal remedies. But many of these products use only trace amounts of the active herbal substances to catch your attention—the product is actually filled with synthetic chemicals. The only way to be sure of what you're using is to make it yourself.

HOW TO PREPARE AN HERBAL BREW

You can buy herbs in many forms: capsules, oil, dried, or fresh. Capsules are not recommended because they are unreliable as to potency and purity. The use of herbal oils is discussed in Chapter 18. The recipes that follow rely on fresh or dried herbs only. You can buy herbs, grow them yourself, or gather them from the wild. If you gather them yourself, be sure they have not been sprayed and that you have identified them correctly.

When shopping for herbs, look for the two-word Latin name on the label. The common names for herbs can vary.

Leaves, flowers, or seeds (fresh or dried) are prepared by the regular tea-making process known as infusion: they are simply steeped in freshly boiled water. Tougher roots, bark, and stems need to be boiled or simmered to release their active ingredients, a process known as decoction.

You will get the best results if you use loose ingredients rather than commercially prepared tea bags and fresh spring or distilled bottled water rather than chlorinated tap water. Also, herbal brews should be made in a ceramic teapot or in glass, enameled, or stainless steel cookware. Never use a container made from aluminum, which can react with an herb. If you like, serve herbal teas with honey or sugar. Strong-flavored teas are even better when sweetened with brown sugar or maple syrup.

If you substitute fresh herbs for dried ones, the general rule is to use two to three times more fresh herbs than the specified amounts for dried.

None of the following recipes can cure disease; they are offered to you as a natural way to relieve symptoms and ease the discomforts of ordinary conditions such as indigestion and the common cold. Never try to substitute an herbal remedy for proper medical attention. A serious or chronic condition should be brought to the attention of your physician. Also, you should use these preparations in moderation. Some herbal teas can be harmful if consumed in large quantities over a long period. But occasionally using a cup of herbal tea to soothe an upset stomach or an herb-filled vaporizer to fill the sick room with healing herbal steam are nature's way of reducing the discomforts of illness.

N INE HERBS TO KEEP IN YOUR "MEDICINE" CABINET

ALOE, *ALOE BARBADENSIS*

Minor burn and wound healing. Aloe is used extensively in modern medicine, especially as a healing emollient. Fluid from the fresh leaves of aloe has been found to promote the attachment and growth of normal human cells. Keeping an aloe plant in your kitchen gives you an inexpensive and effective remedy for minor burns and scrapes. Simply break open the leaf and squeeze the juice directly onto the injured skin.

ANISE, *PIMPINELLA ANISUM*

Carminative (an agent that helps break up and expel intestinal gas), weak diuretic, laxative, and antispasmodic. Anise is one of the most ancient of spices. It is especially effective in treating flatulence. It aids digestion and improves the appetite by promoting gastric secretions.

To make a carminative tea that may relieve intestinal gas, boil $^1/_2$ teaspoon anise seeds in a pint of water, strain, and drink. Some people simply chew the anise seeds.

FENNEL, *FOENICULUM VULGARE*

Indigestion and flatulence. The licorice-tasting fennel has been used since antiquity for relief of digestive discomforts.

To relieve intestinal gas or spasms, steep 1 tablespoon crushed fennel seeds in 1 cup boiling water for 5 minutes. Strain the tea and sweeten to your taste.

GARLIC, *ALLIUM SATIVUN*

Antibacterial, reduction of blood pressure and blood cholesterol levels, and expectorant (an agent that promotes the loosening and expulsion of phlegm). Garlic, a member of the onion family, is commonly used to flavor cooking. But for centuries, garlic has also been used as a remedy for colds and other respiratory infections. In 1858, Louis Pasteur verified garlic's antiseptic properties; further research indicates that it may be effective in lowering cholesterol levels in the blood, in reducing hypertension, and as an expectorant in respiratory ailments.

Fresh garlic is obtained by peeling away the outer protective layer of a garlic bulb and chopping off pieces of the clove, or by squeezing out the oil of the clove with a garlic press. Add the clove and/or the oil directly to your favorite recipes.

Cooking or deodorizing garlic destroys almost all of its antiviral and antibacterial properties. However, cold-pressed aged garlic supplements retain the blood-pressure and blood-cholesterol lowering benefits and the antioxidant, anti-cancer effects of raw garlic. Four 1,000 milligram capsules equal two or three fresh garlic cloves.

GINGER, *ZINGIBER OFFICINALE*

Decongestant, carminative, and antimotion sickness remedy. Ginger was mentioned in Chinese medical books 2,000 years ago, and it is still incorporated in many prescriptions in Oriental medicine.

To relieve the congestion of a head cold, add a pinch of fresh ginger to your tea. Ginger irritates the mucous membranes lining your nose and throat, causing them to weep watery secretions. This can make it easier for you to blow your nose or cough up mucus when you have a cold. Ginger tea is also a carminative (an agent that helps break up and expel intestinal gas).

Ginger taken before travel (fresh in tea, capsule, or oil extract mixed with water) has been found to control motion sickness better than over-the-counter preparations. Take the ginger about half an hour before exposure to motion.

HYSSOP, *HYSSOPUS OFFICINALIS*

Decongestant, cold symptoms, and expectorant. Hyssop has a long history as a folk remedy for stuffed nasal passages, coughs, colds, hoarseness, and sore throats.

To relieve nasal congestion, steep fresh or dried hyssop leaves in hot water and inhale the vapors. Hyssop tea, mixed with a little honey, is said to be effective as an expectorant. You can make your own hyssop cough syrup with this simple recipe:

Steep 1 tablespoon dried hyssop leaves in $1^1/_2$ cups boiled water for 10 to 15 minutes, then strain into a saucepan. Over low heat, gradually stir in about 2 cups of sugar to form a thick syrup. Simmer the mixture for another 5 minutes. Let the mixture cool slightly, then pour the syrup into a sealable container and cover it when cool.

PEPPERMINT, *MENTHA PIPERITA*

Indigestion, flatulence, sore throat, and stuffy nose. To make fresh mint tea for indigestion or flatulence, place about 4 dozen fresh peppermint leaves (4–5 stems of peppermint) in a teapot. Pour 1 cup of boiling water over them and let them steep for 5 minutes. Strain into a cup. (You can also make this tea by substituting spearmint for peppermint leaves.)

Caution: Peppermint tea may be hazardous for very young children who can experience a choking sensation from the menthol.

ROSE HIPS, *ROSA* SPECIES

Mild laxative and diuretic; good source of vitamin C. A cup of tea brewed from 1 ounce of fresh rose hips provides 62 mg vitamin C, 104 percent of the RDA for a healthy adult.

To brew rose hip tea, add 2 tablespoons of fresh or 1 tablespoon dried rose hips to $1^1/_2$ cups of fresh water. Bring the water to a boil, turn off the heat, and let the rose hips steep for 15 minutes. Then strain the tea and use plain, or sweeten to taste with orange juice, apple juice, sugar, or honey.

SAGE, *SALVIA OFFICINALE*

Reduces inflammation of mouth and/or throat. Sage contains volatile oil and tannin, which acts on the mucous membranes as an astringent and also stimulates blood flow by its local irritant properties. These actions combine to make sage useful in treating the pain of a sore mouth or throat.

Throat spray: Pour 8 ounces of boiling water over 5 fresh sage leaves. Cover and steep for 10 minutes. Strain the liquid through a cheese cloth into an 8-ounce glass bottle with a spray top.

For swollen, inflamed throat, apply the spray every 2 hours. For irritated or ticklish throat, apply the spray 3 times a day.

Stored in the refrigerator, the bottle of throat spray will stay fresh for several days. After 3 days, discard the unused portion and make a fresh supply.

Sage vapor: Pour boiling water over the sage leaves. Sit with the bowl in front of you and drape a large towel over your head and shoulder to trap the steam. Lean over the rising vapor. Take slow, deep breaths. Inhale slowly and deeply for 10 minutes or until the water stops producing steam. Repeat the treatment twice a day, morning and evening, to clear your head and dry your sinuses.

❧ *20* ❧

RELAX AND INVIGORATE WITH MANIPULATIVE THERAPIES

You can push, pull, press, and knead your body into good health. Manipulative therapies such as massage, acupressure, and chiropractic are ancient, folk, and modern remedies all rolled into one. They have been known to prevent illness and to treat it. They are Mother Nature's way of realigning, soothing, and balancing the body. If you investigate each one with high hopes and an open mind, you will be pleasantly surprised by the special and unique effect each can work on your body and overall health.

EXPERIENCE THE THERAPEUTIC TOUCH OF MASSAGE

It is difficult to measure all the many benefits of massage. Besides being simply enjoyable and pleasurable, massage is a great way to release stress. On a physical level, massage offers many benefits. It provides stress reduction and deep relaxation, relief from muscle tension and stiffness, better circulation, lowered blood pressure, tension relief, and nourished skin. For thousands of years, massage has been used for healing; yet it is only recently that studies have shown us its enormous effects.

Massage also delivers on a mental level. Massage will promote a calm state of mind, a sense of well-being, reduced levels of anxiety, increase alertness, and reduced mental stress.

Two Types of Massage

There are two main types of massage: shiatsu and Swedish. Shiatsu was developed in Japan at about the same time that acupuncture began to flourish in China. This massage involves finger pressure that stimulates the acupuncture points along the body's meridians. One form of shiatsu firmly massages certain areas of the body to stimulate the flow of energy and restore balance. Another form involves the use of a single fingertip to stimulate acupuncture points. The purpose of shiatsu is to alter the flow of energy within the body, and it works along the same principle as acupuncture. Shiatsu therapists also emphasize the importance of good nutrition and positive mental outlook, and they encourage clients to make lifestyle changes that promote greater health. Shiatsu can be combined with chiropractic to maximize its healing effects.

Swedish massage, which is more common in the West, involves four essential techniques, with the underlying premise that the hands should not lose contact with the body. Swedish massage is effective because of its continual, rhythmic motions. According to The Natural Medicine Collective, who authored the book *The Natural Way of Healing Chronic Pain* (Dell Publishing, 1995), the basic techniques are these:

- **Effleurage:** Rhythmic stroking with open hands, with movements directed toward the heart; this motion soothes and relaxes the body.

- **Percussion:** Brisk rhythmic movements with alternate hands that include cupping, hacking (with sides of hands), pummeling (with fists), clapping, and plucking; this stimulates the skin and circulation.

- **Petrissage:** Deep movement that involves lifting, rolling, squeezing, and pressing the skin; this stimulates muscles and fatty tissues, stretching taut muscles to relax them.

- **Pressure:** As the thumbs, fingertips, or heel of the hand make small, pressured circular movements, friction stimulates superficial tissue.

How to Find an Experienced and Trained Massage Therapist

It's very important that your massage therapist is skillfully trained—so do not use the Yellow Pages as your guide to finding a practitioner. Inconsistencies in national accreditation and licensing make it difficult to obtain a guarantee that everyone listed in the phone book is really a trained therapist. Some states, such as Florida, require that professional massage practitioners earn a certificate from a 500-hour approved school. (A massage certificate may also qualify a practitioner's services for medical insurance reimbursement if the client is referred by a primary-care provider.) Unfortunately, some local governments mistakenly classify massage with escort services and require massage therapists to register with the police and have their fingerprints taken when they apply for a massage business license. Other states have no educational or business regulations at all.

There are two safe ways to find a good massage therapist:

1. Call The American Massage Therapy Association (1-312-761-2682). This association, which promotes massage therapy, has grown from a handful of members in the 1940s to more than 23,000 professionals today with chapters in every state. A representative can put you in touch with therapists who are AMTA members in your area.

2. Use the Yellow Pages to locate a school of massage whose programs are approved or accredited by the AMTA's Commission of Massage Training Accreditation/Approval (COMTAA). A representative from one of these schools can head you in the right direction. Schools are an important source of information, because not all trained and qualified massage practitioners belong to The American Massage Therapy Association.

Be Careful when Choosing Massage for Natural Health

While there are many benefits from therapeutic body massage, there are situations in which particular manipulations may do more harm than good. A medical professional must always be consulted if there is any doubt regarding the advisability of therapy, since contraindications are unique to each client.

The following is a list of conditions, compiled by therapist Julia Cowan (who is a licensed therapist and the teaching staff director at the Atlanta School of Massage), where almost any type of massage is always contraindicated:

- Osteoporosis or brittle bones.

- Abnormal body temperature.

- Acute infectious diseases or systemic infections.

- Acute inflammatory conditions.

- Severe high blood pressure or history of heart failure.

- Skin problems (affected area only).

A primary-care provider should be consulted for advice prior to receiving massage therapy if you have any of these conditions:

- Varicose veins, phlebitis, thrombosis (Superficial massage around these areas may be very helpful.)

- Pregnancy (Massage in low-risk and uncomplicated pregnancies is appropriate if performed by a trained pregnancy massage therapist.)

- Edema (Massage is contraindicated if swelling is the result of heart or kidney disease, obstruction of lymph channels, or toxemia.)

- Specific conditions or diseases (severe asthma, diabetes, cancer, etc.)

- Chronic pain or dysfunction of the muscular or skeletal system.

- Chronic fatigue (Massage over a period of time may help to restore energy once the possibility of disease has been ruled out.)

- During use of medication and drugs.

ADMINISTER HANDS-ON HEALING WITH ACUPRESSURE

Acupressure is a therapy similar to acupuncture in that it uses the same geography of meridians and pressure points. Instead of using needles, however, a practitioner or you yourself use hands or feet to gently apply pressure to the appropriate points. Acupressure relaxes tense muscles, improves blood circulation, and stimulates the body's ability to relax deeply and fall asleep.

The advantage of acupressure's healing touch is that it is safe to do on yourself and others, even if you've never done it before. There are no side effects from drugs, and the only equipment you need are your two hands.

APPLYING ACUPRESSURE

To apply acupressure, use prolonged finger pressure directly on the point. Gradual, steady penetrating pressure for approximately 3 minutes is ideal. You can gradually work up to holding points longer, but do not hold any one point longer than 10 minutes. It's important to apply and release finger pressure gradually because this allows the tissues time to respond, promoting healing. Then slowly decrease the finger pressure, ending with about 20 seconds of light touch.

For best results, you should perform the acupressure routines daily and continue using the same points even after you've obtained relief from your condition or ailment to prevent recurrence. If you cannot practice every day, treating yourself to acupressure two or three times a week can still be effective.

CAUTION

- Use only gentle pressure; it should not cause any pain.
- Pregnant women should use acupressure only under the instruction of a qualified acupuncture or acupressure practitioner.
- Do not use acupressure when taking any drugs or alcohol.
- Do not administer immediately after eating.

AN ACUPRESSURE SAMPLER

Acupressure can be used to treat a vast array of both physical and mental ailments and conditions. If this form of natural therapy sounds like something you'd like to persue in depth, check your bookstore and/or library for one of the assortment of books that can give you in-depth details. Here, you can gain a glimpse into the art of acupressure with a few tried-and-true pressure points that you can try on yourself.

❧ **Allergies:** Acupressure, while not a cure, can be an effective method for relieving many symptoms of allergic reactions. The point called *Joining the Valley* can be pressed to relieve allergy symptoms such as headaches, hay fever, sneezing, and itching.

Location: In the webbing between your thumb and index finger. On the outside of the hand, find the highest spot of the muscle when the thumb and index fingers are brought close together.

Caution: This point is forbidden for pregnant women because its stimulation can cause premature contractions in the uterus.

❧ **Backache and Sciatica:** Acupressure is highly effective for relieving the muscular tension associated with lower-back pain and sciatica. The point called *Sea of Vitality* can relieve both the pain and the fatigue that often results from the pain.

Location: In the lower back (between the second and third lumbar vertebrae) two to four finger widths away from the spine at waist level.

Caution: If you have a weak back, the *Sea of Vitality* point may be quite tender. In this case, a few minutes of light, stationary touch instead of deep pressure can be very healing.

❧ **Colds:** Although acupressure cannot cure a cold, working on certain points can help you get better quicker and increase your resistance to future colds. The point called *Facial Beauty* can relieve stuffy nose, head congestion, burning eyes, eye fatigue, and eye pressure.

Location: At the bottom of the cheekbone, directly below the pupil.

Caution: Because acupressure stimulates your body to expel viral and bacterial germs more quickly, it may seem at first that your symptoms are worsening. But your body is simply progressing through the symptoms faster than usual.

❧ **Constipation:** The best cure for constipation is in a fiber-rich diet and exercise. But acupressure at the point called *Sea of Energy* can be used to relieve the symptoms of abdominal pain, bloating, and gas.

Location: Three finger widths directly below the navel.

• **Headaches:** Headaches are usually a signal from your body that tension in the muscles of the head, neck, and shoulders is constricting blood vessels and reducing the supply of blood to the brain. Aspirins relieve the pain without relieving the muscle tension that causes it. Acupressure at the point called *Drilling Bamboo* can relieve headaches, eye pain, and sinus pain.

Location: In the indentations on either side of where the bridge of the nose meets the ridge of the eyebrows.

READJUST WITH CHIROPRACTIC CARE

Chiropractic is the largest natural primary health-care profession in the world, utilized by more than 25 million Americans each year!

DEFINING *CHIROPRACTIC*

Chiropractic (which means "treatment by the hands, or manipulation") is a system of healing that was developed by David Daniel Palmer in Iowa in 1895. Palmer believed that displacements of the spine caused pressure on nerves, which created pain or symptoms in other parts of the body. Indeed, the purpose of chiropractic care is the adjustment of the spinal column to rehabilitate normal nervous system functioning. Nerve interference does promote sickness and disease. When the vertebrae are misaligned, the flow of messages from the brain to all the other cells in the body is distorted. This type of nerve interference creates disorganization of bodily processes—it robs our vitality and weakens our immune system. Nerve interference is often referred to as a silent killer because it may be present for many years before symptoms arise. It can quietly, painlessly undermine your health before any major warning signs appear. That's one of the reasons why chiropractic is best used to treat pain and disorders before the body has deteriorated into a pathological or disease state.

CAUSES OF NERVE INTERFERENCE

In his book *Chiropractic First*[150] (*The Chiropractic Journal*, 1996), author Terry Rondberg, D.C., tells us that the causes of nerve interference are numerous and often unavoidable. They can be caused at birth, if our delivery is difficult or requires the use of forceps. They can be caused by trauma, such as a fall while learning to walk. In later years, as we grow, we may cause subluxations (misalignment of one or more vertebrae in the spinal column) with activities such as skate boarding or surfing or any other kinds of play or sports. Other spinal problems can be caused by a junk food diet or having poor sleeping positions. Many seemingly harmless activities can disturb the integrity of the nerve system.

In adults, many things can weaken the spine and cause nerve interference. This list includes sports accidents, automobile collisions, falls in the house, bad posture, emotional stress, dental problems, alcohol and drug abuse, or even carrying heavy briefcases or handbags on a daily basis.

THE MANY USES OF CHIROPRACTIC

Chiropractic is primarily used as a therapy for mechanical dysfunctions, such as traumatized muscles and joints. It is especially popular with people who experience low-back pain, slipped disks, and sport injuries. Chiropractic can also be used to treat many physical and emotional conditions, such as allergies, poor posture, stomachache, hearing loss, neck/back pain, sprained muscles and ligaments, numbness, headaches, constipation, skin problems, irritability, nervousness, sinus problems, arthritis, fatigue, neuritis, lumbago, sciatica, neuralgia, and knee, hip, shoulder/ arm, and muscular pains. Some chiropractors also treat dysfunctions with psychosomatic origins, such as migraines and other headaches, neurosis, conditions due to stress, and some asthma conditions.

So what can a chiropractor do for you? Well, chiropractors don't treat symptoms. Their job is to locate the cause of your problem (the nerve interference) and correct it. But don't expect nerve interference to be corrected in a few visits. It will take continued adjusting to be certain the vertebrae have returned to their proper position and your muscles and ligaments can continue to hold them firmly in place. As your condition improves, the number of adjustments will decrease and you'll be placed on wellness care, where through regular checkups, your chiropractor can detect and correct nerve interference early and enhance your body's innate ability to express its maximum health potential.

FINDING A CHIROPRACTOR

It is important to choose an experienced doctor through a medical or personal recommendation because chiropractic treatment involves highly specific adjustment of the spinal tissues. Always be certain that your chiropractor is state licensed and reputable. Never allow a "paraprofessional" or other unlicensed person attempt to manipulate your spine; this could worsen your problem rather than help it. You can get a referral to a trained chiropractor in your area by contacting the American Chiropractic Association at 1701 Clarendon Blvd., Arlington, VA 22209, (703) 276-8800.

ɚ *21* ɞ

FOR WOMEN ONLY

There is one area where men and women are definitely not equal—in their bodies' health needs. But it's only recently that the medical community has recognized this difference and has begun to address it in medical studies, procedures, and products. In the past, female hormonal cycles have been viewed by the health-care profession as an inconvenience, even an anomaly. Until recently, pharmaceutical companies did not take the menstrual cycle into account in their testing of drugs. And only in 1993 did Congress pass the National Institutes of Health Revitalization Act requiring inclusion of women in clinical research. For these reasons, it's not surprising that conventional medicine still regularly treats many women's health problems ineffectively.

But all is not hopeless! To compensate, many women have found a variety of natural methods to treat minor, common problems on their own. These include diet, exercise, herbs, aromatherapy, and an assortment of other natural therapies recommended by Mother Nature.

Easing the Discomforts of Premenstrual Syndrome

About 85 to 95 percent of women suffer from a combination of the physical, mental, and emotional symptoms defined as premenstrual syndrome (PMS). Among the symptoms occurring before or during menstruation are water retention, fatigue, headaches, depression, irritability, joint pain, lack of coordination, muscle aches, intestinal upsets, breast swelling, and food cravings. These problems are caused by cyclic variations in the levels of estrogen and progesterone.

Conventional practitioners prescribe for PMS a variety of medications whose long-term effects are unknown. These include prostaglandin inhibitors, tranquilizers and antidepressants, diuretics, and hormones. But a few natural treatments often work just as well with fewer side effects.

DIET

Many women have found that they can relieve moderate PMS symptoms by simply changing their diet. Many holistic practitioners recommend a diet based on foods high in complex carbohydrates and low in fat, along with reducing the intake of salt, sugar, and alcohol (all of these cause water retention, which is a major factor in PMS discomfort). You should also reduce your intake of refined carbohydrates, such as white bread, cakes, cookies, refined breakfast cereals, crackers, candy, and chocolate. At the same time, avoid all sources of caffeine—even small amounts have been shown to trigger PMS symptoms.

So what can you eat? Well, although it sounds like a contradiction, the best way to eliminate the excess fluids that cause premenstrual discomforts is to drink six to eight glasses of water daily; this washes the fluids through the system with greater speed. It's also a good idea to increase your consumption of natural diuretics, such as watermelon, asparagus, and parsley. In addition, a natural, whole-food diet will greatly reduce the symptoms of PMS. Plan a diet that emphasizes complex carbohydrates (whole-grain bread, brown rice, whole-grain pasta, whole-grain cereals); plenty of fresh fruits and vegetables; low-fat protein sources such as fish, chicken, and vegetarian proteins; and cold-pressed vegetable oils (rich in essential fatty acids).

HERBS

A number of herbs are natural diuretics, offering a safe and natural way to remove the buildup of fluids that can cause PMS discomforts. A good diuretic tea is made of dandelion leaves. Pour 1 cup of boiling water over 2 teaspoons of dried dandelion leaves. Let steep, covered, for 10 minutes, then enjoy.

AROMATHERAPY

There are a number of effective essential oils that can be used to ease the discomforts of PMS. Mindy Green, coauthor of *Aromatherapy: The Fragrant Art of Healing*[73] (Crossing Press, 1995), likes to use a combination of equal parts of chamomile, lavender, and clary sage (which has estrogenic properties), along with neroli (for its sedative effects) and geranium (a hormone normalizer).

For water retention, Green suggests combining equal parts of grapefruit (which is cleansing), juniper (which has diuretic properties), and carrot seed (which helps normalize liver function). See Chapter 18 for the variety of ways you can use essential oil blends.

OTHER THERAPIES

Daily aerobic exercises can burn up stress-related hormones and can stimulate the flow of endorphins (chemicals produced by the body that alleviate depression and create a feeling of well-being). Meditation, yoga, and massage can also help to handle the stress that seems especially unmanageable to women experiencing PMS.

FIGHTING BACK AT MENSTRUAL CRAMPS

Up to 80 percent of women experience discomfort during menstruation. In the western world, this monthly pain (called dysmenorrhea) is one of the most common causes of lost work and school hours for women. Menstrual cramps (which may be accompanied by nausea, diarrhea, backaches, and headaches) are experienced as lower abdominal and lower back pain. These pains can range from a dull, heavy ache to severe cramping similar to labor pains. Cramps occur when prostaglandin-induced contractions of the uterus temporarily cut off the uterine blood supply.

Aspirin medications are often used to reduce the pain, but they can also increase menstrual bleeding, and they don't address the cause of the problem. Several natural remedies may help you fight back.

DIET

Menstrual cramps can be caused by low levels of blood calcium. At least 10 days before menstruation begins, increase your intake of high-calcium foods like dark-green leafy vegetables, cauliflower, peas, beans, molasses, soybeans, sesame seeds, seaweeds, and watercress. A diet rich in calcium also relaxes the central nervous system.

Magnesium deficiency is also a cause of menstrual cramps. This problem is common among women in areas with mineral-depleted soil, and especially so in those who eat a high-meat diet or who take calcium supplements that are not balanced with magnesium. You can get your fill of natural magnesium from dark-green leafy vegetables, nuts, seeds, legumes, brown rice, soybeans, tofu, whole grains, wheat germ, and millet.

HERBS

Drinking a cup of herbal tea is like laying warm healing hands on the discomfort of menstrual cramps. "Women's" herbs—such as raspberry leaf, squaw vine, cramp bark, and blue cohosh—have provided relief for women for hundreds of years. Warm ginger tea is especially useful for its antispasmodic properties. Grate 2 to 3 teaspoons of fresh ginger root and simmer in 2 cups of water for several minutes. Add lemon and honey to taste. Drink as much as desired.

AROMATHERAPY

Essential oils can be used to ward off cramps beginning a few days before menstruation begins. Massage a combination of the following oils into the abdomen once or twice a day, or use them in your bath. Use equal parts of chamomile (an anti-inflammatory), clary sage (for relief of depression), lavender (a relaxant), and tarragon and marjoram (antispasmodics).

OTHER THERAPIES

Locally applied heat often relieves menstrual cramps. Try resting with a hot water bottle or a heating pad on your abdomen. Some women find relief by applying cold to the abdomen. Experiment a bit to find out which works better for you.

A brisk walk three or four times a week throughout the month and during your menstrual period will often lessen or even eliminate menstrual cramps. Exercise improves blood circulation, increases the oxygenation of your cells (including those in your pelvis and uterus), and generally assists in decongesting the pelvic area. Give it a try.

Massage is also very effective in relieving menstrual pain. Ask your partner to massage a bit of oil into your lower back on either side of the spine and over the sacrum (the triangular-shaped bone at the base of the spine). A 10-minute massage will help decongest the uterus and give you prompt and welcomed relief.

GETTING RID OF URINARY TRACT INFECTIONS

When intestinal bacteria make their way up the urethra and into the bladder, you will be faced with a urinary tract infection (also called cystitis). Symptoms include frequent painful or burning urination, the sensation that the bladder is never empty, and pain just above the pubic bone or in the lower back. A more severe infection may be accompanied by fever and blood in the urine.

Conventional medical treatment for urinary tract infections almost always includes antibiotics. Antibiotics usually do the job of eliminating the problem-causing bacteria, but they also target the beneficial flora, resulting in digestive disturbances and yeast infections. If you're not running a fever with your urinary tract infection, try a few natural methods at home. If self-treatment produces no improvement within 5 days—or if symptoms worsen or a fever develops—see a health practitioner.

DIET

Simple water can flush bacteria out of the bladder. At the first sign of a urinary tract infection, drink large amounts of purified water. Cranberry juice can also effectively treat this condition. Cranberries change the pH of your urine, making it more acidic and less hospitable to bacteria. Drink a quart or more of unsweetened cranberry juice every day until symptoms subside. (Avoid cranberry juice sweetened with sugar or other concentrated sweeteners because they feed the bacteria.) Or take three cranberry capsules three times a day.

HERBS

Mucilaginous herbs, such as marshmallow root, can be made into a tea to soothe mild inflammation. To fight the infection itself, you're better off taking two capsules of echinacea or goldenseal three times a day.

Aromatherapy

Aromatherapy treatments, three times daily, can be used to treat urinary tract infections. Use equal parts of sandalwood, bergamot, tea tree, frankincense, and juniper. Add the essential oil mix to a massage oil and rub over the bladder area. Also use it in baths. Continue for 4 to 5 days after the symptoms subside.

Bergamot oil is especially effective for treating cystitis. Take 2 drops diluted in a tiny amount of honey. Repeat twice daily.

Managing Fibrocystic Breasts

Up to 70 percent of women have fibrocystic breasts. Symptoms of this condition include tender, swollen breasts and breast lumps that fluctuate with the menstrual cycle. In the past, this condition was considered a disease and today is often still treated as such. Conventional medicine may prescribe diuretics, anti-inflammatory drugs, and synthetic male hormones, which can cause weight gain, unwanted hair growth, and reduction in breast size.

Excess estrogen may play a role in the development of fibrocystic breasts, so alternative health practitioners focus on natural methods of regulating estrogen. (Although about 85 percent of breast lumps are not cancerous, all breast irregularities should be evaluated by a medical doctor before attempting home treatment.)

Diet

A low-fat diet is the best dietary treatment for fibrocystic breasts because high fat intake helps stimulate estrogen overproduction. (If you must eat meat and poultry, look for sources raised without synthetic hormones, which can exacerbate estrogen-related problems.)

You should also avoid caffeine drinks and products. Although caffeine itself has been linked with fibrocystic breasts, it's the methylxanthine found in these products that has been most closely linked to breast lumps, swelling, and pain. Methylxanthine is a chemical found in coffee, tea, chocolate, cola, and even decaffeinated coffee.

Herbs

Certain herbal combinations can help the liver better process estrogen. Herbs that stimulate liver function—such as yellow dock, burdock, and dandelion roots—can be combined with herbs that help to regulate the hormones, such as vitex and dong quai. Try this tea recommended by Rosemary Gladstar, author of *Herbal Healing for Women*[68] (Simon & Schuster, 1993):

> Combine one part yellow dock root, three parts dandelion root, two parts burdock root, one part ginger root, one part licorice root, one part vitex, four parts pau d'arco. Use four to six tablespoons of the herb mixture per quart of water. Add the herbs to cold water and simmer, covered, over low heat for twenty minutes. Remove from heat and let stand twenty minutes. Drink three to four cups a day to prevent or relieve symptoms.

OTHER THERAPIES

Stimulating circulation facilitates the flow of nutrients and the elimination of waste products. That's why gentle massage of the breasts may relieve symptoms.

TREATING VARICOSE VEINS

Varicose veins are those enlarged, gnarly, bluish veins that appear most frequently on the legs. Normally the veins in the legs contain tiny one-way valves that help the movement of blood back up out of the legs and toward the heart. When these valves become weakened or softened (as often happens during pregnancy), the blood tends to pool in the leg and is unable to return efficiently to the heart. Varicose veins are often painful and can cause leg cramps, fatigue, and ankle swelling.

Conventional medical treatment for varicose veins involves either surgical removal of the weakened veins or the injection of a chemical into the veins that causes them to collapse. Both treatments carry the risk of infection. Natural approaches focus on prevention and treatments that stimulate circulation and restore tone to the venous system.

DIET

A high-fiber diet along with a supplemental fiber product (such as psyllium) can help relieve the problem of constipation, which contributes to the development of varicose veins. Constipation causes straining during bowel movements, increasing pressure in the lower extremities and contributing to a breakdown of the veins.

Foods high in vitamin C and bioflavonoids can reinforce the capillaries and help them heal. Citrus fruits eaten with the white inner rind are an especially rich source of both.

People with varicose veins tend to build up a substance called fibrin, which is deposited in the tissue near the affected veins. Garlic, onions, cayenne pepper, and bromelain (an enzyme found in fresh pineapple and also available in supplemental form) help break down fibrin and keep the blood thinned and moving.

HERBS

Many herbalists in Europe use an extract of horse chestnut to treat varicose veins externally. Apply a topical preparation to the affected area (do not take horse chestnut internally).

OTHER THERAPIES

Apply a topical compress of witch hazel for swelling, inflammation, or a bruised or sore feeling in the veins. The astringent properties of witch hazel can also be massaged into the legs. Each morning and evening, soak a towel with witch hazel and gently rub toward the heart.

Although exercise increases circulation, which is good for varicose veins, high-impact activities such as jogging can cause more problems. Nonstressful exercises such as swimming and bicycling are best.

Whenever possible, elevate the legs to avoid pressure on the veins and capillaries. You might want to keep a footstool under your desk at work and sleep with your feet slightly elevated. Do not cross your ankles or legs. If your veins are really bad, wear support hose.

PREVENTING AND TREATING VAGINAL YEAST INFECTIONS

Vaginal yeast infections are medically known as candida or monilia. This is a common and often infuriatingly stubborn problem to treat. Symptoms include vaginal irritation, a thick white discharge, and itching, itching, and more itching.

Conventional medical treatment tries to eliminate the yeast with antifungal suppositories and creams, but there is quite a high recurrence of infection, usually within 12 weeks. This is probably due to the fact that these drugs do not address the underlying imbalance that caused the infection in the first place. That's why many women find themselves stuck in a chronic cycle of yeast infections.

DIET

The nutritional treatment for vaginal infections is in prevention. Avoid foods that contain molds, fungus, yeasts, sugar, or refined carbohydrates, and also aged or fermented foods. The list of foods to avoid includes yeast breads, aged cheeses, vinegar, beer, cookies, cakes, dried fruits, sweetened fruit drinks, mushrooms, melons, and commercial sauces.

If you get an infection, diet can help return the healthy balance of bacteria in your body. Eat a few cloves of raw garlic and a cup of yogurt containing active *Lactobacillus acidophilus* culture every day. Garlic has potent antifungal properties, and the *Lactobacillus* culture reintroduces beneficial bacteria. Also, build a diet around a wide variety of vegetables, with as much raw food as possible.

AROMATHERAPY

Mindy Green[73] suggests the following mixture of essential oils as a douche:

> Three drops of bergamot, five drops of geranium, five drops of tea tree, and two drops of myrrh to one ounce of carrier oil (preferably calendula oil because of its antimicrobial properties). Immediately prior to use, add five drops of this mixture to a pint of water or yarrow tea and douche. Repeat two to three times a day until the symptoms are relieved.

OTHER THERAPIES

Holistic practitioners often recommend the use of boric acid suppositories for vaginal yeast infections. Fill gelatin capsules with boric acid (available at pharmacies). Insert one capsule vaginally in the morning and another in the evening for 3 to 7 days if treating a mild infection and for up to 2 weeks for a more severe infection.

In her book *Natural Women's Health*[196] (New Harbinger, 1995), author Lynda Wharton explains how you can also treat a vaginal infection with homemade douches. To make a garlic douche, peel two smallish cloves of garlic and blend with a cup of warm water (in a food processor or blender). Leave the thoroughly blended solution to sit for 5 minutes before carefully straining through a piece of cheesecloth. Add another cup of water to the strained liquid. Soak a tampon in the mixture and insert high into the vagina. Leave the tampon in place for several hours. Change the garlic tampon three times daily. The remaining garlic solution can be used to splash the external genitals repeatedly. You can also use a tampon soaked in *Lactobacillus* yogurt. The *Lactobacilli* change the pH of the vagina, making it less hospitable for bacteria.

To avoid vaginal infections and to help speed recovery from one you may already have tried these self-help tips:

- Avoid frequent use of douching and feminine-hygiene products; they tend to upset the pH balance in the vagina.

- Use prescribed antibiotics only when absolutely necessary; antibiotics kill bacteria indiscriminately, and once *Lactobacilli* bacteria are killed off in sufficient numbers, the *Candida* fungus flourishes.

- After a bowel movement, always wipe from front to back to avoid transferring bacteria from the anus to the vagina.

- Avoid tight-fitting pants, nylon underwear, and pantyhose. Always wear cotton underwear and crotchless pantyhose or stockings.

Additional options for natural healing can be found in the author's *Lifetime Encyclopedia of Natural Remedies* (Simon & Schuster, Parker, 1993).

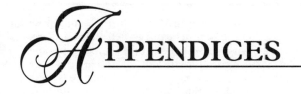

APPENDICES

VITAMIN AND MINERAL CHART
GLOSSARY OF KEY TERMS AND INGREDIENTS
REFERENCES
INDEX

VITAMIN AND MINERAL CHART*

VITAMINS (ingested as food/supplements)	BENEFITS	
	Beauty	**Health**
A (retinol, dry or oil based) **Beta carotene** for conversion to A as needed by the body	essential for healthy, moist, skin; deficiency can cause eruptions or dry, coarse, wrinkled skin; dry hair or dandruff; ridging or peeling fingernails	important for healing, benefits eyes, teeth, mouth, nose and throat linings; beta carotene is an antioxidant, anticancer agent
B COMPLEX (interrelated—a deficiency of one can create a deficiency of all)	essential for healthy skin, hair, and eyes	antistress, energizing, and healing; helps metabolize other nutrients for healthy digestion and nerves
B-1 (thiamine)	important for healthy eyes and hair	helps release energy from carbohydrates; promotes a healthy digestive and nervous system; aids memory and heart function
B-2 (riboflavin—once called vitamin G)	helps eyes, hair, and nails; helps prevent skin dryness and fissures around lips, eye, and mouth corners	same as B complex plus important for respiratory system and vision; helps prevent fatty deposits on artery walls
B-3 (niacin, nicotinic acid; synthetic, niacinamide or nicotinamide)	helps maintain normal skin function, releases trapped sebum that can create skin problems	same as B complex, natural form may cause flushing by stimulating circulation
B-5 (pantothenic acid, panthenol, or calcium pantothenate)	thickens and repairs damaged hair, with PABA and folic acid helps restore color to gray hair	same as B complex, plus aids B-6 and C in allergy relief, benefits colitis
B-6 (pyridoxine)	helps prevent cracks at mouth corners, skin breakouts, and other stress-related skin problems	aids metabolism of protein and fat, brain function, and formation of red blood cells; promotes healthy eyes, tongue, and nervous system; alleviates PMS and "morning sickness"

298

PRINCIPAL FOOD SOURCES	RDA	TOXICITY (unless per MD)
dairy products, eggs, green and yellow fruits and vegetables	5,000 IU	50,000 IU for extended periods; excessive amounts of carotene may yellow skin
brewer's yeast, liver, whole grains	(see individual listings)	excess of one can create a deficiency of the others
same as B complex plus dried legumes; fish; lean beef, pork and poultry; nuts	1.5 mg (more if exercising)	rare
same as B complex plus brussels sprouts, dairy products, and nuts	1.7 mg (more if exercising)	rare
same as B complex plus beef, pork, and poultry; dairy products; nuts, rhubarb, seafood	20 mg	1,000 mg
same as B complex plus kidney, legumes, milk, raw fruits and vegetables, salmon	7 to 15 mg (estimated)	rare
same as B complex plus avocado, banana, beef, cauliflower, chicken, corn, dark leafy green, eggs, nuts, potatoes, salmon, and tuna	2 to 2.2 mg	rare

VITAMIN AND MINERAL CHART *(continued)*

VITAMINS (ingested as food/supplements)	BENEFITS	
	Beauty	Health
B-9 = folic acid, folate, or folacin (once called vitamin M)	delays hair graying when used with B-5 and PABA, promotes healthy skin	acts with B-12 for hemoglobin production; energizing, promotes healthy nerves
B-12 (cobalamin or cyanocobalamin)	necessary for healthy skin, hair, and nails	anti-anemia; maintains healthy nerves, blood, and tissues
Biotin (co-enzyme R, once called vitamin H)	helps prevent hair loss, premature wrinkles, scaly skin rash	helps circulatory system and release of energy from carbohydrates
Choline	helps maintain healthy hair	aids memory function, lowers cholesterol, soothes nerves; necessary for storage of vitamin A
Inositol	needed for healthy hair and skin; helps prevent eczema and falling hair	aids memory function and fat metabolism; lowers cholesterol
PABA (para-aminobenzoic acid)	keeps skin smooth and healthy; with B-5 plus folic acid helps restore gray hair	aids blood cell formation and protein utilization; internal supplements augment sunscreens
VITAMIN C COMPLEX (ascorbic acid, plus the bioflavonoids—once called vitamin P—citrus flavons, hesperidin, quercetin, and rutin); bioflavonoids assist utilization of C and strengthen capillaries; vitamin C alone, natural or synthetic, is a cold remedy	regulates sebaceous glands to keep skin from drying out; helps prevent facial lines, wrinkles and spider veins; hair tangling or breaking	essential for collagen synthesis, healthy bones and cartilage; promotes healthy eyes, gums, and teeth; helps heal wounds and repair damaged cells; burned up by stress and tobacco use

PRINCIPAL FOOD SOURCES	RDA	TOXICITY (unless per MD)
same as B complex plus dairy products, leafy greens, orange juice, oysters, salmon, and tuna	400 to 600 mcg	rare
animal foods	3 to 6 mcg	rare
same as B complex plus dried legumes, egg yolk, kidney, milk, most fresh vegetables, nuts	300 mcg (estimated)	rare
same as B complex plus egg yolk, leafy greens, lecithin supplements, legumes, nuts	none established	rare
same as B complex plus backstrap molasses, citrus fruit, lecithin supplements, lima beans, milk, nuts	none established	rare
bran, brewer's yeast, molasses, organ meats, unpolished rice, wheat germ, whole grains	none established	rare (excess may cause nausea)
citrus fruits (with white membrane for flavons); broccoli; cabbage; cantaloupe; green peppers; kiwi, strawberries and other fruits; potatoes; raw, leafy greens; tomatoes; (black currants, blackberries, buckwheat, cherries, and grapes for bioflavonoids)	60 mg C (ratio of 5 to 1 for ascorbic acid to bioflavonoids)	rare (excess may cause temporary diarrhea, burning urine, or itchy skin)

VITAMIN AND MINERAL CHART *(continued)*

VITAMINS (ingested as food/supplements)	BENEFITS	
	Beauty	**Health**
D (calciferol, ergosterol, or viosterol)	promotes healthy eyes, skin, and teeth	aids absorption of calcium for healthy bones and nervous systems; best utilized when taken with vitamin A
E (tocopherol, alpha or 7 mixed; dl = synthetic)	helps form muscles and tissues to prevent wrinkles and premature aging of the skin; helps prevent dry, dull, or falling hair	antioxidant to protect essential fatty acids and cells from destruction; vasodilator, energizer and anticoagulant
K (K-1 and K-2 are synthesized by the body, K-3 is chemically manufactured)	helps prevent bruising and premature aging of the skin	helps maintain bone metabolism, reduces excessive menstrual flow, necessary for blood clotting; vitality and longevity factor

MINERALS (ingested) as foods/supplements)	BENEFITS	
	Beauty	**Health**
CALCIUM (carbonate, gluconate, lactate, orate, trialcium phosphate—balance with twice as much phosphorus and half as much magnesium; accompany by vitamins A, C, and D)	helps clear blemished skin and revitalize lifeless, tired-looking skin	strengthens bones and teeth, calms tense nerves, helps regulate heart beat and muscle contractions
CHROMIUM (accompany supplements with brewer's yeast to increase absorption)	improves circulation for healthy skin and hair	helps maintain blood sugar level; activates enzymes for carbohydrate, fat, and protein metabolism

PRINCIPAL FOOD SOURCES	RDA	TOXICITY (unless per MD)
fortified milk, beef liver, salmon, and tuna; produced by the body from the action of sunlight on the skin; synthetic D manufactured from fish liver oils	400 IU	excess stored in the liver but less toxic than excess vitamin A
asparagus, broccoli, brussels sprouts, butter, dried legumes, egg yolks, leafy greens, liver, olives, soybeans, sunflower seeds, vegetable oils, wheat germ, whole grains	10 to 30 IU	nontoxic under normal conditions; check with doctor if have high blood pressure, diabetes, or overactive thyroid
egg yolk, fish liver oils, leafy greens, lentils, raw cauliflower, safflower and sunflower oils, yogurt	140 to 500 mcg (estimated)	500 mg of synthetic
dairy products, dark leafy greens, dried legumes, peanuts, salmon, sardines, shellfish, soybeans, sunflower seeds, walnuts	800 to 1,500 mg	over 2,000 mg may cause drowsiness or calcium deposits in soft tissues
brewer's yeast, cheese, clams, corn oil, liver, meat, whole grains	200 mcg (estimated)	rare

VITAMIN AND MINERAL CHART *(continued)*

MINERALS (ingested as food/supplements)	BENEFITS	
	Beauty	**Health**
COPPER	helps prevent hair-color loss, pale or blotchy skin, and easy bruising	necessary for formation of bones, connective tissues, and red blood cells; assists healing and normal functions of brain and nervous system
FLUORINE— **FLUORIDE** (calcium fluoride, synthetic sodium fluoride)		helps prevent tooth decay and osteoporosis; strengthens bones
IODINE (iodide)	promotes healthy hair, nails, skin, and teeth	energizes, helps thyroid burn excess fat, improves mental alacrity, prevents goiter and hypothyroidism
IRON (ferrous citrate, ferrous fumarate, ferrous gluconate, and ferrous peptonate)	essential for healthy nails, skin color, and hair growth	builds red blood cells to prevent iron-deficiency anemia; bolsters energy and disease resistance, helps offset stress
MAGNESIUM	prevents skin disorders	helps metabolize calcium, C, and carbohydrates; promotes healthy teeth, nerves, and muscles; energizes, and fights depression
MANGANESE	helps maintain healthy hair	assists utilization of B-1, biotin, C, and E; aids nervous system and thyroid gland function; energizes, helps memory and is needed for normal bone and tendon structure

PRINCIPAL FOOD SOURCES	RDA	TOXICITY (unless per MD)
beef and pork liver, chicken, leafy greens, mushrooms, nuts, raisins, shellfish (especially oysters), whole grains	2 to 4 mg (estimated)	rare
fluoridated drinking water; traces in gelatin, seafood, tea, and whole grains	4 mg (estimated)	excess can cause mottled teeth, osteoclerosis, and calcification of soft tissues
iodized salt, kelp, onions, seafood, vegetable oils	150 mcg	rare from natural sources; excess supplements can trigger thyroid dysfunction
egg yolks, blackstrap molasses, dark leafy greens, dried fruits and legumes, lean meat, liver, whole wheat	18 mg	rare from natural sources; supplement only under medical supervision
almonds, apples, apricots, bananas, bran, corn, dairy products, figs, grapefruit and lemons, meats, raw leafy greens, soybeans	300 to 400 mg	can be toxic if not balanced with calcium and phosphorus
bananas, beets, bran, coffee, egg yolks, leafy greens, legumes, nuts, pineapple, tea, and whole grains	2 to 7 mg (estimated)	rare

VITAMIN AND MINERAL CHART *(continued)*

MINERALS (ingested as food/supplements)	BENEFITS	
	Beauty	**Health**
PHOSPHORUS (must be balanced with calcium in order to function)	promotes healthy teeth and gums	aids bone and cell growth and repair; carbohydrate and fat metabolism; energizes
POTASSIUM	helps maintain healthy skin and prevent puffiness	controls fluid balance in tissues; aids mental alacrity and muscle strength; helps regulate blood pressure and heart rhythm, has tranquilizing effect
SELENIUM	maintains skin elasticity, helps prevent and correct dandruff	alleviates menopausal distress; complements vitamin E to prevent cell damage by oxygen
SULFUR	helps maintain healthy hair, nails, and skin; helps prevent dermatitis, eczema, and psoriasis	facilitates collagen synthesis and tissue formation
ZINC	helps prevent hair loss, brittle or spotted nails; aids formation of collagen to prevent wrinkles; improves acne conditions	essential for protein synthesis and brain function; important for healing; sense of taste and smell

*This table is not intended to be used for diagnostic or prescriptive purposes. For any diagnosis or treatment of illness, please see your physician. The RDAs shown for some nutrients reflect the results of current studies and are higher than those previously published.

PRINCIPAL FOOD SOURCES	RDA	TOXICITY (unless per MD)
dairy products, dried legumes, egg yolks, fish, poultry, meats, and grains	800 to 1,200 mg	excess reduces calcium absorption
bananas, citrus and dried fruits, coffee, fresh vegetables. kiwi fruit, lean meats, legumes, peanuts, potatoes, tea	1,500 to 6,000 mg (should equal sodium consumed)	excess of supplements can cause muscle weakness and heart disturbance
asparagus, bran, broccoli, chicken, egg yolks, milk, onions, red meat, seafood, tomatoes, whole grains	200 mcg (estimated)	rare
bran, brussels sprouts, cabbage, cheese, clams, eggs, fish. mushrooms, nuts, peas and beans, wheat germ	not established	rare
brewer's yeast, eggs, lean red meat, legumes, mushrooms, nonfat dry milk, pumpkin and sunflower seeds, shellfish (especially oysters), spinach, whole grains	15 mg (estimated)	150 mg from supplements

GLOSSARY
OF KEY TERMS
AND INGREDIENTS

acupressure: a generic term encompassing any number of massage techniques that use manual pressure to stimulate energy points on the body.

almond meal: blanched, pulverized almonds. Available in health food stores or can be made in an electric blender or food processor. (To blanch: bring shelled almonds to a boil in water to cover. Let stand until cool. Drain. Remove skins.) Used for facial scrubs and as an ingredient in many skin-care products.

aloe vera: a plant used since Biblical times to treat burns and skin damage, and condition hair. Easily grown indoors or out, or available as a bottled gel from health food stores.

alum: crystalline potassium-aluminum sold in supermarkets, primarily for pickling. As a cosmetic ingredient it refines pores and tightens skin.

aromatherapy: the use of aromatic essences extracted from wild or cultivated plants for beauty treatments or therapies.

astringent: a liquid, usually containing either alcohol or acetone. Used after cleansing to remove excess oil or makeup residue, tighten pores, restore pH balance, and inhibit the growth of bacteria.

benzoin: a fragrant resin first used as a temple incense in Sumatra; now available from pharmacies as tincture of benzoin. It serves as a preservative and skin toner in natural beauty products.

biofeedback: a technique for learning to monitor and gain control over automatic, reflex-regulated body functions by using information obtained from various types of machines.

borax: a mineral containing magnesium chloride. Used in natural beauty products for over a century; now sold in supermarkets as Boraxo.

brewer's yeast: originally a brewing byproduct, now grown on molasses for a food supplement. Used externally to activate circulation, chase wrinkles, and tighten pores.

chiropractic: a health-care technique in which practitioners manipulate the skeletal-muscular system of the body, usually by hand. Its central modality is adjustment of the spinal column to rehabilitate normal nervous system functioning.

cocoa butter: (or *oil theobroma*), obtained by separating the fat from the cacao beans used for chocolate; has been a favored skin softener for hundreds of years.

comedones: *whiteheads* (closed comedones) are underskin bumps of trapped sebum. *Blackheads* (open comedones) form when the pores become so clogged they burst and the sebum oxidizes in the air to turn black.

emollient or moisturizer: a substance that locks in moisture to keep the surface of the skin soft and supple.

epidermabrasion: sloughing off of dead skin cells by means of friction or exfolliant substances.

epsom salt: magnesium sulfate, marketed as a cathartic or pain-relieving soak. May be used half-and-half with table salt to equal sea salt in homemade beauty products.

exfolliant or scrub: sloughs dead cells from the skin's surface.

glycerin: a byproduct of soap manufacture available from pharmacies. Long used as a humecant to soften skin by drawing moisture and preventing its evaporation, it also keeps cosmetic products moist and makes them spread more easily.

herbalism: the use of any plant part—leaf, seed, stem, flower, root, bark—for the relief of certain complaints, conditions, or ailments.

humectants: water-loving compounds that latch on to moisture and help hold it on the skin's surface.

kelp: mineral-rich seaweed available as granules or powder from health food stores. Used as a salt substitute and as a beauty-product enhancer.

keratolytic: skin peeling agent.

lanolin: a fatty substance obtained from sheep's wool. Used in commercial cosmetics and available from pharmacies—test before using if you are allergic to wool.

lecithin: a natural emulsifier made from soybeans. Available in capsules, granules, liquid, or powder for internal or external use.

loofah: the fibers of a special type of gourd formed into friction gloves, bath mitts, or sponges. When lightly rubbed over the body, a loofah stimulates circulation anal carries away dead cells and debris.

massage: the systematic, therapeutic stroking and kneading of the body.

mayonnaise: commercially bottled or homemade, it is excellent for skin or hair. Cosmetic mayonnaise may be made by omitting the seasonings from any standard recipe, or made in an electric blender from these room-temperature ingredients:

1 whole egg

1 teaspoon honey

1¹/₄ cups vegetable or nut oil

3 tablespoons fresh lemon juice

Whir egg, honey, and ¹/₄ cup oil until combined. With blender running, slowly add ¹/₂ cup oil, then the lemon juice, then the remaining oil. Blend until thickened; store in the refrigerator.

mineral water: marketed as a bubbly beverage, the trace minerals it contains are absorbed by and benefit the skin when applied as a skin freshener or as an ingredient of other natural beauty products.

occlusive: an oil, cream, or lotion applied as a protective film to trap moisture and prevent its evaporation from the surface of the skin; and to prevent contaminants from makeup or airborne pollutants from seeping into the skin (See also emollient).

papules and pustules: inflamed, pus-filled bumps on the skin's surface resulting from an under-skin infection and the body's defensive effort of sending white blood cells to the area.

petroleum jelly: a derivative of petroleum, once called *petrolatum*, now marketed as Vaseline®.

pH: the pH scale (0 to 14) shows the acid/alkaline balance: 0 to 6.9 indicates acidity, 7.0 is neutral, 7.1 or above is alkaline. Contact with an alkaline substance such as soap necessitates an acid-containing toner to restore the healthy skin and hair balance of between pH 3.0 and pH 5.5.

phytochemicals: naturally occurring chemicals that help fight cancer and other diseases.

sebum: a combination of oil and wax carried to the skin surface by the sebaceous glands.

toner: an acid-containing liquid used as a skin freshener or astringent to restore a normal pH balance.

white vegetable shortening: vegetable oils hydrogenated into a creamy solid that can be used as a makeup remover or beauty-product ingredient. Marketed as Crisco®.

witch hazel: a liquid commercially extracted with alcohol from the bark and leaves of the witch hazel shrub for use as a mild antiseptic and astringent. Also available as a dry herb.

REFERENCES

1. Adams, Rex. *Miracle Medicine Foods*. West Nyack, NY: Parker Publishing Company, Inc., 1977.

2. Aero, Rita. *The Complete Book of Longevity*. New York: Perigee Books, 1980.

3. Albrecht, Karl. *Stress and the Manager*. Englewood Cliffs, NJ: Prentice-Hall, Inc., 1979.

4. Allen, Oliver E., and editors of Time-Life Books. *Building Sound Bones and Muscles*. Alexandria, VA: Library of Health/Time-Life Books, 1981.

5. Arnold, Caroline. *Too Fat? Too Thin? Do You Have a Choice?* New York: William Morrow and Company, 1984.

6. Arpel, Adrien, with Ronnie Sue Ebenstein. *Adrien Arpel's 3-Week CRASH Makeover/Shapeover Beauty Program*. New York: Rawson Associates Publishers, Inc., 1977.

7. _____. *How to Look Ten Years Younger*. New York: Rawson, Wade Publishers, Inc., 1980.

8. Atkinson, Holly, M.D. *Women and Fatigue*. New York: Putnam's Sons, 1986.

9. Bailey, Adrian. *The Blessings of Bread*. New York: Paddington Press Ltd., 1975.

10. Bailey, Covert. *Fit or Fat?* Boston: Houghton Mifflin Company, 1978.

11. Beeton, Mrs. Isabella. *Beeton's Book of Household Management*. London: S.O. Beeton, 1861.

12. Begley, "Beyond Vitamins." *Newsweek*, April 25, 1994: 45–49.

13. Begoun, Paula. *Blue Eyeshadow Should Be Illegal*. 2nd edition. Seattle, WA: Beginning Press, 1986.

14. Benson, Herbert, M.S. *Beyond the Relaxation Response*. New York: Times Books, 1984.

15. _____. *The Relaxation Response*. New York: William Morrow and Company, Inc., 1975.

16. _____. *Your Maximum Mind*. New York: Times Books, 1987.

17. Bernhardt, Dr. Roger and David Martin. *Self-Mastery Through Self-Hypnosis*. Indianapolis/New York: Bobbs-Merrill Company, Inc., 1977.

18. Birnes, Nancy. *Cheaper and Better*. New York: Harper & Row, Publishers, 1987.

19. Bland, Jeffrey. *Medical Applications of Clinical Nutrition*. New Canaan, CT: Keats Publishing Co., 1983.

20. Blaurock-Busch, Eleanor, Ph.D., with Bernd W. Busch, D.C. *The No-Drugs Guide to Better Health*. West Nyack, NY: Parker Publishing Company, Inc., 1984.

21. Bloomfield, Harold H., M.D., and Robert B. Kory. *Happiness*. New York: Simon & Schuster, 1976.

22. Brenton, Myron. *Aging Slowly*. Emmaus, PA: Rodale Press, Inc., 1983.

23. Bricklin, Mark. *The Practical Encyclopedia of Natural Healing*. Emmaus, PA: Rodale Press, Inc., 1976.

24. _____. *Rodale's Encyclopedia of Natural Home Remedies*. Emmaus, PA: Rodale Press, Inc., 1982.

25. Bricklin, Mark, editor. *The Natural Healing Annual, 1986*. Emmaus, PA: Rodale Press, Inc., 1986.

26. _____. *The Natural Healing Annual, 1987*. Emmaus, PA: Rodale Press, Inc., 1987.

27. _____. *The Natural Healing Annual, 1988*. Emmaus, PA: Rodale Press, Inc., 1988.

28. Briggs, George M., and Doris H. Calloway. *Bogert's Nutrition and Physical Fitness*. 11th edition. New York: Holt, Rinehart and Winston Co., 1984.

29. Brody, Jane E. *Jane Brody's Nutrition Book*. New York: Bantam Books, Inc., 1982.

30. Cameron, Myra. *Treasury of Home Remedies*. Englewood Cliffs, NJ: Prentice-Hall, Inc. 1987.

31. Campbell, Greg. *The Joy of Jumping*. New York: Richard Marek Publishers, 1978.

32. Carroll, David. *The Complete Book of Natural Medicines*. New York: Summit Books, 1980.

33. Castleton, Virginia. *The Handbook of Natural Beauty*. Emmaus, PA: Rodale Press, Inc., 1975.

34. Chang, Dr. Stephen T. *The Complete System of Self-Healing*. San Francisco, CA: Tao Publishing, 1986.

35. Chang, Edward C., Ph.D., translator. *Knocking at the Gate of Life and Other Healing Exercises from China*. Emmaus, PA: Rodale Press, 1985.

36. Chase, A.W., M.D. *Dr. Chase's Recipes; or Information for Everybody*. Ann Arbor, MI: Published by the author, 1863; 1866 editions.

37. Chenault, Alice A. *Nutrition and Health*. New York: Holt, Rinehart and Winston Co., 1984.

38. Child, Mrs. Lydia Marie. *The American Frugal Housewife*. Boston: American Stationers' Company, 1836.

39. Clark, Linda. *Face Improvement Through Exercise and Nutrition*. New Canaan, CT: Keats Publishing, Inc., 1970.

40. _____. *Handbook of Natural Remedies for Common Ailments*. Greenwich, CT: Devon-Adair Company, 1976.

41. _____. *Secrets of Health and Beauty*. New York: Pyramid Books, 1974.

42. _____. *Stay Young Longer*. New York: Devon-Adair Company, 1962.

43. Clement, Brian. *Living Foods for Optimum Health*. Rocklin, CA: Prima Publishing, 1996.

44. Connor, Sonja L., M.S., R.D. and William E. Connor, M.D. *The New American Diet*. New York: Simon & Schuster, 1986.

45. Consumer Guide Editors. *Flatten Your Stomach*. New York: Beekman House, 1979.

46. Craig, Marjorie. *Miss Craig's 21-Day Shape-Up Program*. New York: Random House, 1968.

47. Crenshaw, Mary Ann. *The Natural Way to Super Beauty*. New York: Dell Publishing Co., Inc., 1974.

48. Cross, Jean. *In Grandmother's Day*. Englewood Cliffs, NJ: Prentice-Hall, 1980.

49. Daché, Lilly. *Lilly Daché's Glamour Book*. Philadelphia and New York: J. B. Lippincott Company, 1956.

50. Davis, Adelle. *Let's Eat Right to Keep Fit*. New York: Harcourt Brace Javanovich, Inc., 1970 revised edition.

51. _____. *Let's Get Well*. New York: Harcourt Brace Javanovich, Inc., 1965.

52. Davis, Phyllis B. *Looking Good, Feeling Beautiful*. New York: Simon & Schuster/Avon Products, Inc., 1981.

53. DeBakey, Michael E., M.D. *The Living Heart Diet*. New York: Simon & Schuster, 1984.

54. Dick, William B. *Dick's Encyclopedia of Practical Receipts and Processes or How They Did It in the 1870's*. New York: Funk & Wagnalls, reprint edition prepared by Leicester and Harriet Handsfield, 1977.

55. Eaton, S. Boyd, M.D., Marjorie Shostak and Melvin Konnor, M.D., Ph.D. *The Paleolithic Prescription. A Program of Diet & Exercise and a Design for Living*. New York: Harper & Row, 1988.

56. Edelstein, Barbara, M.D. *The Underburner's Diet*. New York: Macmillan Publishing Company, 1987.

57. Faelten, Sharon, David Diamond & the editors of Prevention Magazine. *Take Control of Your Life*. Emmaus, PA: Rodale Press, 1988.

58. Failes, Janice McCall, and Frank W. Cawood. *Natural Healing Encyclopedia*. Peachtree City, GA: FC&A Publishing, 1987.

59. Ferri, Elisa, with Mary-Ellen Siegel. *Finger Tips*. New York: Clarkson N. Potter, Inc./Publishers, 1988.

60. Fitzgibbon, Theodora. *The Food of the Western World*. New York: Quadrangle/The New York Times Book Co., 1976.

61. Frank, Dr. Benjamin S. *Nucleic Acid Therapy in Aging and Degenerative Disease*. New York: Psychological Library, 1974 revised edition.

62. Franklyn, Robert A., M.D., and Marcia Borie. *A Doctor's Quick Way to Achieve Lasting Beauty*. New York: Information Incorporated, 1970.

63. Fredericks, Carleton. *Eat Well, Get Well, Stay Well*. New York: Grosset & Dunlap, 1980.

64. Fredericks, Carleton, and Herbert Bailey. *Food Facts and Fallacies*. New York: Arco Publishing Company, Inc., 1978.

65. Gardner, Joseph L., editor. *Eat Better, Live Better*. Pleasantville, NY: The Reader's Digest Association, Inc., 1982.

66. Garrison, Robert H., and Elizabeth Somer. *The Nutrition Desk Reference*. New Canaan, CT: Keats Publishing Co., 1985.

67. Gilmore, C. P. *Exercising for Fitness*. Alexandria, VA: Library of Health/Time-Life Books, 1981.

68. Gladstar, Rosemary. *Herbal Healing for Women*. New York: Simon & Schuster, 1993.

69. Goldbeck, Nikki and David. *The Dieter's Companion*. New York: Signet, 1977.

70. Goodenough, Josephus, M.D. *Dr. Goodenough's Home Cures and Herbal Remedies*. (Revised edition of *The Favorite Medical Receipt Book and Home Doctor*, 1904). New York: Avenel Books, 1982.

71. Goodman, Harriet Wilinsky, and Barbara Morse. *Just What the Doctor Ordered*. New York: Holt, Rinehart and Winston, 1982.

72. Gormley, James. "Non-Organic Coffee Provides False Hope If You Want an Energy Boost." *Better Nutrition*, May 1996: 18.

73. Green, Mindy. *Aromatherapy: The Fragrant Art of Healing.* Freedom, CA: Crossing Press, 1995.

74. Grossbart, Ted, Ph.D., and Carl Sherman *Skin Deep: A Mind/Body Program for Healthy Skin.* New York: William Morrow & Co., Inc., 1985.

75. Guinness, Alma E., editor. *ABC's of the Human Body.* Pleasantville, NY: The Reader's Digest Association, Inc., 1987.

76. Hamilton, Eva M., and Elinor N. Whitney. *Understanding Nutrition.* 4th edition. St. Paul, MN: West Publishing Co., 1984.

77. Harris, Ben Charles. *The Compleat Herbal.* New York: Larchmont, 1972.

78. _____. *Kitchen Medicines.* New York: Weathervane Books, 1968 edition.

79. Hauser, Gayelord. *Gayelord Hauser's Treasury of Secrets.* New York: Farrar, Straus and Company, 1963.

80. _____. *Look Younger, Live Longer.* New York: Fawcett World Library, 1971 revised edition.

81. Heimlich, Henry J., M.D., with Lawrence Galton. *Dr. Heimlich's Home Guide to Emergency Medical Situations.* New York: Simon & Schuster, 1980.

82. Hern, Wayne. "Studies Create Confusion, But Eating Greens Is Good." *American Medical News,* May 9, 1994: 20.

83. Hill, Ann, editor. *A Visual Encyclopedia of Unconventional Medicine.* New York: Crown Publishers Inc., 1979.

84. Hirschhorn, Howard H. *Pain-Free Living: How to Prevent and Eliminate Pain All Over the Body.* West Nyack, NY: Parker Publishing Company, Inc., 1977.

85. Holistic Health Center staff. *The Holistic Health Handbook.* Berkeley, CA: And/Or Press, 1978.

86. Hupping, Carol, Cheryl Winters Tetreau, and Roger B. Yepsen, Jr., editors. *Hints, Tips and Everyday Wisdom.* Emmaus, PA: Rodale Press, Inc., 1985.

87. Hutchinson, E. *Ladies' Indispensable Assistant.* New York: Published by the author, 1852.

88. Imber, Gerald, M.D., and Stephen Brill Kurtin, M.D. *Face Care.* New York: A & W Publishers, Inc., 1983.

89. Jackson, Carole. *Color Me Beautiful.* New York: Ballantine Books, 1981 edition.

90. Jarvis, D.C., M.D. *Folk Medicine.* New York: Henry Holt & Co., Inc., 1958.

91. Kingsley, Philip. *The Complete Hair Book*. New York: Grosset & Dunlap, 1979.

92. Kirschmann, John D. *Nutrition Almanac*. New York: McGraw-Hill, 1979 revised edition.

93. Kloss, Jethro. *Back to Eden*. Santa Barbara, CA: Woodbridge Press Publishing Company, 1975.

94. Korth, Leslie O., D.O., M.R.O. *Some Unusual Healing Methods*. Surrey, England: Health Science Press, 1960.

95. Kounovsky, Nicholas. *Instant Fitness*. New York: Paragon Books, 1979.

96. _____. *The Joy of Feeling Fit*. New York: E. P. Dutton & Co., Inc., 1971.

97. Lamb, Lawrence E., M.D. *What You Need to Know About Food & Cooking for Health*. New York: The Viking Press, 1973.

98. Lawrence, Herbert, M.D. *The Care of Your Skin*. New York: Gramercy Publishing Company, 1955.

99. Lawson, Donna. *Looking Fit & Fabulous at Forty Plus*. Emmaus, PA: Rodale Press, 1987.

100. Lesser, Gershon M., M.D. *Growing Younger*. New York: St. Martin's Press, 1987.

101. Leyel, Mrs. C. F. *Herbal Delights*. New York: Gramercy Publishing Company, 1986.

102. Liebman, Bonnie. "The Salt Shakeout." *Nutrition Action Health Letter*, March 1994: 1.

103. Lillyquist, Michael J. *Sunlight and Health*. New York: Dodd Mead & Co., 1985.

104. Lindsay, A.H., E.A. Oddoye, and S. Margen. "Protein-Induced Hypercalciuria: A Longer Term Study." *American Journal of Clinical Nutrition* (32) 1979: 741–749.

105. Loewenfeld, Claire, and Philippa Back. *Herbs, Health and Cookery*. New York: Gramercy Publishing Company, 1965.

106. Lubowe, Irwin I., M.D. *New Hope for Your Skin*. New York: E. P. Dutton, 1963.

107. Lucas, Richard. *Nature's Medicines*. West Nyack, NY: Parker Publishing Company, Inc., 1966.

108. Maltz, Maxwell, M.D., F.I.C.S. *Psycho-Cybernetics*. Englewood Cliffs, NJ: Prentice-Hall, Inc., 1960.

109. McDougall, John A., M.D., and Mary A. McDougall. *The McDougall Plan*. Piscataway, NJ: New Century Publishers, Inc., 1983.

110. McKee, Alma. *To Set Before a Queen*. New York: Simon & Schuster, 1964.

111. Meyer, Clarence. *American Folk Medicine*. New York: New American Library, 1973.

112. _____. *Vegetarian Medicines*. Glenwood, IL: Meyerbooks, 1981.

113. Miller, Fred D., D.D.S. *Open Door to Health*. New York: The Devon-Adair Co., 1959.

114. Miller, Peter M., Dr. *The Hilton Head Metabolism Diet*. New York: Warner Books, Inc., 1983.

115. Mindell, Earl. *Earl Mindell's Quick and Easy Guide to Better Health*. New Canaan, CT: Keats Publishing, Inc., 1982.

116. _____. *Earl Mindell's Shaping Up with Vitamins*. New York: Warner Books, Inc., 1985.

117. _____. *Earl Mindell's Vitamin Bible*. New York: Warner Books, 1979.

118. Mitchell, Curtis. *The Perfect Exercise: The Hop, Skip and Jump Way to Health*. New York: Simon & Schuster, Inc., 1976.

119. Morris, Freda. *Self-Hypnosis in Two Days*. New York: E.P. Dutton & Co., 1975.

120. Morrison, Marsh, D.C., Ph.C., F.I.C.C. *Doctor Morrison's Miracle Guide to Pain-Free Health and Longevity*. West Nyack, NY: Parker Publishing Company, Inc., 1977.

121. Munson, Marty, and Greg Gutfeld. "Pressure Drain: The Official Way to Cut Hypertension Without Drugs." *Prevention*, April 1994: 20.

122. Murphy, Wendy, and editors of Time-Life Books. *Touch, Taste, Smell, Sight and Hearing*. Alexandria, VA: Library of Health/Time-Life Books, 1982.

123. Nagler, Willibald, M.D. *Dr. Nagler's Body Maintenance and Repair Book*. New York: Simon & Schuster, 1987.

124. Norfolk, Dr. Donald. *The Habits of Health*. New York: St. Martin's Press, 1976.

125. Notelovitz, Morris, with Marsha Ware. *Stand Tall! The Informed Woman's Guide to Preventing Osteoporosis*. Gainesville, FL: Triad Publishing Company, 1982.

126. Nudel, Adele. *For the Woman Over 50*. New York: Avon Books, 1979.

127. Null, Gary and Steve. *Complete Handbook of Nutrition*. New York: Dell Publishing Co., Inc., 1972.

128. Osmond, Marie, with Julie Davis. *Marie Osmond's Guide to Beauty, Health, and Style*. New York: Simon & Schuster, 1980.

129. Palm, J. Daniel, Ph.D. *Diet Away Your Stress, Tension, and Anxiety*. New York: Pocket Books, 1976.

130. Parrish, John A., Barbara A. Gilchrist, Thomas B. Fitzpatrick. *Between You and Me*. Boston: Little, Brown, 1978.

131. Pauling, Linus. *How to Live Longer and Feel Better*. New York: W.H. Freeman and Company, 1986.

132. Pearson, Dr. Leonard, Lillian R. Pearson, M.S.W., and Karola Saekel. *The Psychologist's Sensational Cookbook*. New York: Peter H. Wyden Publisher, 1974.

133. Pearson, Durk, and Sandy Shaw. *Life Extension*. New York: Warner Books, 1983.

134. People's Medical Publishing House Staff. *The Chinese Way to a Long and Healthy Life*. New York: Random House Value, 1987.

135. Petulengro, Leon. *The Roots of Health*. New York: New American Library, 1968.

136. Pfeiffer, Carl C. *Zinc and Other Micro-Nutrients*. New Canaan, CT: Keats Publishing Co., 1978.

137. Pinkham, Mary Ellen. *How to Become a Healthier, Prettier You*. Garden City, NY: Doubleday & Company, Inc., 1984.

138. Prevention Magazine editors. *The Complete Book of Vitamins*. Emmaus, PA: Rodale Press, 1984.

139. _____. *The Encyclopedia of Common Diseases*. Emmaus, PA: Rodale Press, 1976.

140. _____. *Herbs for Health*. Emmaus, PA: Rodale Press, 1979.

141. _____. *The Natural Way to a Healthy Skin*. Emmaus, PA: Rodale Press, 1972.

142. Principal, Victoria. *The Beauty Principal*. New York: Simon & Schuster, 1984.

143. Prudden, Bonnie. *Bonnie Prudden's Fitness Book*. New York: The Ronald Press Company, 1959.

144. Pugh, Katie. *Baldness: Is It Necessary?* Richmond, VA: Mailing Services, Inc., 1967.

145. Randolph, Vance. *Ozark Magic & Folklore*. New York: Dover Publications, Inc., 1964.

146. Registein, Quentin, M.D. *Sound Sleep.* New York: Simon & Schuster, 1980.

147. Reilly, Harold H. and Ruth Hagy Brod. *The Edgar Cayce Handbook for Health Through Drugless Therapy.* New York: Macmillan Publishing Company, 1975.

148. Riedman, Sarah. *The Good Looks Skin Book.* New York: Julian Messner, 1983.

149. Rodale, J.I. and Staff. *The Complete Book of Minerals for Health.* Emmaus, PA: Rodale Press, 1972.

150. Rondberg, Terry. "Chiropractic First." Chandler, AZ: *The Chiropractic Journal*, 1996.

151. Rose, Jeanne. *Herbs and Things.* New York: Grosset & Dunlap, 1972.

152. Rossiter, Frederick M., M.D. *Face Culture.* New York: Pageant Books, Inc., 1956.

153. Roth, Beulah. *The International Beauty Book.* Los Angeles: Price/Stern/Sloan Publishers, 1970.

154. Royal, Penny C. *Herbally Yours.* Payson, UT: Sound Nutrition, 1982.

155. Rutledge, Deborah. *Natural Beauty Secrets.* New York: Hawthorne Books, 1966.

156. Saffon, M.J. *The 15-Minute-A-Day Natural Face Lift.* Englewood Cliffs, NJ: Prentice-Hall Inc., 1979.

157. Sassoon, Beverly and Vidal, with Camille Duhe. *A Year of Beauty and Health.* New York: Simon & Schuster, 1978.

158. Saunders, Rubie. *The Beauty Book.* New York: Julian Messner, 1983.

159. Schoen, Linda Allen, editor. *AMA Book of Skin and Hair Care.* Philadelphia, PA: J.B. Lippincott Company, 1976.

160. Schorr, Lia. *Lia Schorr's Skin Care Guide for Men.* Englewood Cliffs, NJ: Prentice-Hall, Inc., 1985.

161. Schurmann, Petra. *Be Beautiful!* Tucson, AZ: H P Books, Fisher Publishing Inc., 1984.

162. Schwartz, Alice Kuhn, Ph.D. and Norma S. Aaron. *Somniquest.* New York: Harmony Books, 1979.

163. Sehnert, Keith W., M.D., with Howard Eisenberg. *How to Be Your Own Doctor (Sometimes).* New York: Grosset & Dunlap, 1981.

164. Selye, Hans, M.D. *The Stress of Life.* New York: McGraw-Hill Book Company, Inc., 1956.

165. Shames, Richard, M.D. and Chuck Sterin, M.S., Ph.D. *Healing with Mind Power*. Emmaus, PA: Rodale Press, 1978.

166. Shute, Evan V. *Common Questions on Vitamin E and Their Answers*. New Canaan, CT: Keats Publishing Co., 1979.

167. Shute, Wilfrid E. *Health Preserver*. Emmaus, PA: Rodale Press, 1977.

168. Siegel, Bernie S., M.D. *Love, Medicine and Miracles*. New York: Harper & Row, Publishers, 1986.

169. Smith, Ann. *Celebrity Exercise*. New York: Walker and Company, 1976.

170. Soglow, M. H. *Relax Your Way to Health*. Englewood Cliffs, NJ: Prentice-Hall, 1958.

171. Stabile, Toni. *Cosmetics: The Great American Skin Game*. New York: Ballantine Books, 1973.

172. Stein, Laura. *The Bloomingdale's Eat Healthy Diet*. New York: St. Martin's Press, 1986.

173. Sternberg, Thomas H., M.D. *More Than Skin Deep*. New York: Doubleday & Co., Inc., 1970.

174. Swarth, Judith. *Skin, Hair, Nails, and Nutrition*. San Diego, CA: Health Media of America, Inc., 1986.

175. Tannahill, Reay. *Food in History*. New York: Stein and Day/Publishers, 1973.

176. Tapley, Donald F., M.D., Robert J. Weiss, M.D., and Thomas Q. Morris, M.D., medical editors. *Complete Home Medical Guide*. New York: Crown Publishers, Inc., 1985.

177. *The Brown University Long-Term Care Quality Letter*. "Even Moderate Exercise Can Improve Health." Nov. 13, 1995: S2.

178. The University of California, "The Energizer." *Berkeley Wellness Letter*, August 1995: 4.

179. Thomas, Mai. *Grannies' Remedies*. New York: Gramercy Publishing Company, 1965.

180. Time-Life Books consultants. *Eating Right*. Alexandria, VA: Time-Life Books Inc., 1987.

181. _____. *The Fit Body*. Alexandria, VA: Time-Life Books Inc., 1987.

182. _____. *Getting Firm*. Alexandria, VA: Time-Life Books Inc., 1987.

183. _____. *Managing Stress*. Alexandria, VA: Time-Life Books Inc., 1987.

184. _____. *Restoring the Body*. Alexandria, VA: Time-Life Books Inc., 1987.

185. _____. *Staying Flexible*. Alexandria, VA: Time-Life Books Inc., 1987.

186. _____. *Wholesome Diet*. Alexandria, VA: Library of Health/Time-Life Books Inc., 1981.

187. *Tufts University Diet & Nutrition Letter.* "No Grounds Found for Breaking the Coffee Habit." April 1996: 6.

188. Van Fleet, James K., D.C. *Extraordinary Healing Secrets from a Doctor's Private Files*. West Nyack, NY: Parker Publishing Company, Inc., 1977.

189. Vaughan, Beatrice. *The Old Cook's Almanac*. New York: Gramercy Publishing Company, 1966.

190. Veyne, Paul, editor. *A History of Private Life*. Cambridge, MA: The Belknap Press of Harvard University Press, 1987.

191. Wade, Carlson. *Health Secrets from the Orient*. West Nyack, NY: Parker Publishing Company, Inc., 1973.

192. _____. *Helping Yourself with New Enzyme Catalyst Health Secrets*. West Nyack, NY: Parker Publishing Company, Inc., 1981.

193. _____. *Natural Folk Remedies* Greenwich, CT: Globe Communications Corp., 1979.

194. Wagonvoord, James, editor. *The Man's Book*. New York: Avon Books, 1978.

195. Weiner, Michael A., Ph.D., and Kathleen Goss. *Nutrition Against Aging*. New York: Bantam, 1983.

196. Wharton, Lynda. *Natural Women's Health: A Guide to Healthy Living for Women of Any Age*. Oakland, CA: Harbinger Publications, Inc., 1995.

197. Wurtman, Judith J., Ph.D. *Managing Your Mind and Mood Through Food*. New York: Rawson Associates, 1986.

198. Zak, Victoria, Chris Carlin, M.S., R.D., and Peter Vash, M.D., M.P.H. *The Fat-to-Muscle Diet*. New York: G. P. Putnam's Sons, 1987.

INDEX

A

Acidophilus
for acne, 66
for athlete's foot, 145
for bad breath, 160
for cold sores, 151
for vaginal yeast infections, 295
Acne, 64-70
causes of, 64-65
and diet, 65-66
herbal teas for, 66
and hormone levels, 6, 65
natural treatments for, 67-70
nutritional supplements for, 66
soapless cleansers for, 67
and sunlight, 70
Acne rosacea, 70-71
nutritional supplements for, 71
prevention of, 70-71
Acupressure, 281-284
ailments treated by, 283-284
cautions about, 282
method for, 282
Aerobic exercise, 228-239
aerobic dance, 235
benefits of, 229-231
cool-down, 232
cross-country skiing, 235
cycling, 236
guidelines for success, 232-234
heart rate monitoring, 231
jogging/running, 236
jumping rope, 236-237
rowing, 237
swimming, 237-238
walking, 238-239
warm-up, 232
water workouts for, 241
After-shave, recipe for, 29-30
Aging skin
photoaging, 106-107
sagging skin, 84-89
wrinkles, 76-84

Alcohol
for acne, 67, 68
alcohol-based toners, 29-30
for athlete's foot, 145
as deodorant, 92
as skin cleanser, 16
soapless shampoo, 177
for sunburn, 155
Alcoholic drinks, 209-211
and breast cancer, 209-210
calories in, 211
and heart disease, 209
and medications, 210
moderate drinking, 210
Allergies, acupressure for, 283
Almond flower milk, as skin toner, 32
Almond meal
for blackheads/whiteheads, 62
dry shampoo, 175
as exfoliant, 17-19
as facial masque, 51
hand care, 127
soap made from, 15
for sunburn, 115
Aloe vera
for acne, 67-68
for athlete's foot, 146
for burns/wound healing, 274
for cold sores, 151
for sunburn, 116
tanning lotion, 112
as vaginal douche, 92
Alpha hydroxy acids, for wrinkles, 80
Alum
eye compress, 167
for sunburn, 155
Ammonia
hand care, 127
as skin cleanser, 16
Anise, health benefits of, 275
Antioxidants, 217
Apples
as facial masque, 51-52
as skin toner, 30

Presented to:

_____

From:

_____

Date:

_____

WWJD

Stories for Teens

Honor Books
Tulsa, Oklahoma

2nd Printing

WWJD Stories for Teens (black gloss edition)
ISBN 1-56292-570-9
Copyright © 1998 by Honor Books
P.O. Box 55388
Tulsa, Oklahoma 74155

Compiled by Karen DeSollar

Introduction

Being a teen in today's world isn't easy. The gray area between right and wrong seems to have grown, and decisions are harder to make. Even as you struggle to win trust, freedom, and a chance to prove yourself to the world, the really important decisions become harder to make.

But the truth is that everyday you do have to make decisions—some that could seriously affect the rest of your life.

People expect a lot from you these days, and the pressure can really add up. You are expected to use your head, work hard, stay out of trouble, and still have fun.

How do you find answers that really make sense?

How can you get the help you need?

Where do you turn?

Look no further!

This book is for you. It is written about the real issues you face.

You will read about teens just like yourself, who had to face tough issues and make those hard decisions. And they did it the right way by taking time to stop, think, and ask—WHAT WOULD JESUS DO?

The good news is you can live your life the same way, with incredible grace and poise, if you will also ask *yourself*—WWJD?

Table of Contents

What Would Jesus Do regarding...

What Would Jesus Do regarding...

The Payoff

By Alan Cliburn

Marty Davis stared at me. "You mean you aren't gonna do anything?" he demanded.

"I didn't say that," I replied, drinking my orange juice.

"Steve Harper rips you off for over four hundred bucks and you act like it's nothing!" Marty hissed. "If he did that to me, I'd thrash him!"

I gave Marty a look. "You would not."

"Well, maybe not," he conceded. "But at least I'd try to get my money back."

"I thought about it," I admitted, "but then I took a look at what the Bible says."

"So in other words, Steve's getting away with it and you're letting him," Marty surmised.

"He's not getting away with anything," I corrected.

I couldn't blame Marty for being confused.

Actually the whole episode with Steve Harper started last Monday afternoon. I was in a hurry to get to work and backed out of my space in the student parking lot too fast, scratching Steve's car in the process.

It wasn't much of a scratch, especially since his door was all dinged up anyway, but I saw Steve coming and waited for him. Naturally he blew up. Anybody else would've shrugged it off or acted halfway rational, but that isn't Steve's style.

"You're gonna pay for this, Holloway," he informed me.

"I'm willing to pay for it," I said. "It was my fault. Just get an estimate and let me know how much it'll cost."

That calmed him down a little bit. "Yeah, okay. I'll bring the estimate tomorrow."

I felt slightly sick about scratching his car, but the next morning I felt a whole lot worse. The estimate from the body shop was all official and everything and the total was $396.78!

I stared at it without saying anything.

"They want the money ahead of time," Steve said. "How about tomorrow?"

I swallowed. I had been expecting maybe $200, tops. That scratch couldn't have been more than two or three inches long and a fraction of an inch wide. "Yeah, sure," I agreed.

So I took the money from my savings and had a check made out to the body shop.

Thursday afternoon I was making a delivery for my job and parked near the front of the body shop where Steve had taken his car. His blue Mazda was just sitting there, so after I finished my delivery, I decided to take a closer look.

"What do you need?" a man in dirty white overalls asked.

"Just looking at this car," I explained. "Belongs to a guy I know at school. In fact, I'm the reason it's here!"

"Yeah?"

"You sure did a good job on this door. Must have cost plenty," I continued.

"About $400," he answered, "give or take a couple bucks."

"No, I mean for the whole door," I said.

"That's what I mean, too," he answered.

I frowned. "How about the little scratch that was down here?" I asked. "How much would that have been?"

He shrugged. "Maybe $150 or $200. But it made more sense to do the whole door. Hey, there's my phone!"

Somehow I got through the rest of my deliveries, but it was hard. Steve made me pay for the whole door!

"So what are you going to do about it?" Dad wanted to know.

"I know what I'd like to do," I muttered. "Dad—"

"We could drive over to his house tonight and discuss it with his parents," Mom suggested.

"Would you like to do that, Matt?" Dad asked.

"I don't know," I said. "He's not getting away with it, though; that's for sure!"

"We already know that," Dad replied.

I frowned. "What do you mean?"

"Pastor Gibbons' sermon dealt with this last Sunday," he reminded me.

"Vengeance is mine," Mom said, quoting Romans 12:19. "God has His own way of dealing with people like Steve Harper, Matt."

I read some Scripture verses for myself and prayed about it before I went to sleep that night. *Okay, I'll do what God says,* I decided.

Marty just couldn't understand, though, no matter how many times I tried to explain it to him.

"You're still entitled to your money back," he insisted as we drove to school one morning. It was pouring down rain. "There's nothing unchristian about standing up for your rights, you know."

"Maybe not," I conceded.

Then suddenly there he was! Steve Harper! He was standing next to his car, getting soaked. There was a big puddle right near him, too.

"Splash him!" Marty told me.

But I didn't. Can't say I didn't think about it, but I just pulled over to the curb and asked Marty to open the door.

"Thanks a—" Steve began. Then he saw who he was talking to and froze.

"Get in," I invited. "We're gonna be late."

He did, and the look on his wet face was classic.

"What's wrong with your car?" I asked.

"Went through some deep water and got the points wet," he replied.

"Too bad," Marty said, looking straight ahead and trying to keep from laughing.

Steve couldn't get out of my car fast enough when we reached school. "Thanks," he managed.

"Okay," I called after him.

I gave him a ride back to his car after school, too. Marty had to stay late, so it was just the two of us.

"Looks like the rain's stopped," I said.

"Hope so," he replied.

We rode in silence for a few blocks.

"School year's really going fast, isn't it?" I asked.

"Uh huh."

I pulled up across from his car. "Shouldn't have any trouble starting it now," I told him.

He looked at me like he was going to say something, but instead he ran across the street, hopped into his car, and tried to start it. It caught on about the third try, so I waved and drove off, unable to describe the way I felt.

Happy seemed inadequate; joyful was a little vague. But I felt at peace about Steve. Even losing the money didn't seem to matter. Somehow I knew God would work things out in His own way and time and I didn't need to worry about it anymore.

w w j d   p o w e r   s t a t e m e n t

As Christians, we are to give everything to God, including our anger. He's big enough to hear about it, so feel free to tell Him how you really feel. He's also big enough to be trusted with it. He will work out all of the situations of our lives if we will allow Him to, in a way that brings glory to Him and benefits us too.

s c r i p t u r e

Losing your temper causes a lot of trouble,
but staying calm settles arguments.

PROVERBS 15:18 CEV

A Springtime Christmas

By Micah Stevens

You've probably heard someone say, "Wouldn't it be nice if it could be Christmas all year long?" I agree; it would be nice. But it seems like once the tree is down and all the decorations are packed away, that old "Christmas feeling" disappears too. This year, I don't think I even got into the spirit of Christmas while it was going on.

So no one was more surprised than I was to see the true meaning of Christmas unfold before my eyes during a work project I went on in Appalachia over spring break.

What happened that week helped me understand that God still uses unlikely people and sends them to unlikely places to bring us closer to Himself—just like He did two thousand years ago when He sent a baby to save the world. That's what He did when He sent Derek Armstrong to Appalachia.

Derek's the last guy you'd expect to see getting his hands dirty helping others. He has everything— money, good looks, good grades, athletic ability. While all the girls at youth group trip over themselves to talk to Derek, the guys would rather trip him up.

Even though Derek shows up almost every week, we guys know he's only doing it to look good. If there's something more interesting to do, Derek's out the door in a minute.

Like the four Sundays Derek missed because of the city-wide basketball tournament.

Nick and I saw Derek one Saturday practicing with his team at the basketball court. We talked with him a while and asked him if he was coming to the youth group on Sunday.

"I'd love to, but we made the final four in the tourney and I have to play tomorrow. But tell everyone 'hi' for me."

"That guy has absolutely no sense of what's important in life," I said as we went to the other end of the gym.

The Sunday after the tournament ended, Derek strolled into youth group wearing this bright red t-shirt that said, "City Basketball Champions."

From then on he wore it to youth group every Sunday. He wore it to school. He wore it to hang around in. If you saw Derek, you saw the t-shirt. With everything Derek owned, I was amazed at how important that shirt was to him.

All the guys in the youth group were surprised when Derek signed up to go on the missions trip. "Maybe a week of living with poor people will teach Derek what's important in life," I whispered. Nick nodded. We both knew what this guy needed was to get his priorities straight.

So a couple of weeks later when the bus rolled out of the church parking lot, Derek Armstrong was sitting in the back wearing his red basketball t-shirt and trying to act like one of the guys. We were all nice to him, but there was a sense of holding back our friendship until we saw if he and his new-found "servant attitude" was for real.

During the next week, there wasn't time to worry about Derek because we were all too busy working. We dug trenches for water pipes, built an addition to the school house, fixed roofs, and taught vacation Bible school. It was strange to see Derek knee-deep in mud digging a ditch while proudly wearing his basketball t-shirt over another thermal shirt to ward off the chilly April breeze.

We had a big party at week's end to dedicate the school addition, and people came from miles around. All the kids were excited about the games and treats they'd get. At the end of the day, we pulled out a big box of t-shirts our church had sent to give to the kids. You'd never seen so many happy faces as everyone lined up to get their shirts.

I guess it all went better than anyone had expected because when Mark, our youth pastor, handed out the last t-shirt, there was still one little boy standing in line—Samuel.

Samuel hadn't missed one event over the past week. He'd come to vacation Bible school, worked on the school addition, and generally helped whoever needed him. Everyone had grown to love Samuel.

Mark didn't know what to do. The rest of us just stood there looking at the sky or at the ground— anywhere but at Samuel.

But then Derek stepped forward. With a quick movement he pulled his red "City Basketball

Champions" t-shirt over his head and slid it over Samuel's. The red t-shirt swallowed Samuel, and it really stood out in the sea of sky-blue shirts our church had sent.

"This t-shirt is especially for you, Samuel," Derek said. "It's our thanks for all your help this week."

Everyone applauded as Derek stood there with his arm around Samuel. I thought Samuel was going to pop with happiness.

As I watched Derek, I knew I was seeing God's reason for having him on that work project. It wasn't so much for his benefit as it was for mine. God reminded me that He uses unlikely people in unlikely places to bring us closer to Him.

w w j d   p o w e r   s t a t e m e n t

So much of life has to do with our attitudes. With God's help, we have the power to choose to think the best about others, to not make judgment calls that are not ours to make, and to remember that each person is made in God's image.

s c r i p t u r e

You are God's children whom he loves, so try to be like him. Live a life of love just as Christ loved us.

EPHESIANS 5:1-2 NCV

Leroy and the Peaches

By Dennis C. Gerig

I stared at Leroy's grandmother. She wasn't making any sense at all.

"You don't have any peaches?" I repeated.

"Not anymore," Mrs. Kincaid replied.

Something just didn't add up. All I did was casually mention to Mrs. Kincaid how much we were enjoying her peaches. I mean, it was mostly just making conversation.

That's when she told me she didn't have peaches anymore. Something weird was going on. *Not that you should be surprised,* I reminded myself. *Not if it has something to do with Leroy!*

Leroy Kincaid had been going to our church for as long as I could remember, but somehow he never seemed to fit in, if you know what I mean. He wasn't stupid or anything; he was just—well, Leroy. He was dependable about coming, but he was shy and awkward and kind of nerdy-looking.

When we had a sports night at church, everyone hoped Leroy would be on the other team. No kidding, he was just so clumsy we couldn't believe it!

The youth pastor frequently made comments about how we should treat our Christian brothers and sisters and for a while, that seemed to make a difference, but then we'd go right back to leaving Leroy out of things.

17

Especially on Sunday nights after church. A bunch of us liked to go out to get something to eat after the service. It wasn't a youth group activity or anything; we just liked to do it. Giving Leroy the slip before he could ask for a ride became a weekly game for us.

"I feel sorry for Leroy," Lauren Nelson said one Sunday night as about ten of us surrounded a table, waiting for pizza. "He wants to be a part of us so bad."

"Well, I guess I could go back to the church and get him," I offered, starting to get up.

"That's all right," Lauren assured me quickly.

Then, about two months ago, everything changed. The choir director brought some peaches to Wednesday night rehearsal and they were really good.

"Enjoy them while you can," he said. "Our tree didn't produce a very big crop this year."

Suddenly, a soft, nasal voice which could belong to only one person spoke up.

"My grandmother has lots of peaches on her trees," Leroy announced. "I could bring some."

"That'd be great, Leroy," Mr. Anderson said, "if it's not too much trouble."

And he did. They were the big, juicy kind, too, and tasted fantastic after we had been singing for an hour.

"All right, Leroy!" Trevor exclaimed, slapping him on the back. "Best peaches I ever ate!"

"I'll bring some more next week," Leroy said.

Week after week Leroy brought those peaches and it definitely made a difference in how we treated him. We used to just sort of tolerate him and hope he would find some place else to sit with that annoying voice of his, but when he walked in with those peaches everybody cheered.

It never occurred to me that most peach trees have very short harvest periods. To be honest, I didn't give it a second thought. Or at least I didn't until this one Wednesday afternoon when I ran into Leroy's grandmother and found out the truth about her peach trees.

I was still thinking about it when I reached the store and started my shopping.

Just as I approached the produce section, I saw him. Leroy, I mean. He didn't see me, though, so I ducked behind a display of paper towels to watch him.

He was buying peaches! Not just a little sack of them, like I usually did, but a whole box! It was a flat box and Leroy was carefully sorting through the peaches, selecting only the biggest ones.

What a weirdo! I thought. Peaches weren't exactly cheap, after all. Of course it was Wednesday and he was apparently planning to take them to choir practice later on. No wonder the peaches hadn't tasted quite so good the past few weeks; store-bought fruit never tastes as good as fruit right off the tree.

I considered confronting Leroy right then, just to see what he'd say, but then I changed my mind. The kids at church would find it amusing that Leroy was trying to buy their friendship! In a way, it was an insult.

As I stood in line I contemplated how I would tell the other kids. "These are great peaches," I might say, "almost as good as the ones at Food Barn." I could just see Leroy's face. Or I could say, "By the way, Leroy, I saw someone who looks just like you at Food Barn this afternoon, buying peaches." Or, "Strangest thing happened today, Leroy. I ran into your grandmother and she told me her peach trees stopped producing fruit about a month ago."

I wasn't sure what approach I would take, but expose him I would. What kind of a guy would spend his hard-earned money on peaches? As the answer to that question began to sink in, I swallowed hard. A very lonely guy, that's who. Also a very insecure guy who was willing to do just about anything to be accepted.

The dumb thing about it was that it had sort of worked, at least on the surface. As long as Leroy kept bringing those peaches, we had treated him better. He was our "brother in the Lord," yet, he had to buy our acceptance. I felt really bad as I realized that I was as guilty as anyone—maybe guiltier, in fact. *God, forgive me,* I prayed.

Leroy was still selecting peaches when I came up next to him.

"Hi, Leroy," I began.

He looked at me, then back at the peaches—which he tried unsuccessfully to hide—and blushed. "Uh, hi, Brad," he managed.

"You don't need to bring any peaches tonight," I said.

"But everybody likes them—"

"Just bring yourself this time," I interrupted. "Okay?"

He was putting the peaches back by then, but he looked at me. "Will you tell the others—"

"That you were buying peaches?" I finished. "No. Anyway, these aren't nearly as good as your grandmother's."

He nodded. "I know."

"See you tonight," I said, heading for the checkout stand again.

I doubted that Leroy Kincaid and I would ever become good buddies or anything, but I vowed to treat him as my brother in Christ, not like some misfit; and that included Sunday night after church, too.

I wouldn't bother to explain my change of attitude to the others, though. My example would say it all.

w w j d   p o w e r   s t a t e m e n t

Jesus loves and accepts each of us just the way we are, even those of us who aren't the most popular or attractive. His church is the place where everyone should be able to find that kind of love and acceptance.

s c r i p t u r e

*If two or three people come together in my name,
I am there with them.*

MATTHEW 18:20 NCV

21

Like a Piece of Raw Meat

By Derek Graham

I don't know who ever said there was nothing competitive about church basketball games, but I think they lied, er, rather, exaggerated.

Or at least that's how I felt after the game against Southside church. They tromped over us so badly that I felt kind of like a piece of steak after Mom's taken her meat pounder to it and tenderized it—only we endured their pounding for an hour and a half. Fortunately, by the time I helped put up the equipment and got to the locker room, no one was left from their team. When I got out of the shower, only Michael was in the room. He just sat on the bench, socks in hand, looking at his feet.

The shower washed away a lot of gloom, but I still didn't feel like talking; so since Michael didn't say anything, neither did I. By the time I started to pull on my shoes and fresh socks, Michael was a little farther along. He had his sock half on one foot and was staring at his heel, like his mind was in a galaxy far away.

I was so sore I couldn't help but moan as I sat down. He looked at me mutely—his eyes full of misery. *He must be taking this worse than I expected,* I thought. Maybe if I looked on the bright side, it would help.

"Hey, Michael, it's not really that bad. It's not like it's the end of the world. By this time tomorrow, you'll have forgotten all about it." I gave him a weak grin, but he just stared.

"It's no use," he plied hopelessly, "I feel lousy."

"Okay, so we were slaughtered. Their guys were twice as tall as ours and their guards blocked like football players."

"Huh?" He asked, looking at me as if I was crazy. "What are you talking about?"

"The game. What else?"

Something seemed to snap in Michael's brain. "Oh . . . I was thinking about something else," he lamely explained.

"Wanna' talk about it?" I offered.

"Derek, every since I became a Christian last year, I've tried so hard to do everything that would please God. But no matter how hard I try, I just can't seem to control my temper."

I nodded. Michael and I had discussed his temper before. "You've come a long way. I remember when we used to have to walk on eggshells around you." At 6'2", he wasn't a good person to mess with.

"Yeah, but I haven't come far enough. I blew up at my mom before I came tonight. I was hotter than I've ever been—let alone since becoming a Christian. I said things to her that were horrible—especially for a Christian to say. How can I ever read my Bible or come to Bible study or pray again? God must be totally disgusted with me."

"We all blow it sometimes . . ." I reassured him.

"Not like I did," Michael moaned, "and not just tonight. It seems like I'm always failing. I might as well give it up. God must be sick of me by now."

"God isn't like us," I said carefully. " We get tired of forgiving someone when they keep doing the same stupid things. We may get mad with the person, but God . . . Look, when you blow it in a basketball game, you don't just throw down the ball, walk off the court and quit the team. You don't figure the coach is mad at you for failing, and the coach doesn't kick you off the team just because you blew it."

"Unless it's Coach Eisele." Michael interrupted with a grin.

"Yeah," I grinned. Coach Eisele, our school coach, was well known for his ruthless punishments. "But fortunately, God's not like Coach Eisele. The Bible says that God's understanding is unlimited. He understands when we blow it, and why we blow it. That doesn't mean He wants us to mess up or that we can do any old thing we want, figuring He'll forgive us. But failures will come. Remember what we studied in Bible study last Wednesday night?"

"In Hebrews?" Michael asked.

"Yeah," I said as I pulled my Bible out of the locker. We have Bible studies before the games, so I had mine with me.

"This is what stuck with me." I thumbed through it for a minute and then showed it to Michael. "For we do not have a high priest who is unable to sympathize with our weaknesses, but we have one who has been tempted in every way, just as we are—yet was without sin."

"I must have missed that the other night." Michael admitted.

"You were too busy studying Stacy," I teased. He grinned sheepishly.

"Yeah, but even though God understands, I still feel pretty horrible about it."

"Then let's read on. 'Let us then approach the throne of grace with confidence, so that we may receive mercy and find grace to help us in our time of need.' Because He understands our temptations, we can know He'll welcome us when we come to Him to admit our sins. Not only does He welcome our confession, but He promises to forgive us." I commented.

"Yeah, I remember studying that in discipleship class after I got saved. It's John 1:9," Michael filled in. "But if we have to come to Him to forgive us over and over again, well, doesn't He ever get sick of it? Doesn't our sin ever add up enough that he won't forgive us anymore, where we could be put on probation or something?" he questioned.

"He promises when we confess our sins, He will remember them no more. When we confess a sin and He forgives us, it's like we've never sinned—we get to start out again with a clean scoreboard. And since He's promised to forget them, there's no need for us to keep reminding ourselves."

He sighed. "Well, I guess besides asking God to forgive me, I need to ask Mom to forgive me, too. I wish her understanding was as unlimited as God's. I'm afraid she rates closer to Coach Eisele."

"It won't be so bad," I reassured. "She'll give you the benefit of the doubt. After all, you're her kid. And

25

she'll be glad you've matured enough to admit you were wrong."

"Maybe the Lord will make it into an opportunity to share more about Him with Mom."

"I wouldn't be surprised. C'mon. Let's stop by for a hamburger. My treat," I offered.

As I stood up, pain shot through my limbs. I groaned. "Man, just wait until we play those guys again. I'm going to make them feel like a piece of raw meat."

Michael finished tying his shoes and stood up, stretching his long arms to the ceiling. Looking down at me, he grinned and shook his head. "Where's your level of forgiveness, Derek?"

"About even with Coach Eisele's," I admitted leveling a basketball at his stomach. "Let's go."

w w j d   p o w e r   s t a t e m e n t

Jesus understands the confusion we feel, but He doesn't want us to live in it. We can trust His Word to tell us the truth so we don't have to rely on our feelings or on our ability to understand.

s c r i p t u r e

Trust GOD from the bottom of your heart;
don't try to figure out everything on your own.
Listen for GOD's voice in everything you do,
everywhere you go; he's the one
who will keep you on track.

PROVERBS 3:5-6

Geronimo!

By Marlys G. Stapelbroek

Cold wind pushed past Ryan's face. *Faster,* he chanted silently. The fastest downhill ever. The finish line flashed past. Skidding to a halt, Ryan pushed up his goggles, then skied over to his coach.

"Top 15 for sure," Coach Myers assured him with a pat on the back. "You'll get some points."

Ryan blinked quickly. Rating points. He always won some, but what he wanted was a medal.

"You're racing A league now," the coach reminded him. "You can't expect to win every week."

"How about once in a while?" Ryan grumbled.

The coach sighed. "You're a good racer, but you ski with your head. To win, you have to let yourself go."

The loudspeaker crackled. "Girls' Class A Downhill, Jeanie Zell on course."

The coach patted Ryan's arm. "I've got to watch Jeanie. Don't worry about it, okay?"

Ryan tried to smile as he watched a red streak flash across the finish line. She didn't race with her head. She flew down the mountain.

Stopping beside him, she tugged off her white racing helmet. "Whew! I almost bought it on that transition gate." Before he could answer, she pointed behind him. "The lifts are still running. Let's hit Logger's Run one more time!"

They skied over to the chairlift, but as it carried them up the mountain, Ryan found himself thinking back to the race.

27

"Why do you do it?" he blurted out.

"What?"

"Push so hard?"

She grinned. "With three older brothers, I was always complaining about being left behind. Finally Dad told me to quit bellyaching and use that energy to keep up instead."

But aren't you afraid? Ryan didn't ask the question. He knew where it would lead. Somehow they'd end up arguing about the fact that Jeanie didn't believe in God.

God's just an excuse for people afraid to live their own lives.

That's how she'd ended their last discussion, and right now, Ryan didn't feel like arguing.

But the question wouldn't go away. Why wasn't she afraid? Because he sure was. Deep inside ran a thread of fear that kept his head in control and stopped him from winning.

"Heads up," Jeanie called, pushing off the chair and onto the exit ramp. Ryan followed, skating hard to catch up.

"Hey!" he shouted as Jeanie headed toward a narrow path. "The runs on the north face close at four."

"It's only 3:59," she shouted, then let out a whoop as she plunged onto Logger's Run. "Geronimooooo!" Her cry echoed as Ryan watched her attack the steep slope.

Sucking in a cold breath, he started after her. He could feel his own skiing, the precise rhythm, the smoothness. It had none of the abandon that made people gasp as Jeanie flew down a slope. Safe skiing meant that he rarely fell and never got hurt, but it also meant that he never won.

Below him, the red figure of his friend suddenly disappeared into a cloud of snow. She'd fallen. Changing course, Ryan headed toward the snowy red heap.

"Jeanie?" he called, stopping beside her.

"Ohh," she moaned. "My leg. I think it's broken!"

"Broken?" Ryan whispered glancing at the deserted slope above them.

Jeanie groaned again. "Coach'll kill me."

"If he gets the chance."

"What?"

Stooping, Ryan slid his jacket beneath her. "The sun's below the mountains. The north face gets dark fast."

"The ski patrol—"

"They'll find us on their final sweep, but they'll have to ride back up to get a toboggan and then carry you down in the dark." Not to mention the possibility of exposure and shock. The temperature was dropping fast as the sun's warmth seeped out of the air. But Ryan kept those fears to himself. "I'm going for help."

"Don't leave. . . . It hurts bad."

He was sure of it. Jeanie never complained, and the strange angle of her leg made his throat tight.

"I have to go, Jeanie. Now." He controlled his voice; hid his fear. "If I get to the bottom before the patrol starts down, we can phone the top, tell them where you are and to bring a toboggan. It'll save time—lots of it."

She nodded slowly, but her fingers tightened around his wrist. "Ryan?" she whispered, "Geronimo."

He frowned. Why had she said—? And then he understood. She was asking him to ski fast, super fast. The way she'd ski.

"Geronimo," he promised, but as her hand fell away and he pushed off, he knew he couldn't ski like that. Not during a race and not now, with deep shadows stretched across the mountain.

His skis twisted as he hit a bump. Wrenching his body, he found his balance. But every second made it harder to see . . .

Hurry, hurry, hurry.

He had to get to the bottom before the patrol started down. But the thick gloom of dusk caught at his fear. He could barely see. If he hurried, he'd fall—

Yea, though I walk through the valley of the shadow of death, I will fear no evil: for thou art with me.

The words surfaced from his memory. Squinting down at the shadowed slope below him, Ryan understood. Fear. The fear that kept him from winning. But this time victory meant helping Jeanie. Jeanie who didn't believe in God, who might die not knowing Jesus.

For thou art with me. The whispered words were gone before Ryan heard them, but they echoed in his heart. Thrusting his fear toward God, he pushed his skis into the fall line and headed down the mountain.

Unweight, his head ordered. *Turn.* His brain worked faster and faster as his skis pounded over the moguls.

"Shut up," he shouted, wishing he could turn off his head. His right leg flew up. Throwing his body to the side, he landed on his feet and plunged on down the slope.

Be with me—

Another bump! His leg twisted, but as if a switch had been thrown, his thoughts remained silent. His knees sucked up the bump. Beneath his skis he felt the mountain. His body flowed with the roll of the land.

"Geronimo!" The wind caught the word, dissolving his cry as he slid over a patch of ice. Trees and signs flew past. He couldn't see them, but he knew they were there. Skiing blind. But a part of him seemed in touch with the mountain, warning him when to turn, when to ride his skis flat.

The bottom. Beside the chairlift he saw the rust-colored jacket of a ski patrol—

"Jeanie!" he shouted, skidding to a halt beside the man.

"Hey, watch where you're—"

"She's hurt," Ryan gasped, "up on Logger's Run. Jeanie's hurt!"

With a quick nod, the man skied to the lift house and the phone. Leaning over his poles, Ryan sucked deep breaths.

God's just an excuse for people afraid to live their own lives. Jeanie's challenge echoed softly, and Ryan smiled. Finally, her own brand of courage had pushed her too far. Maybe, just maybe, she'd need a little of God's courage to come back. If she did, he'd be ready to tell her about it.

w w j d   p o w e r   s t a t e m e n t

Jesus wants His followers to live with courage; to not be afraid of what the world dishes out because He has overcome the world. We can have a spirit of boldness because of the confidence we have in Him.

s c r i p t u r e

Light, space, zest—that's GOD! So, with him on my side I'm fearless, afraid of no one and nothing.

PSALM 27:1

The Invitation

By Kent Phillips

You're late," Mom said as I walked into the house after school.

"I know. Danielle needed a ride."

Mom didn't say anything, but there was that disapproving look again. I saw it whenever I mentioned Danielle's name.

"Any calls?" I asked.

"No, but there's some mail on your desk."

Most of the mail I got was ads and other junk, and I seemed to be getting more of it as high school graduation came closer. But this one big square-shaped white envelope caught my eye right away.

It was a wedding invitation, the first I'd ever received. My parents usually got them and I was just included in the words "and family" on the envelope.

"Mr. and Mrs. Henry Caldwell request the honor of your presence at the wedding of their daughter, Amanda Renee, to Mr. Jared A. Burnett Jr." It gave the time and date.

Jared used to live right across the street, and, even though he was a year oler than I, we were really good friends.

In fact, it was Jared and his parents who started my family going to church, where all of us eventually accepted Christ. Jared and I became even better friends after that.

The Burnetts moved about two years ago, but that didn't change a thing between Jared and me. Since I didn't drive yet, Jared would pick me up for youth group on Sunday nights.

I was with Jared the day he met Amanda Caldwell. It was last year, right after school got out for the summer, and we were at the beach.

"I wish I was finished with high school," I told Jared while we were stretched out on the sand.

"Yeah, it's a good feeling," he agreed. "I'm looking forward to college, too."

"Have you decided where you're going yet?"

"I've been praying about it a lot," he said. "I want to go to a Christian college."

I nodded in agreement.

"Hey, check this out!" Jared whispered suddenly poking me in the ribs.

I sat up just as a girl walked by and spread her blanket about three feet in front of us.

"Guess she couldn't find her own bathing suit," I snickered. "Had to borrow her little sister's!" No kidding, it was barely there.

The next thing I knew, Jared and this girl—who turned out to be Amanda—started talking. I had been to the beach with Jared lots of times, but he had never talked to strange girls before.

Jared and Amanda got along really well from the very beginning. It turned out that she had just graduated too, so for starters, they had that in common. Come to think of it, they seemed to have everything in common.

Well, almost everything, as Jared soon discovered.

"Do you go to church?" he asked casually

"I have better things to do with my time," she replied. "Oh, I've been a couple times, and what a bore!"

They talked the whole time we were there, and before we left he had written down her phone number.

"Are you really going to call her?" I asked on the way home. "I thought you didn't date non-Christians," I said.

"This is different," he interrupted. "She needs Christ, and it's obvious that she isn't going to start going to church on her own."

"You mean you'll bring her to church?" I wondered a little suspiciously.

"I'm sure going to try," he said.

And he did bring her, twice, I think. He and Amanda started dating a lot after that, and I began to see less and less of Jared, except at church. Then one Sunday he called and said he wouldn't be able to pick me up because he was going to a barbecue at Amanda's house.

"It's a family thing," he explained, "and really important to her."

After that I hardly saw him at all. I got my driver's license about that same time and didn't really miss him very much. Sure, Jared and I had been good friends, but I had gotten used to not being with him after he met Amanda.

I guess the last time I saw Jared was by accident— or at least it wasn't planned. I pulled into a service station to get some gas one Friday night and there he was in the cashier's booth.

"That'll be $12.60," he said before he saw who it was. "Hey, Mike, how're you doing?" he exclaimed. "I keep planning to get over to see you, but working two jobs—"

"Two jobs?" I repeated, frowning. "Aren't you in college, Jared?"

He looked a little embarrassed. "Couldn't swing it this year. Costs money, you know."

"Jared, where are you going to church now? I haven't seen you in over—"

"If the boss catches me talking instead of working, I'll get canned," he interrupted. "Good to see you again, Mike!"

Meeting Danielle didn't exactly increase the free time I had available either. She was in my senior English class and really great. We became friends right away and I found her easy to talk to. I even got up enough nerve to invite her to church.

"I don't believe in religion," she replied, "But thanks anyway."

I was really stunned when she said that, because she was such a nice girl. For some reason I expected non-Christian girls to be completely different. Danielle didn't smoke or drink or swear or cheat on tests, or anything like that.

"The only difference is that she doesn't believe in Jesus," I told my mother when she wanted to know about Danielle.

"Only?" my mother repeated. "Mike, do you realize what you're saying? The Bible makes it clear that a Christian should not marry a non-Christian."

I stared at her. "Marry? Mom, I've only taken her out a couple of times! I'm not even out of high school yet!"

I was writing down the date of Jared's wedding on my calendar when Mom came in.

"I see you opened your invitation," she said.

"Yeah. I can hardly believe he's getting married, though. Jared's barely a year older than I am."

"His parents can hardly believe it either," Mom replied.

I frowned. "Are they against it?"

"I talked to Mrs. Burnett just yesterday They are really struggling with the idea."

I swallowed. "Amanda isn't . . . ?"

Mom looked at me. "Oh no, nothing like that and they do like her. It's just that—"

"She's not a Christian," I surmised.

"Right?"

"But maybe she'll become one later," I began.

"That's what they thought when Jared first started dating her, but it hasn't worked out that way. In fact, it's just the opposite. Jared seldom goes to church, and seems to have no interest in spiritual things."

She spoke of Jared and Amanda, but her eyes were directed at me.

"Wait a minute," I said, suddenly getting the message. "Is this the reason you're against my dating Danielle?"

"Well, she isn't a Christian," Mom replied.

"Yeah, but I don't love her or anything," I insisted.

"Jared didn't love Amanda at first," she reminded me.

"But Danielle—"

"Why did you miss the youth group party last Saturday?" Mom asked.

"Danielle wanted to go horseback riding instead," I answered. "But—" I stopped to think. The party was just one thing I missed because of her. There had been a couple of other things. And I had done them willingly, just because I wanted to be with her.

I thought about Danielle for a long time after Mom left the room. Without my even realizing it, she was becoming more and more important to me. I didn't even eat lunch with the kids from church anymore. I usually ate with Danielle and her friends. They were nice, but they didn't pretend to be Christians.

So what are you going to do now? I asked myself. It was a good question. It would be hard to break up with Danielle. I had grown used to having her at my side, and I liked the feeling.

I hadn't talked to her about my faith for a while. We talked about everything else instead. That would have to change. If our relationship was going to go any further, she'd have to start going to church and learning more about Christianity. My relationship with Christ was the most important thing in my life and I wasn't about to lose it, not even for a girl like Danielle.

It took Jared's invitation to open my eyes.

w w j d   p o w e r   s t a t e m e n t

To become emotionally attached to a non-believer is dangerous. Your reason and spirituality can be clouded by emotion, which can create a painful no-win situation. It is far wiser to date those whose lives are centered around the same Jesus you serve.

s c r i p t u r e

Don't become partners with those who reject God. How can you make a partnership out of right and wrong? That's not partnership; that's war. Is light best friends with dark?

2 CORINTHIANS 6:14

The Silver Death

By Marlys G. Stapelbroek

I was asleep when the mountain first rumbled. My sister shook me awake. "Lana, it's thunder!"

"No, Puni," I murmured, clinging to sleep, "the sunset was clear."

"I heard it!"

Opening one eye, I peered at her in the moonlight. Rubbing my eyes, I realized it was getting lighter, not slowly like dawn, but quickly like the tail wind of a hurricane sweeping clouds off into the Pacific.

A cold fear exploded inside me. Grabbing Puni's hand, I pulled her from our room, running toward the door.

The roar of thunder was louder this time, the flash of light longer and brighter. Mother met us by the door. It was open, and Daddy stood on the lawn, staring toward Kilauea.

"The Silver Death," Mother murmured, her face ashen. "Grandmother warned it would come again."

Puni gripped my hand. "What's the Silver—?" The thunder of explosions came again as a stream of fire arced across the sky. Golden light warmed the darkness. Or was it the heat of the fire? It was miles away, but my face seemed to burn as fireworks shot skyward again.

Mother trembled. "The mountain will kill us all."

Grabbing her arm, I shouted, "We have to leave."

"No. No, Grandmother stayed and saved the house."

Father's voice came from the doorway. "Lana's right. We have to get out. We'll stay with your sister." He stood silhouetted against the fiery sky, his face in shadows, but I heard the fear in his voice. Even my father, who was never afraid, was scared. My stomach knotted.

A thunderous clap cracked the air—an explosion inside the volcano. The ground shook as a fireball rained flames onto the hillside. Instantly fires sprang up, trees and bushes flaring into torches. Moments later only their smoldering skeletons remained. Golden streams of lava cut paths down the mountainside, flowing toward the cluster of homes that stood between Kilauea and the sea.

"We have to go!" Father shouted. "Grab small things we can put in the car!"

Puni nodded, then fled to our room. I know what she wanted. The stuffed bear she'd had forever and probably the new pink dress Mother had finally bought her yesterday.

"Mother!" I shook her, pulling her back from the door. "Get your jewelry. And the pictures. The family albums."

It took me less than a minute to dress, jeans, tennis shoes, and a long-sleeved shirt. I looked around. What should I take? I saw my Bible, with its worn cover and two years of thoughts and lessons scratched in the margins. Grabbing it, I fled into the fire-lit night.

Mother was shaking and Daddy pushed me behind the wheel of the car. "Drive," he ordered "and don't

stop until you get to Aunt Kai's. I'm going to help the
Hales. With Emma's bad hip, they might need help."

My hands shook on the wheel, but the soft pressure
of Daddy's kiss calmed me. Blowing a kiss back, I
pulled out of the driveway.

Already cars jammed the road, using both lanes to
flee the Silver Death. We had driven nearly two miles
when an explosion deep within the earth rocked the
car. My hands tightened on the wheel. The mountain's
roar rang in my ears. The lava became a night sun.

Daddy! Fear welled up inside me, but I said nothing.
There was no going back. Two streams of cars moved
relentlessly forward, away from the mountain, away
from death.

For hours we sat in Aunt Kai's kitchen, waiting,
praying, hoping. It was morning before the rangers
finally came and told us. The Hale's house had been cut
off by the lava. Before they could help, it had burned.

Mother's wail rose into the cool morning air. I
buried my cries deep inside. *How could God have taken
everything from us?* First our home, everything we
owned, and then, most horribly, Daddy. Why?

There was government aid for the families who'd
lost homes. We bought a small house on the outskirts
of Hilo. We bought new dishes and chairs and clothes.
But I was haunted by the death of my father. God held
all life in His hands. Why would He choose death for
us, His children?

It was a month before the rangers allowed us to
visit our land. The Silver Death was everywhere. The
golden lava that had shot from Kilauea had cooled

into a silver sea sliding over the land, hot enough to consume anything in its path. There was nothing left, not a building or tree or bush. The hard crust of the lava had sealed the land within a silver tomb. I cried.

I started walking, knowing only that I had to get away. I followed the road back to the edge of the lava flow, then kept walking. The land around me was still barren, consumed by the Silver Death years before when I'd been only a child. But as I walked, I was drawn to a twisted crevice where a pair of flowering plants had pushed through the hard crust. They at least were alive, in spite of the Silver Death.

Or maybe, because of it.

I don't know where the thought came from, but instantly I knew it was true. A million years ago the big island of Hawaii had not existed. A thousand eruptions, each bringing death, had created the island, giving it life.

I had always thought of death as the end of life, but was it? The Silver Death of the volcanoes had given life to my island. Christ's death had meant spiritual life for me.

And what of my father's death? Was the death of his body also a gateway to a brand new life?

"For God so loved the world . . ." How many times had I repeated John 3:16? It was the verse every Christian knew, but now I really heard the words. ". . . that whosoever believeth in Him should not perish, but have everlasting life."

Death was the gateway to eternal life. The Silver Death had taken Daddy to the streets of gold.

Bending down, I picked the flower that had defeated the Silver Death. I would put it on my father's grave.

w w j d   p o w e r   s t a t e m e n t

The death or loss of someone you love can be so devastating that it doesn't feel like you will ever be able to fill the void. But God is in the habit of making things new and, in time, He will heal your heart if you trust in Him.

s c r i p t u r e

He[God] will destroy death forever. The Lord GOD will wipe away every tear from every face.

ISAIAH 25:8 NCV

Like Geese Flying South

By Walt Carter

Grandpa was raking leaves when Eric turned the corner and hurried up Chestnut Lane. Just seeing his grandfather made Eric feel a little better and he quickened his pace slightly.

"Hi, Grandpa," he said a moment later, entering the yard.

"Well, this is a pleasant surprise!" his grandfather exclaimed. "Thought you and the other boys were playing football."

Eric swallowed. "Can I help you rake?"

"I need the exercise," his grandfather answered. "Think I've corralled enough leaves for today, though. Maybe I can get your grandmother to make us some hot chocolate if I ask her real nice."

"Sounds good to me," Eric admitted.

"I'm glad to see you, Eric," his grandfather went on, leading the way to an old-fashioned porch swing.

At least somebody wants me around, Eric thought, bitterly recalling what had happened at the park less than fifteen minutes earlier. But he forced a smile. "Thanks, Grandpa."

"Your grandmother just doesn't appreciate the finer things of life," the old man continued.

Eric frowned. "The finer things?"

43

"Like watching geese fly south for the winter," his grandfather explained, pointing. Eric looked up to see a giant "V" passing overhead, made up entirely of birds. "Would you believe she'd rather stay inside working on a quilt than come outside to watch the geese?"

"That's hard to believe, all right," Eric agreed, grinning. He observed the birds as they continued on, maintaining their perfect formation, one of them the undisputed leader. His grin faded as quickly as it had come; Eric knew that feeling. Or at least, he had known it.

He had always been a leader. Even when they moved and he was new in the neighborhood, Eric soon had the other boys playing the games he wanted to play and asking for his help to build things. He just always knew how to take charge.

It was the same at school. If there was a class election, Eric was automatically nominated for president. Even substitute teachers picked him as line leader or team captain in elementary school. It had been happening so long that Eric expected it.

"Runs in the family," his father had told him when Eric ran for student council in seventh grade and won by a landslide. "Some people just naturally have more leadership ability than others."

"That's me, all right," Eric agreed, still excited about his latest triumph.

"But it's also a God-given gift," his father added, "and it's important that you use it to glorify Christ instead of yourself."

"I know," Eric replied, and he meant it, too. He wasn't ashamed of his faith in Jesus and had invited lots of kids to church.

His leadership ability extended into other areas, too. Due to a budget cut, after school sports had been eliminated at the junior high Eric attended. "Well, good-bye to football," one of the guys muttered when the coach announced the cutback.

"Yeah," somebody else agreed.

"Wait a minute, you guys," Eric began when the coach had finished. "If we want to play football after school, we don't have to do it here. Let's meet at the park at 3:30. I'll bring the football."

Enough guys for two teams showed up for practice at 3:30, so they spent the rest of the afternoon running plays and having a great time. Eric had grinned to himself. *And I set this up*, he thought, satisfied.

Everything was going okay until "he" showed up, Eric thought grimly, remembering the afternoon a tall boy with dark hair and long arms had suddenly appeared. For a few minutes he just stood on the sidelines watching.

"Hey, can I play?" he asked finally.

The other boys looked at Eric, as usual. "Sure," Eric decided, "go out for a pass."

He threw the ball as hard and as far as he could, but somehow the new guy was there in time to catch it. Then he sent it back, the ball spiraling beautifully as it went straight to Eric.

"What a pass!" one of the guys standing near Eric exclaimed.

At first, Eric was glad to have someone like David on the team, but that feeling was quickly replaced by one of apprehension and uncertainty when the other guys started looking to David for advice. He was more than willing to give it, too. Some of the plays he suggested were pretty good, Eric admitted.

"My dad's the new football coach at State University," David explained when someone asked how come he knew so much about the game. "I've been playing all my life. I think I had a football in my crib instead of a rattle!"

Everybody laughed; even Eric. But it had been a forced laugh for him. The guys were getting better, there was no doubt about that, but he always hoped and prayed that David wouldn't show up for practice. Oh, he was still the leader—until David arrived. David even brought extra footballs for the guys to practice with when they weren't running plays.

Eric hadn't liked it, but he had been willing to live with it—up until this afternoon.

They were getting ready to run a few plays when the park director arrived on the scene with a clipboard in his hands.

"Listen, I've been watching you guys lately and I think you're ready for a little competition," he said. "The director of Northside Park thinks he has a pretty tough team, but I told him I had a team over here that's twice as tough. How about this Saturday afternoon at two? Right here."

"That would be great," Eric replied quickly. "Okay with you guys?"

They all nodded agreement.

"We'll have to put together some sort of roster," the park director went on. "Who's the captain of this team?"

"We've never picked one," Eric had answered.

"Maybe we'd better do that right now then," the park director decided.

"I nominate Nicholson," a voice said.

"I second it," another added.

The voting had been almost unanimous, Eric thought, looking up as more geese flew over. Only a few of his really loyal friends had voted for him. Angry and hurt, he had slipped away when no one was looking, with no plans to return.

"Here's the hot chocolate," his grandfather said suddenly, handing a cup to Eric. "My, those geese have been flying south all day. Remember when you were first learning your letters and used to cry out 'V!' when you saw the geese?"

"No, not really," Eric said. "How do they know to fly in that 'V' formation?"

"I used to think it was just instinct," his grandfather replied, "and to some extent, it is. But it's also aeronautically sound. By flying in a 'V' formation, they somehow encounter less friction and make the trip much faster. Teamwork has a lot to do with it, too. If each bird set out by itself, a lot of them wouldn't make it."

Eric didn't answer. At that moment he didn't appreciate hearing about teamwork.

"And see that bird at the very front?" Grandpa asked.

"Sure," Eric answered, "he's the leader."

"One of the leaders," his grandfather corrected.

Eric frowned. "One of the leaders? There's only room for one bird in the lead position. See?"

"One at a time," his grandfather said. "But when you've watched geese fly south for as many years as I have, you'll discover that pretty soon the lead bird drops back and another one takes its place."

Eric looked up again just as the lead bird in the formation passing overhead did indeed drop back.

"One bird could never stand the strain of leading the formation all the way south," Grandpa continued. "There's a time to lead and a time to rest. Every leader must be a follower sooner or later."

Eric glanced at his grandfather quickly. Did he know what had happened at the park? But the old man was gazing at the sky, obviously enjoying the migration of the geese.

Is that it? Eric wondered. *Had he been a leader so long he didn't know how to be a follower?* He wouldn't even admit to himself that David was a better football player. Or at least he hadn't admitted it up to now.

"I'd better get back to the park, Grandpa," he said suddenly, standing up. "We have a football game Saturday at two o'clock. Want to come?"

"Wouldn't miss it," his grandfather replied, smiling. "See you then."

Geese flying south for the winter, Eric thought as he hurried back to the park. *God could use anything to teach a guy a lesson!*

wwjd power statement

Discouragement can come from many places and in many forms. It helps to remember that we have God to lean on when we are down. We have His unlimited resources and power to help us.

scripture

Why are you down in the dumps, dear soul?
Why are you crying the blues? Fix my eyes
on God—soon I'll be praising again. He puts
a smile on my face. He's my God.

PSALM 43:5

Nobody Knew Me

By Alan Cliburn

Nobody knew me. It was a strange sensation after growing up in a sleepy little village in the Midwest where everybody knew everything about everybody but I liked the anonymity of city living—instantly.

Yeah, there were some people back home I missed—kids I had grown up with, for example. But I sure didn't miss living under a microscope. I couldn't spit back home without Mrs. Crousemeyer telling my mom about it. Suddenly nobody cared what I did or said. I closed my locker before removing my thumb one morning, and a short, very explicit word escaped my lips. It was what is known as an "involuntary response," and I got really embarrassed after I said it.

I glanced around, ready to apologize. Nobody standing nearby expected me to. Only one or two people acted like they heard me, and they smiled approval. There were no shocked expressions.

But I'm a Christian, I reminded myself. *That makes a difference, or shouldn't it?*

I stood in the middle of the quadrangle during lunch hour and looked around me. There were kids all over the place. The high school back home was a fraction the size of this one, and all the kids knew each other.

"You're to set an example for the others, Todd," my father had told me. "You understand your responsibility?"

"I understand," I had replied.

There had been many times when I didn't feel like setting an example, but I seldom gave in to that desire. The consequences were too great when you live in a small town. My dad wasn't mean, but he was strict.

Despite the pressure, I really didn't want to move when Dad accepted the responsibility to edit a monthly Christian magazine. Of course I didn't realize how much pressure I had been under until it was lifted. It was the only lifestyle I had known.

"How're you doing, Blakely?"

I smiled as some guy from one of my classes—English, I think—walked up to me. "Barkley," I corrected. "Todd Barkley."

"Sorry."

"That's okay," I assured him. I meant it, too. Blakely! These kids didn't even know my name!

"Were you looking for somebody?"

"Oh, no. Just looking around, checking the place out." He grinned. "Checking out the women, you mean!"

I blushed in spite of myself, even though I really hadn't been looking at the girls at all. Not the way he meant anyway.

"I'm Jeremy Freeman. Interested in coming to a party at my house Friday night?"

"I was thinking of going to the game," I replied.

"This is after the game," he said. "Think about it. I'll be talking to you again before Friday. See you later."

"Thanks a lot, Jeremy," I called after him.

I had seen Jeremy a few times since transferring; he seemed pretty popular. He'd be a good guy to know, I decided. Anyway a party would be a good way to get acquainted.

I went to the basketball game, as scheduled, and then to the party even though I wasn't planning to stay long.

"How long will you be gone?" my dad had asked as I was leaving.

"Can't say," I replied. It was the usual question, and I had answered it willingly before, but now I resented it.

"Well, what time will the game be over?" he wanted to know.

I shrugged. "Ten o'clock, I guess. But I've been invited to a party afterward."

My parents looked at each other. "What kind of party?" Mom asked.

"Just a party" I told her, annoyed.

"It's not at the church, is it?" Dad questioned.

"No. Look, I have to go, or I'll be late."

"Get home early, Todd," Dad called after me.

Maybe there was nothing wrong with parents interrogating a twelve-year-old kid before he left the house on a Friday night, but when that same kid is nearly seventeen, it's slightly hard to take.

The game was really good. With so many more students, I guess there was a lot more competition to make the team than there had been at my old school. I sat with Jeremy and some of his friends.

"Coming to the party?" Jeremy asked during a time-out.

"Yeah, for a little while," I replied. "You'll have to give me directions, though."

"I'll just have somebody ride with you," Jeremy said. "How about you, Shannon?"

"Fine," she agreed, smiling at me.

I smiled back. Shannon was nice-looking, a lot better looking than anyone I had dated back home. I kind of assumed that she was with Jeremy, but some other girl seemed glued to him. It occurred to me that I had never been out with a non-Christian girl before. *So what?* I thought. I can handle it.

Our team won by two points, and we left pretty soon after that.

"See you at my place as soon as you can get there," Jeremy yelled as we reached the parking lot. "By the way, bring your own if you're particular!"

"Right!" I yelled back. Then I frowned. "What did he say?"

"Bring your own booze," Shannon explained. "Unless you like punch."

The party was going full blast when we arrived; so was the music. The room was dimly lit, and cigarette smoke—I guess it was from cigarettes—formed crazy white patterns before joining the cloud hovering near the ceiling. In the middle of the floor several couples bobbed and weaved in time to the music.

"Make yourself at home," Jeremy shouted as Shannon and I moved through the mass of bodies.

"Thanks," I replied.

"Stick with Shannon," he hissed in my ear. "You'll have a good time!"

I nodded, fascinated and ill-at-ease simultaneously.

"Let's get something to drink," Shannon told me, pulling me past the dancers into the dining room.

"I don't drink," I heard myself reply. My honesty surprised me a little bit, but being a nondrinker was no crime.

"Just a little punch?" she asked.

"Sure," I agreed, smiling.

I took one swallow, and my throat was on fire! It looked like ordinary punch, but it was spiked.

"Hmmm, good!" Shannon exclaimed, emptying her cup and getting another. It didn't seem to phase her.

"Where are Jeremy's parents?" I asked.

"Vegas," Shannon said, "They go at least once a month. It'll take poor Jeremy the rest of the weekend to put the house back in shape before they get home!"

"I wouldn't doubt it," I answered, shaking my head.

"Of course, some of us help him out," she went on. "Maybe you could join us Sunday afternoon, Toddy."

"Sunday?" I repeated. "I might be busy" I didn't bother to mention that I'd be in church in the morning and attending a reception that afternoon.

For the next thirty minutes or so I wandered around, more curious than anything else. Back home there would've been a shocked look on everyone's face if I walked into a party like this. But nobody seemed surprised to see me at Jeremy's house. I even got a friendly nod or smile from some kids I vaguely knew from school.

Of course, why should they be surprised? I reminded myself. Nobody knew me. Not the real me, anyway. They didn't know my father was a minister and that I had been raised in the church and was saved when I was ten years old. As far as they were concerned, I was just as lost as they were.

Only they probably don't even know they are, I thought, frowning. My eyes were starting to smart a little from all the smoke, and I couldn't see most of the faces too clearly; but it was apparent from those I could see that they were feeling no pain.

"Having fun?" a thick voice behind me questioned.

I turned and saw Jeremy standing behind me, a glass in his hand and a glazed look in his eyes.

"Jeremy—"

"Wait till later," he went on, sipping the drink. "Things get really wild!"

I didn't know exactly what Jeremy had in mind, but I knew I wanted no part of it. Was this what I had supposedly been missing? I felt stupid and out of place and was experiencing none of the excitement I had anticipated, just disappointment and guilt.

"Oh, there you are!" Shannon exclaimed, grabbing me around the waist. "Thought you went bye-bye!"

"I did," I told her. "I mean, I am. I really have to go now."

She looked at me through eyes that weren't quite focusing. "So soon?"

"Yeah. Can you get home okay?"

"Oh, sure. No problem. Sorry you have to go, though. We barely got acquainted, Toddy."

I left her standing there, mumbling at some other guy, and headed for the door. The night air was cold and cut through my jacket, but I was so glad to breathe oxygen again instead of smoke that I didn't care.

Nobody knew me, I thought as I drove home alone. They had met a guy named Todd Barkley, but they didn't really know me. I wasn't sure I knew myself anymore.

The Todd Barkley I knew back home may have felt the pressure of being a preacher's kid and of having to set an example for everyone else to follow, but at least he didn't feel guilty when he went home from a party.

Maybe that Todd is still around, I decided. Anyway, he was worth looking for. I kind of wanted everyone to know him, especially people like Jeremy and Shannon. There was more to life than getting drunk at parties.

The real Todd Barkley could tell them.

w w j d   p o w e r   s t a t e m e n t

It is a wise person who can see through the lie that drugs and drinking are the way to a good time. Pray that God will keep your eyes open and able to see the reality of the devastating effect of drinking and drugs.

s c r i p t u r e

Run away from the evil young people like to do. Try hard to live right and to have faith, love, and peace, together with those who trust in the Lord.

2 TIMOTHY 2:22 NCV

Fallen Hero

By Mike Chapman

I stood alone on the front porch aware of the music and laughter inside the house, but not really hearing it. The party was in my honor too; at least that had been the original idea. Pretty funny, huh? Who wants to honor a fallen hero?

The screen door opened, but I didn't turn to see who it was, preferring to remain hidden in the shadows.

"Curt?" Dad's voice began. "Why don't you come in, son?"

"Maybe later."

"Nobody blames you."

I didn't reply, hoping he'd just leave me alone. Eventually he did.

It didn't seem fair, not after the way I had trained so hard. I had just about lived at school for the last two months, working out every day, weekends included. Well, maybe not on Sundays, but even the coach thought I should take one day off.

There was a time when I would have worked out seven days a week, but that was before I accepted Christ last fall. One of the churches in town had a youth rally especially for athletes, so I went. There were some crazy skits and music that was all right, but it was the guest speaker that made the whole thing worthwhile. He was a professional athlete, yet he said that his life had been empty until he invited Jesus Christ into his heart.

I didn't understand the part about inviting Jesus into your heart, but I knew what he meant about life being empty. Just a few months before that I had broken the state track record for high hurdles, and the local paper made a big deal out of it. People recognized me on the street and everything, and the kids at school treated me like I was a star.

It was great, but sure didn't last long. For some reason I expected to feel a whole lot different, but inside I was the same old me and something was missing. So when that football player said that Jesus could fill the "God-shaped vacuum inside each one of us," I ate it up. I asked Jesus to forgive my sins and come into my heart that very night.

"The Christian life is like anything else," he told those of us who made decisions. "You get out of it what you put into it. If you want to grow as a Christian, you need to pray regularly, join a church, get baptized, and study God's Word daily. If you do, I guarantee there'll be changes in your life."

And he was right. I knew something had happened that night. As I read the Bible and prayed, I really could feel an inner strength. Joining a church and being around other Christians helped too.

It may sound weird, but I even ran better after I accepted Christ. Maybe I had more purpose or was running because I felt God wanted me to run; I don't know, but when the track season started this year I won every race I entered.

I made sure I didn't let it go to my head, though. I even prayed that the Lord would be glorified. And he was. I had a chance to share my testimony and parts of it even wound up in various sports columns.

My pastor was pleased that I was bringing so many kids to church with me, but I wouldn't take any credit for that. "I just invite them to come," I said with a shrug. "Jesus means a lot to me; why shouldn't I tell people?"

I meant it—up until this particular night, that is. The regular track season was over, and our school made it to state finals for the first time in the history of the school.

I had worked out extra hard that week before the finals, and prayed like anything too. "God, you know I'll be able to reach more people with your Word if we win," I told Him.

I woke up that morning feeling fantastic. I just knew I was going to win my event.

The other guys on our team were in good shape too, and we were holding our own going into the high hurdles. For some reason, they saved that for last. Whichever school won that event would win the meet. The crowd was going wild and started chanting my name when we got into position on the track. I had the inside lane, which was my favorite place to be.

I glanced up at that sea of faces and grinned.

"Keep smiling, Superstar," the guy next to me said, "and you'll get a mouthful of dust!"

I looked at him. "Yours?"

I felt like reminding him that I had the best time for high hurdles in the history of the state and had beat my own time from the previous year, but I didn't. Instead I closed my eyes briefly and prayed for strength to accept whatever happened as God's will. It was a standard prayer I said before every race.

The shot was fired and we were off, my legs carrying me out in front almost from the beginning.

The others weren't far behind, though, especially that smart-mouthed guy in the next lane.

As we approached the first set of hurdles, I was suddenly blinded by something in my left eye! I couldn't see a thing for a split second and my foot caught the top of the hurdle, sending me to the ground. By the time I got up and resumed the race, it was too late and I finished last.

I replayed that part of the meet a million times in my mind as I stood on the porch, but it always came out the same, of course. When I fell, I cost our school the state championship. I tried to explain about getting something in my eye, but nobody seemed too interested.

Even the coach shrugged it off. "Probably a cinder from the track," he said. "Don't worry about it, Curt."

I felt sick though. Sick and confused. *Why, God?* I wondered. *I was willing to give all the glory to you!*

Other guys on the team patted me on the back and said it was okay, but I knew they were just going through the motions. The more honest ones avoided me like I had some rare disease.

All I wanted to do was go home, but then Mom reminded me about the party. I hadn't wanted a party in the first place, even if I won, but she said I had no right to deny her and Dad the opportunity to show how proud they were.

"But I lost!" I protested.

"Only this once," she replied. "Think how many times you won!"

"Mom, it was the state finals," I went on.

"It's too late to cancel it anyway," she informed me. "Besides, it'll be mostly family, plus a few neighbors and friends from church."

I tried to be friendly as our guests arrived, but after I heard "Too bad about today," about ten times, I retreated to the porch. I wasn't used to losing and I didn't like being reminded that I had.

"Curt, you out here?" a voice asked.

"Getting a little air," I replied, turning to face Pastor Wilson from church.

"Sorry I had to miss the meet today," he went on.

"You didn't miss much," I assured him.

"Don't forget, you're scheduled to give your testimony in the evening service this Sunday," he said.

I swallowed. "After what happened today? I don't think I'd better."

"Curt—"

"Pastor Wilson, telephone!" Mom announced from the doorway.

Give my testimony? I thought after he had gone in. *And say what? That I had asked God to help me win for His glory and He answered by letting me lose?*

Except that isn't what you prayed for all, I reminded myself. I had prayed for strength, sure, but I had also prayed that I would accept whatever happened as God's will.

"Hi," a voice began. It came from the front lawn.

"Who's there?" I asked.

"It's me—Del."

Del Mullins lived across the street, and we had never been exactly buddies, even though he was on the track team, too. I guess we just traveled in different circles.

"Your parents are inside," I told him.

"Yeah, I know. Too bad about the meet today."

"One of those things," I said.

"I lost my event, too," he answered, coming up onto the porch. "Same as usual."

I looked at him. Del wasn't kidding. He never won a race, yet he hung in there and kept trying.

"Well, losing's no fun, that's for sure," I admitted. "I found that out today."

There was silence for a moment. "You always give God the credit when you win," Del continued finally. "Do you blame Him when you lose?"

"No, of course not," I said, surprised by the question. "Christians don't operate like that. You have to trust the Lord no matter what happens. There's a reason why I didn't win today; I just don't know what it is yet. But I didn't lose my faith just because I lost a race." I grinned in spite of the way I felt. "It's a lot easier when I win, though!"

"I wouldn't know," Del replied. "I've never won anything in my whole life."

I could barely see his face as we stood on that dark porch, but it was as if a light went on inside my head. There were a lot more losers—or at least people who had experienced defeat at some point in their life— than there were people who did nothing but win! In fact, eventually everyone loses at something.

But a Christian is a winner regardless because of what Christ did through his death and resurrection! It suddenly occurred to me that my loss at the state finals might give me a better chance to relate to others than I had ever had before! I also realized that a lot of people—especially non-Christians like Del, who had heard me share my faith when I won—would be watching to see how I handled losing. So far I hadn't been much of an example.

"How about going to church with me this Sunday?" I asked Del. It was strange, but somehow I had never invited him before, always choosing the popular kids at school.

"Yeah, maybe," Del agreed.

"Let's get something to eat," I went on, heading for the door. "If I know my mom, there's all kinds of food inside! Besides, I have to see my pastor about Sunday night's service."

Don't get me wrong. I wasn't suddenly glad I had lost that afternoon or anything, but I was ready to accept what had happened as God's will and go on from there. Believe me, that made all the difference in the world.

wwjd power statement

Jesus' style was to take the value system of the world and turn it upside-down. Winning and success are highly prized in our world but God can use failure and defeat to make us more like Himself.

scripture

When a persons's steps follow the LORD,
God is pleased with his ways. If he stumbles,
he will not fall, because the LORD holds his hand.

PSALM 37:23-24 NCV

Not Quite "Dear Abby"

By Julie Berens

My best friend Candace and I lay in the shade of the big oak tree in her backyard. While I stared at the sky, Candace hunted the paper for the advice column.

"Here it is," she said triumphantly, folding the paper back. "Dear Abby. . . ."

Even as Candace began to read, I tuned her out. Candace loves the advice columns and reading about other people's problems. It's like an obsession with her. Candace tells people she has a healthy curiosity, but Candace's mom tells her that she's just plain nosy. I'm not sure which of them is right.

Well, if Candace is the reader, I'm the writer. Sometimes when we're in my room and Candace starts reading the paper, I'll sit at my desk and peck away at the old manual typewriter I found for $5.00 at the flea market. I write a lot of different things—stories, plays, poetry. Lately though, Candace's advice has inspired me. I've been writing some letters of my own.

It never seems to bother Candace that she doesn't have my full attention while she's reading to me. Maybe she just likes the sound of her own voice. Yesterday when she asked what I was writing about, I told her it was a science fiction romance written in the neo-gothic style—whatever that means. She didn't pry.

So as Candace lay in the sun and read this latest letter to "Dear Abby," I composed my own letter in my head. *Dear God,* I typed secretly in my heart, glad that today there was no clacking of typewriter keys to arouse Candace's ever-present curiosity.

It's me again with the same old problems. Seems like I've been writing You an awful lot these last few days, doesn't it?

Craig banged out of the house late last night after a terrible argument with Mom. She found a bottle of rum under his bed when she was cleaning. He just told her to mind her own business, and he walked out. I could tell by the look on Mom's face that she wishes Dad was still around.

Marie still can't figure out long division, and so she sits and cries through her math homework every night. Before she left for work, Mom told me to help Marie but I had enough homework of my own to do.

And me? Well, I'd just like to leave town until all these problems go away. What I hate most about being the oldest is that everyone expects you to act like an adult. With Dad gone and Mom working all the time, I know I have responsibilities, but sometimes I'd just like to be as carefree as Candace and other sixteen-year-olds I know.

"You must be writing your neo-gothic science fiction romance again," Candace teased, interrupting my thoughts. "You seem kinda spaced out."

"Very funny," I said, "but for your information, I'm on chapter four."

As I looked at Candace, I realized how glad I was that she's my friend, and also how much I envy her— two parents at home, a great older sister, good grades.

What a life, I thought. *I'm lucky if I read my Bible every few weeks, much less memorize it.*

"Candace, do you think God really hears our prayers?" I asked out of the blue.

"I know He does," Candace said, as if this was a subject we talked about all the time. "In the Psalms it says that the Lord receives our prayers" (Psalm 6:9 NAS).

"So if God hears, why doesn't He always answer?" I persisted.

"But He does," Candace said.

I looked skeptical.

"It's like this." Candace picked up the newspaper and pointed to the "Dear Abby" column. "I have a problem, so I write a letter to 'Dear Abby.' Well, I might get an answer to my letter when I open the newspaper one day and see my letter and Abby's answer typed out in black and white on page 14. Or I might see someone else's letter in the paper and that person's letter is so much like mine that I get my answer. Or I might get a letter back from Abby in the mail. Either way, I get my answer. It's the same with prayer."

Candace made the whole process seem so logical that I wondered why I hadn't been writing to "Dear Abby" all this time instead of to God.

"So God is like 'Dear Abby?' I asked with a giggle in my voice.

"Well, He's not quite 'Dear Abby,'" Candace admitted. "I mean, you're probably not going to get an answer back from Him typed out in black and white in the daily newspaper. But you will get an answer."

That night before she left for work, Mom asked me again to help Marie with her long division. I don't know why but this time I didn't balk like I usually do.

It was kind of fun working with Marie, and I think after a few problems she caught on. While she kept working, I sat down at my typewriter.

"Dear God," I typed. Then I stared at the words. Candace had said God answers our prayers, but He hadn't answered mine yet. *Why not?* I wondered. So that's exactly what I typed in big, bold letters, "WHY DON'T YOU ANSWER ME!!!" Then I waited.

I'm not sure what I expected. I think I wanted God to type back His reply in letters as bold as the ones I'd used. I think I wanted an immediate response. I think I wanted a Heavenly "Dear Abby."

Then I remembered Candace's explanation of how "Dear Abby" worked. You might get your answer in the newspaper, she'd said, or the answer to someone else's letter might solve your problem, or you may get a reply back in the mail.

If there were different ways for "Dear Abby" to respond, I wondered, *shouldn't God have the option of responding in different ways too?*

It was then I realized I'd been limiting how God could respond in my life. I searched my mind for one of the few Scriptures I'd ever memorized and remembered it talked about being still so that you could hear God's voice (Psalm 46:10). God wasn't like "Dear Abby" who responded through letters in a newspaper or personal responses in the mail. God's answer was more likely to be heard in a still, small voice or seen when one person reached out to someone else—like me helping Marie tonight.

As silly as it seemed, I had expected some sort of printed response from God. What I hadn't expected was for God to show me that I could be part of the solution to the problems at home. In that way, I guess God did write His answer back to me. He had shown me it was time to start pitching in and stop retreating from my problems in my room.

I knew I needed to go downstairs to help Marie finish her long division, but before I did I put a new sheet of paper in the typewriter. "Dear God," I typed, "*THANK YOU!* Love, Charlotte."

I know God got my message just as clearly as I had gotten His.

Your faith may be small, but the God in Whom you have placed your faith is huge.

It's impossible to please God apart from faith. And why? Because anyone who wants to approach God must believe both that he exists and that he cares enough to respond to those who seek him.

HEBREWS 11:6

Dear Abby is a registered trademark of Abigail Van Buren.

Curb-side Chat

By Dennis C. Gerig

My younger brother Jeff was sitting on the curb when I came home from work. A neatly tied sleeping bag and my worn-out old suitcase were beside him. I waved and he waved back. But instead of looking excited about going to camp, he wore a sad expression.

"What's wrong with Jeff?" I asked Mom when I entered the kitchen.

"Wrong?" she repeated.

"Mom, he looks like he's going to Devil's Island instead of church camp!" I explained.

"He's been impossible all day," Mom replied. "First, he thought he was coming down with a fever, so I took his temperature; then he was afraid Trixie would miss him too much—"

"You mean he doesn't want to go to camp?" I asked. "But that's all he's talked about for weeks!"

Mom smiled. "He wants to go, yet he doesn't want to go. Don't you remember how you felt the first time you went to camp? You were worse than Jeff!"

I frowned. "You mean I didn't want to go to camp?" It hardly seemed possible. I loved camp.

"Oh, you wanted to go," Mom corrected, "until the time to go actually arrived. Then you changed your mind. You thought up one excuse after another."

"I don't remember any of that," I said. "Well, I'd better shower and change. I have to pick Anne up early tonight."

"We'll be ready to eat soon," Mom assured me.

"Good. What about Jeff?"

"He ate a sandwich before I sent him out to wait for the Belmonts. He'll be fine."

I nodded and hurried upstairs. From my bedroom window I could see my brother sitting on the curb. His head was down and his shoulders were drooping. Trixie raced around him, barking furiously but unable to get a response.

My mind traveled back seven years to the first summer I had gone to camp. I had been separated from my parents before then, of course, but never for more than a night or two, and on those occasions I stayed with my grandparents. A week away from home was quite different.

When the time to go came, I did everything but cry and lock myself in the bathroom. After a while though, I admitted to myself that there was something babyish about being afraid and made up my mind to go.

Is that what Jeff is going through right now? I wondered.

I glanced at the clock on my nightstand. I had to pick Anne up in forty-five minutes. I needed every second to shower, eat, and dress.

But a moment later, despite all my rationalizations, I headed toward the curb. Jeff didn't hear me walk up behind him.

"Ready for camp?"

He forced a brave smile. "Uh-huh."

"That poor old suitcase! I wonder how many more trips it will last!"

He didn't answer.

"You know, I was just your age the first time I took that suitcase to camp," I went on. "Wouldn't it be something if you had the same cabin?"

He nodded. "Which cabin was it?"

I laughed. "You know, I don't remember the number. But it was the closest one to the dining hall. I liked that, because you really get hungry up in the mountains. You'll love it."

He swallowed. "I will?"

"Can I tell you a little secret?"

"Sure."

"Well, I didn't want to go to camp that first year."

He looked at me with new interest. "You didn't? But I thought you loved camp! You've always said—"

"Oh, I do love it now," I agreed, "and part of me wanted to go then too. But part of me wanted to stay home. I know this'll sound silly, but I was scared because I didn't know what it would be like up there."

No response.

"I didn't realize we'd have interesting speakers, go on camp-outs, and go to the lake every afternoon for swimming, boat rides, and water skiing."

"You really liked it" he asked cautiously. "That first time, I mean."

"Would I have gone back every year after that if I hadn't?" I replied. "And we had so much fun in the cabin too. The other guys and I were just like brothers by the end of the week. Our counselor was fantastic, and we had devotions every night before we went to bed. In fact, it was at camp that I became a Christian."

"But I'm already a Christian," Jeff began.

"Then you'll learn even more about Jesus and how to put Him first in your life," I explained. "I'm so glad you're going, Jeff."

"I wish you were going too," he said.

"High school camp won't be for another month," I told him. "But I'll write you."

He smiled. "You will?"

"Sure. Now the Belmonts should be here any minute and I have a lot to do."

"Will you wait with me until they get here?" Jeff asked. "Please?"

I almost turned him down, but since I was hopelessly behind schedule already, Anne would have to understand. So I nodded. "I haven't even eaten yet—but I will."

"How is the food at camp?" Jeff asked.

"Better than you'd expect," I told him.

"Do you have to water ski if you don't want to?"

"No, of course not! It might be fun to try though— especially since you're such a good swimmer. They also have horseback riding, basketball, and softball."

"You know, I have a little secret," Jeff said. "Do you want to hear it?"

"Only if you want to tell me," I replied.

"Well, this morning I changed my mind about going to camp," Jeff admitted. "I even pretended I was sick. But I wasn't really pretending because just thinking about camp made me feel sick inside. Only I didn't have a temperature and the money was already paid, so I decided I had to go whether I wanted to or not."

I put my arm around his shoulder. Just then the Belmonts drove up in their station wagon and Jeff's friend Bob jumped out to help with the suitcase and sleeping bag. Mom came out on the porch to say good-bye. "Ready to go?" Bob asked Jeff.

Jeff gave me a special look. "Sure am."

Jeff was getting into the station wagon when he suddenly turned and ran over to me. "Thanks for everything," he whispered, "and I mean everything!"

"I'll be praying for you," I whispered.

Then they were gone and I hurried toward the house to get ready for my date with Anne. If I skipped dinner, I could pick her up on time, so that's what I decided to do. Sure, I was hungry but in a way I was full, with a very special feeling that only two brothers can have for each other. Jeff had left for camp a different guy, and that made the time I spent with him well worth it.

w w j d   p o w e r   s t a t e m e n t

Showing love for family members takes effort and sometimes means you have to shelf your own plans. But it's worth the effort. Think of it as a deposit in an emotional bank account that you have with each member of your family. Those deposits add up.

s c r i p t u r e

How wonderful, how beautiful,
when brothers and sisters get along!
PSALM 133:1

The Look

By Marlys G. Stapelbroek

I don't usually get nervous before a basketball game, but tonight was different. We were playing Division, and they have a big center. I'm a big center too, which is why I'm the only sophomore playing varsity.

I was in the locker room putting on my socks when the yelling started. "Look out, David!" Glancing up, I saw Pete with a bucket of water. Then Todd raced past.

Splash. Pete flung the water at Todd, but most of it hit me.

"What'd you do that for?" I shouted. "Now I'm all—"

Coach Myers walked in. He didn't yell. He just pinned me with the look. "Whose idea was the shower?"

I stared at the floor. This wasn't the first dumb thing Pete had done, but I wasn't a rat. Then I noticed my shoes sitting beside the bench. They were soaked.

"Great," I muttered. "Thanks a lot, Pe—" I tried to stop, but it was too late. Coach turned the look on Pete.

"Twenty extra laps, every day after practice for a month. Everyone out on the court and loosen up." Seconds later the locker room was deserted. Coach shook his head. "Some people need to be the center of attention, David. That's not an excuse for Pete, but it might help you understand him."

I nodded even though understanding Pete was the last thing on my mind. My stomach was already in knots, and now I was cold and wet too.

Coach handed me his keys. "Get an extra uniform from my office."

"What about my shoes?" I turned them upside down and water poured out.

Coach shook his head. "I should have made it thirty laps. You have an extra pair?"

"At home. My dad could get them."

I didn't have any trouble finding a uniform and socks, but I felt dumb walking across the court without any shoes to ask Dad to run home for my other pair. It didn't help to watch Pete warming up.

"Coach should have made it forty laps," I muttered. Then Pete ran over and slapped me on the back.

I pulled away. "Leave me alone."

"Come on, man. It was a joke."

"Not to me." Or the team. Our first-string center was out with mono, and now I had no shoes.

Coach waved us into a huddle. "Larry, you're going to have to play center until David's dad gets back."

Larry groaned, then nodded toward the other center. "And how am I supposed to handle Rambo?"

"Just get out there and hustle!" Coach ordered.

I turned to sit down, but Pete was behind me. I glared at him. I was tired of his jokes and tired of him.

He coughed. "Hey, man, I didn't mean. . . ."

"Leave me alone."

"If that's the way you want it."

Slumping into my seat, I tried to keep my stocking feet out of sight.

Actually, Larry played pretty well, except he used a little too much elbow. He had three fouls by the time Dad got back with my shoes.

They were old and had a tear in one side, but I would have worn slippers to get in the game. We were down by eight points with two minutes left in the half.

Coach put me in, but I wasn't warmed up. Division's center got around me with a hook. When I tried to shoot over him, he blocked it.

"Nice try, kid," he taunted, passing the ball off to a teammate.

The locker room was quiet at half-time. Coach didn't even need to settle us down for his pep talk, but I couldn't help thinking that without Pete, we'd be ahead by ten and wouldn't need a talk.

When I squared off against Division's center for the tip-off, he glanced down at my shoes. "Great tennies, kid."

I clenched my jaw. On Division's first trip up the court I stole a pass. Looking around, I saw our only player open was Pete.

I turned away, then back when their center reached in—

Tweet. The ref's whistle cut through the jumble of sounds. "Jump ball."

I groaned. How could I have lost the ball?

It was the end of the third quarter before I got the rhythm of the game. Then Larry fouled out.

"Great," I muttered. And it was Pete's dumb stunt that had gotten him in foul trouble.

We hung in there even without Larry, chipping away at their lead. With twenty seconds to go, and only two points behind, we got the ball. I was open at the top of the key and took the pass. I dribbled once, then went up for a turnaround jumper.

Tweet. Division's center had fouled me. He grinned. "Make 'em from the line, kid."

"No problem." I was the best free-throw shooter on the team. Trouble was, I hadn't been all that hot today.

Coach called a time-out. When I got to the side, he gave me the look. "You ever heard of forgive and forget? What Pete did was stupid, but you're letting it eat you up. It's history, David. Get out there and make those free throws."

Nodding, I jogged back onto the court, but his words echoed in my head. *Forgive and forget. . . . Forgive. . . .*

"We'll get 'em in overtime," someone shouted from the crowd. Probably Dad. But to get into overtime, I had to make both free throws.

I shot the ball. It bounced off the rim. A massive groan filled the gym.

Forgive and for— Suddenly, I knew why Coach's words sounded familiar, except it wasn't forgive and forget. It was forgive...and be forgiven! Jesus' words.

I glanced at Pete standing along the free-throw lane. Jesus had already forgiven me for every sin I'd ever committed. How could I hold a grudge against Pete for a joke that had gone wrong?

Maybe Pete felt me watching because he looked up. It took a second, but finally, I smiled. About the time he smiled back, I got an idea, and gave him a tiny nod.

He answered with a questioning glance, just as the ref motioned for me to shoot my second shot.

I aimed for the backboard, just behind the left rim. The ball hit the backboard and bounced off the rim and up. Pete had understood my signal and was ready. His right hand met the ball about two feet from the rim and tipped it back in, tying the game.

The points hadn't even registered on the scoreboard when the buzzer went off.

The gym exploded and the other guys surrounded Pete, giving him high fives and pounding him on the back. As soon as he could break free, he ran over to me. "We don't make a half-bad team, you and me," he shouted over the pandemonium.

When I hugged Pete there in front of everybody, I suppose they thought I was congratulating him on his shot. I shouted into his ear, "I guess we won pretty big today, huh?"

Puzzled, Pete glanced up at the scoreboard showing the tie score, with the clock reset for overtime. Then his eyes lit up. "Yeah," he said with a grin. "I guess we did."

w w j d   p o w e r   s t a t e m e n t

True forgiveness can be achingly difficult. To forgive is not to pretend that nothing happened; it's to acknowledge what did happen and respond in grace as God does to us.

s c r i p t u r e

In prayer there is a connection between what God does and what you do. You can't get forgiveness from God, for instance, without also forgiving others. If you refuse to do your part, you cut yourself off from God's part.

MATTHEW 6:14-15

Darcy's Decision

By Teresa Cleary

Darcy Holmes lay on her stomach and stared at her algebra book while her feet did a midair tap dance to the radio. She wasn't sure if it was the music or the steady drone of her friend Charlotte's voice from across the room that prevented her from concentrating. She'd been looking at the same problem for ten minutes.

Why couldn't I have finished this in study hall like Charlotte did? Darcy asked herself.

She studied her friend from over the top of her algebra book—curly red hair pulled back in a headband, braces, and freckles galore. But Charlotte's eyes were the first thing you noticed about her. They were as green as emeralds, and they could sparkle like the sun or darken with anger or tears. They were the kind of eyes that were hard to look into and tell a lie— but lying to Charlotte was exactly what Darcy was thinking about.

After all, I have a right to make new friends besides ones from church, don't I? Darcy asked herself. *I don't have to go to every youth group party, do I? How am I ever going to be popular at school if I don't make an effort?*

And so Darcy was considering skipping this weekend's youth group overnighter to go to a party with her new friend, Lisa—one of the most popular girls at school. She was even considering lying to her parents and saying she was going on the overnighter and instead staying at Lisa's. The only problem was she wasn't sure how she'd pull it off.

Darcy threw down her pencil. *What should I do?* she wondered.

"Darcy!" Charlotte's voice interrupted. "You're not listening."

"Sorry. I have a lot on my mind," Darcy admitted.

"Got enough problems of your own that you don't want to hear other people's, right?" Charlotte said with a laugh.

Darcy felt like Charlotte had read her mind, until she realized her friend was talking about the algebra homework.

Darcy shut her book and sat up on the bed. "What's up?"

"Well, my problem is there's this girl I know who's really nice, but all of the sudden she wants to be part of the in crowd at school. That never used to matter to her, but now—well—it's all she thinks about."

Darcy was having a hard time meeting Charlotte's eyes. She could relate perfectly well to how this girl felt.

"I think this girl may do something dumb this weekend like give up a great overnighter at church to go to a party where there's sure to be drinking and stuff. I don't think she should go, but I'm not sure how to tell her. What do you think?" Charlotte asked a little too innocently.

As Darcy realized Charlotte already knew all about her plan, her temper flared. She knew her friend was trying to look out for her, but this was too much.

"I think you should just butt out and let this girl do what she wants," Darcy retorted. "She's a big girl."

"But is she a smart girl?" Charlotte flung back.

"I can make my own decisions," Darcy said.

"Can you?" Charlotte asked. "Like when we were kids and you decided you'd be cuter with short hair, so you cut all your hair off about two inches from your head. Then you looked so bad you tried to convince me to do it so at least you wouldn't be miserable alone. Great decision, Darcy."

Darcy couldn't help but smile. It had taken years for her hair to grow back in. "Okay, that was a bad decision, but I was only seven."

"Well, you're fifteen now, and you're about to make another bad decision. A major one. I think you should reconsider your priorities."

When Charlotte left later, Darcy called Lisa. "What time will the party start?" she asked.

"Right after the game," Lisa replied. "But we'll let things get going before we arrive."

"Will there be beer?"

"Of course. Troy's brother got a keg."

"I guess his parents aren't going to be around?"

"Are you crazy? They left town for a trip to Hawaii. Troy and Geoff are on their own. Hey, you aren't getting cold feet, are you?" Lisa asked.

"I—I have to go, my mom's calling me," Darcy said, glad to get off the phone. "I'll call you later."

When she hung up, Darcy was more confused than ever. As much as she wanted to be part of the in crowd, she wasn't sure this was the way to do it. But then again, it might be her only chance.

81

"Darcy, time for dinner!" her mom called again.

After dinner Darcy headed back to her room. Almost immediately, the phone rang.

"Darcy, it's for you," her mom called.

"Darcy, it's Pam. I'm in charge of refreshments for this weekend. Can you bring a bottle of pop and a bag of chips? It would help a lot."

"Uh, I'm not sure if I'm going, Pam. Can I let you know?"

Darcy was back in her room when the phone rang again. It was Jill calling to say she hoped Darcy would make the overnighter. Jill's phone call was followed by one from David, then Ellen, then Scott, then Luke, then Terri.

When Darcy hung up with Terri, the doorbell rang. She heard Charlotte's voice as her dad let her in. "I came to talk to Darcy."

Darcy walked out into the hallway and crossed her arms.

"Did anyone call?" Charlotte asked innocently.

Darcy couldn't help it. She burst out laughing. "Yes, someone called. Someone named Pam, and David, and Ellen, and Scott, and Luke, and Terri. Should I expect any more pressure to sway my decision?"

"Well, there won't be any more calls," Charlotte said, her green eyes dark. "Just a visit—from a friend who wants to see you do the right thing."

"You really outdid yourself," Darcy said. "Did you ask everyone from youth group to call?"

"Just the ones who care," Charlotte replied.

"That's a pretty convincing argument," Darcy said quietly.

"Darcy, I don't know why being popular is such a big thing with you lately, but I wanted you to see how popular you already are. Maybe it is with youth group and not with the crowd at school, but we all really care about you. I know we're pressuring you to go with us this weekend, but I didn't know what else to do. I felt like since Lisa and her friends were pulling you in one direction, I needed to start pulling you in the other."

"A tug of war, huh?" Darcy asked.

"Kind of," Charlotte admitted.

"Well," Darcy said, looking into Charlotte's eyes, "call it a victory. Your side won."

"Great!" Charlotte said, pulling Darcy toward the phone. "C'mon, you have a lot of calls to return."

Darcy looked at her friend and smiled. She was glad to see the sparkle back in Charlotte's green eyes.

w w j d   p o w e r   s t a t e m e n t

Friends can make all the difference in the world. You become like the people with whom you spend your time, so it's important to find friends who not only honor your faith in Christ but help you live for Him.

s c r i p t u r e

A truly good friend will openly correct you.
You can trust a friend who corrects you,
but kisses from an enemy are nothing but lies.

PROVERBS 27:5-6 CEV

Sticks and Stones

By Julie Berens

Who would have thought that a copy of *Gone With the Wind* could teach me a lesson about honesty and respect. That's what happened though when I lent my copy of the novel to my best friend, Christine.

"Please, Katie, I'll take good care of it," Christine said. Pleeeease!"

I'll admit I'm crazy about my book collection, which includes an old copy of *Gone With the Wind* that my grandmother gave to me.

"Well, okay," I reluctantly agreed, knowing books weren't that important to Christine. But she's my best friend, and I felt like I had to say "yes."

Over the next few days, Christine kept me filled in on her progress through the story.

"Scarlett just married that wimp Charles!" she told me as we boarded the school bus one morning. "How could she?"

"Take good care of the book," was my usual reply every time she came to me with a report. She'd nod, but I wondered if she really heard me.

Christine not only kept me up-to-date about what page she was on in *Gone With the Wind*, but she also filled me in on the latest happenings at school.

"How do you find out this stuff?" I'd asked her in shock one day after hearing the latest story about Patty Speers, a cheerleader at our school. Christine shrugged. "I just keep my ears open."

Sometimes I wondered why my Christian friend was so interested in other people's lives. "I don't hurt anyone," Christine would say when I questioned her about the gossiping. "Besides I only tell a few people."

I wasn't sure who those few people were or exactly how many "a few" included, but I learned to shrug off Christine's wagging tongue even though I continued to listen to her. *There are worse sins,* I reasoned. Or so I thought.

A few weeks later Christine called me on the phone with more news about Patty. "She's pregnant!"

"What!" I could believe it about some other girls at our school, but not Patty. She went to my church and showed up at youth group meetings about twice a month. She'd made a stand for Christ at last spring's retreat and told the whole group how she wanted her life to make a difference. "You must have heard wrong," I told Christine.

"No, I didn't," she insisted. "Suzanne and Marcia were in the restroom talking about Patty and about babies. I distinctly heard her and Marcia say that Patty was expecting."

"What else did they say?"

"I don't know. I couldn't hear anything else."

I hung up with Christine and decided to call Robin, another girl in my youth group who's good friends with Patty. As I was dialing, my older brother Mark walked through the family room and into the kitchen to get a snack. He stood there as I talked to Robin.

"I heard that Patty's pregnant. Do you think it could be true?"

Robin said that she hadn't spent much time with Patty in the last few months because Patty was so busy with her new boyfriend. We talked a while longer and then I hung up. I still didn't have my answer.

"What are you doing?" Mark asked. I told him about Christine's call.

"Do you really think you should be calling these people?" he asked in that know-it-all voice that older brothers use.

"I'm trying to find out if the story's true." I dialed another number.

Mark looked at me funny but didn't say anything else. He left the room shaking his head.

The next day as we got on the bus, Christine told me she had about fifty pages to go. My thoughts were on Patty, but it didn't stop me from reminding Christine to be careful with my book.

That day at school the halls were full of whispers about Patty's pregnancy. "Is she or isn't she?" The question seemed to bounce off the walls and echo in the stairwells. The fact that Patty was absent only fueled the speculation.

Right before dinner that night, Christine showed up with my copy of *Gone With the Wind.* "What a fantastic book!" she said as she handed it to me.

As soon as I took it I could tell there was something wrong. The book fell limply backwards as I opened it.

As I turned the pages I could see where Christine had turned down corners to help her keep her place. The back cover of the book held a big coffee ring. "My dad couldn't find a coaster, so he set his mug down on the book," Christine explained. "The bottom of the mug must have been wet. I'm sorry about that."

"Christine, I asked you a million times to take care of this book!" I said. As my voice rose, Mark came out of his bedroom to see what the commotion was about. "If you can't take care of other people's things, you shouldn't ask to use them. You know how much my books mean to me."

Christine looked stunned. "I-I-I'm sorry," she stammered and hurried out the door to escape my tirade.

"Some people have no respect for other people's things," I muttered under my breath as I headed for my room.

"It's funny hearing you say that," Mark commented.

"And what's so funny about it? I told her to take care of my book, and she ruined it."

"Kind of like the two of you ruining Patty's reputation with your story about her being pregnant."

"Now wait a minute, I didn't spread that story. Christine called me, and I just called a few people to see if it was true."

"If that's what you were interested in, why didn't you call Patty and ask her? " Mark demanded. "No, you didn't care enough about her to do that. You're just trying to hide your gossiping by acting like you care about Patty's welfare. Well, you're not fooling anyone."

I stood there taking in what Mark was saying. "Maybe you need to think about it," he said coming over and taking the book out of my hand. "This is just a thing, a book. So what if Christine turned some pages down or tore some of them or even spilled coffee on it. That's no big deal. But spreading rumors about someone being pregnant and hurting her reputation—now that is!"

Mark handed the book back to me. "I talked to Patty's mom today after school. Apparently Patty's expecting a new niece or nephew in the next few days. Her sister, Tina, is pregnant with her second child. Apparently Christine didn't hear the whole conversation."

I went to my room and closed the door. I laid on my bed and opened *Gone With the Wind*. Mark was right. A brown mark on a few pieces of paper shouldn't matter but the stain of doubt and suspicion that I'd left on Patty's reputation did.

I closed the book and put it back on the shelf, resolving that tomorrow I'd talk to Patty. On paper or in life, stains are hard to remove.

wwjd power statement

When you talk, you speak volumes about yourself.

scripture

When you talk, do not say harmful things,
but say what people need—words that will
help others become stronger. Then what
you say will do good to those who listen to you.

EPHESIANS 4:29 NCV

Date with a Romeo

By Teresa Cleary

"Oooh! There he is," my friend Nicole squealed in her best teenybopper voice as Nathan Grant walked by our locker. "Isn't he the biggest hunk you've ever seen?" I nodded, oblivious to Nicole's teasing. At our school, every girl in the junior class was madly in love with this guy who not only was tall, dark, and gorgeous but also played varsity football and drove a red sports car. Every girl, that is, except Nicole. While she only pretended to be awestruck by Nathan's mere presence, I had a bad case of "Nathanitis."

"He sits next to me in study hall, and yesterday . . ." I paused dramatically, "he asked to borrow my pen."

"Lucky you," Nicole replied. "So when do you get his class ring?"

"Oh, quit!" I said as I jabbed her with the corner of my English book. "I plan on getting to know him a lot better."

"Do you think that's such a good idea?" Nicole asked. "He may be cute, but he doesn't have the best reputation."

"I can handle it," I replied. "I just need him to ask me out."

"I see a scheme boiling," Nicole said with a laugh, "though I think you're making a big mistake."

I sighed. Deep down inside, a small voice was telling me the same thing. *But I really want to go out with Nathan, I told the voice. What harm is there in that?*

I knew Nathan had a reputation for being a "love 'em and leave 'em" kind of guy but I thought that as a Christian, I was the person to change that. I'd just do a little "missionary dating" and WHAM! our youth group would expand by one very handsome guy.

So, despite that small voice telling me that missionary dating didn't wash as a method of evangelism, and Nicole's constant badgering that this wasn't the kind of relationship for a Christian to get involved in, I pursued Nathan.

After two months of "accidentally" showing up outside the door of his classes, sitting near his table in the cafeteria, and going out of my way to be friendly in study hall, I got my wish—Nathan asked me out for pizza after that Friday's football game.

"The whole team is going;" he explained. "It'll be fun."

I sat with Nicole at the stadium on Friday, though I was too nervous to watch the game. "I still wish you weren't going," Nicole told me for the hundredth time that night. I ignored her and the increasing volume of the voice inside of me saying I should cancel the date.

Nicole waited with me after the game until Nathan found me.

"You ready to go?" he asked as he slid his arm easily around my shoulders. I waved to Nicole and walked off with Nathan.

We arrived at the restaurant, ordered our pizza, and then got absorbed in conversation about the game. It had been a 21-20 victory for our team, and part of that was due to a pass that Nathan had intercepted.

Nathan was friendly and attentive. He wanted to know about my other interests ("You go to church every Sunday?" he teased) my family, and my other classes at school. Before we left, he asked if I wanted to go to a party that one of his teammates was throwing.

"No, thanks," I said, realizing that there would probably be a lot of drinking at the party. "I'd rather just be with you."

Nathan grinned. "You got it!" he said. We drove around for a while and I talked about school, the game, and anything else that came to mind. After about forty-five minutes of aimless driving, Nathan pulled off on a side street. Warning lights went off in my brain. *What have I gotten myself into?* I wondered.

"You're different than I thought you'd be," Nathan said as he slid toward me across the front seat. "I thought all you churchy types were real straight-laced and boring. Looks like you're going to prove me wrong."

And you're just the same as I heard you'd be, I thought. Why hadn't I listened to that little voice inside of me and done what I knew was right all along? I realized now in hindsight that my uneasy feelings were the Holy Spirit working to open my eyes to a situation that I shouldn't have let myself get involved in.

"Nathan," I began in a rush, "I'm afraid I've misled you. I can't do this. I don't think it's right." Nathan looked at me in astonishment. "You mean you've hounded me to ask you out for two months, and now you're going to sit here and tell me you don't want to make out?"

"I-I'm sorry," I told him, close to tears.

"Man!" Nathan said, as he started the car and headed to my house. "You're really something, you know that?" I scrunched down in the seat. All I wanted right now was to be spending a typical, boring Friday night with Nicole. The car tires screeched as Nathan backed out of my driveway. I tried to apologize once more, but he waved away my words like they didn't matter.

I went in the house and crept up to my room, hoping that no one knew I was home. Minutes later there was a light knock on the door, and my mom stuck her head in. "You're home early," she said. "How did the date go?"

"Just as I should have expected," I said truthfully. "That's why I'm home."

Mom smiled. "I'll leave you alone," she said.

"Thanks," I called as she shut the door.

I reached for the phone on my nightstand and started to dial Nicole's number. I stopped halfway through and put the receiver back on the hook. It wasn't Nicole I needed to talk to, I realized. For months before this date, God had used the Holy Spirit in my life to try to make me see the folly of pursuing Nathan, yet I had ignored Him. No, it wasn't Nicole I needed to talk to.

I got on my knees beside my bed. "God, it's me . . ." I said in a quiet voice, almost hoping the Lord wouldn't hear. Suddenly I felt like a child who had to confess to her father that she'd done something wrong. "I'm sorry," I continued, my voice growing stronger. "Sorry for ignoring those feelings You've put in my heart that let me know when I'm doing something wrong; sorry for disobeying You, sorry for . . . for everything."

I paused to catch my breath. "Lord, I'm just sorry," I whispered. "Please forgive me."

As I knelt there I could feel God's love spread over me like the comfort of a father's hug. I knew God had accepted my prayer, and I could now accept His forgiveness.

w w j d   p o w e r   s t a t e m e n t

We not only have the power of God's Word to help us know right from wrong, but God will guide us through His Holy Spirit and our conscience, if we will only pay attention to His voice.

s c r i p t u r e

If you don't know what you're doing, pray to the Father.
He loves to help. You'll get his help, and won't be
condescended to when you ask for it.

JAMES 1:5

Dime Store Romance

By Julie Berens

Jacey Marshall settled herself in the bay window seat in the family room and opened her Bible. Just outside, the leaves of the maple tree were turning bright red. During the summer, Jacey had often sat under the maple for her quiet time, but the cooler weather had driven her inside today. She pulled her sweater a little tighter around herself, picked up the apple she'd brought to munch on, and turned her attention to the Book of Ruth. She'd made a deal with herself over the summer that her devotions came before any other reading she did for fun.

When she finished her devotions, Jacey picked up the romance novel she'd checked out of the library last week. Soon she was lost in the story of Amber and Kent, two high school students who found love and romance while working on a cruise ship for the summer. Even though the plot was far-fetched and the characters were too perfect to be real, she found herself caught up in the romance.

"Jacey," came her mom's voice from the next room. "I left some papers at work. Want to ride along with me?"

"No thanks, Mom! I'm reading," Jacey called back. Her mom worked downtown, and the drive would take at least an hour. In that amount of time, she'd be halfway through the book.

Jacey could just see her mom shaking her head. She thought her daughter read entirely too many of those "dime-store romances," as she called them.

After dinner, Jacey called her friend Beth. "How do you like *Love on the High Seas?*" Beth asked.

"It's good but I can already tell you how it's going to end."

"That's because those romances you read are so predictable. I've got a book I want to give you tomorrow. You'll love it. There's a little more to it than those silly romances you read. I'll bring it to your locker."

Jacey was just getting her books together for her first class when Beth showed up. "Take a look at this," she said, handing Jacey a book whose cover made her eyes widen. The woman's dress was cut so low that she might as well have not been wearing anything.

Jacey tried to give the book back. "No thanks, Beth, I don't think—"

"Take it, take it," Beth insisted. "It's really a good story. Not at all like those yawners you read."

"I don't know," Jacey hesitated.

"Let me show you one of the really good parts." Beth took the book and flipped through the pages. "Here, page 180."

As Jacey started to read, she could feel her cheeks reddening. She quickly shut the book. "I can't read this," she stammered. "It's—"

"Hot?" Beth supplied.

Jacey giggled nervously at her friend's choice of words. "That wasn't exactly what I was going to say, but yes," she replied, then added, "I don't think this is something I want to read."

"Just keep it," Beth said, waving away the book as Jacey tried to hand it back. "Maybe you'll change your mind."

Jacey hesitated. "Well, okay," she finally said, tucking the novel between her English and American history books. "But I'm not going to read it."

Beth didn't say anything, but her look said she doubted her friend's words.

At home that afternoon, Jacey hunted for *Love on the High Seas*, but she couldn't find it. She picked up the book Beth had given her. *Maybe it's not as bad as it looks*, she thought as she carried it and her homework downstairs to the window seat.

Yet before she started to read, Jacey took the novel and slid it between the pages of the English book. *That way there won't be any need to explain things if Mom gets home early*, she thought.

An hour later, she was so absorbed in her novel, she didn't hear her mom come in from work.

"What are you reading?" Mom asked as she passed by on her way to the kitchen with a sack of groceries.

"Something for school," Jacey replied, holding up the English book. She was surprised at how easily the lie came. She tried to return to her book but her mom interrupted again. "How about some help?" she called. Jacey set her book aside with a sigh. It figured, just as she was getting to a really good part.

Jacey rushed to meet Beth the next morning at school. "I was up past midnight reading *Love's Passionate Destiny*. I couldn't put it down."

"See I told you you'd like it," Beth said. "I've got another one when you're finished with that."

"Well, that would probably be okay," Jacey said, ignoring the funny feeling in her stomach.

Jacey rushed home from school in the rain to get back to her book as quickly as possible. The darkness of the afternoon made her usually sunny window seat a little less inviting, but she didn't let that bother her as she sat down to read.

The further into the novel Jacey got, the racier it seemed to get. Unlike the romances she usually read, there weren't any long, loving looks or tender kisses stolen in the moonlight in this book. Instead, the love scenes were intimate and graphic, and they made Jacey uncomfortable. She still had about half the book to read when she put it down and went to the kitchen for a snack.

She sat at the table with the package of Oreos open in front of her, thinking about the book and about a talk her youth pastor had recently given. "Everything you do should be held up to the light of Jesus Christ," Jess had said. "If Jesus wouldn't approve of what you're doing, you shouldn't be doing it at all."

Jacey knew Jesus wouldn't be pleased with the book she was reading. She prayed a short but sincere prayer for forgiveness. Then she pushed aside the Oreos and returned to the family room, knowing full well what she needed to do. This was one book she couldn't finish.

As Jacey reached for the novel, her hand brushed against something that had fallen between the cushions of the seat. She pulled out her copy of *Love on the High Seas*. Jacey smiled as she realized how innocent it was compared to the book Beth had given her. She didn't think Jesus would have a problem with this one.

Yet before Jacey sat down to finish her novel, she kept a promise to herself. She reached deeper into the seat cushions and pulled out the Bible she had left there only yesterday. She'd forgotten her devotions then, but she wouldn't do it again today. She smiled as she turned to the Book of Ruth. Before anything else, she had this romance to finish.

w w j d   p o w e r   s t a t e m e n t

Living in the world we do, it is next to impossible to protect our minds from images, ideas, words and actions that are impure. What makes us different from the world is that even though we are exposed to those messages, God's Holy Spirit will keep them from taking root in our lives, if we are committed to Him.

s c r i p t u r e

*Summing it all up, friends, I'd say you'll do best
by filling your minds and meditating on things true,
noble, reputable, authentic, compelling, gracious—
the best, not the worst; the beautiful,
not the ugly; things to praise, not things to curse.*

PHILIPPIANS 4:8

The Birthday Present

By Teresa Cleary

The minute my friend Jenny and I got to the mall, I knew I shouldn't have come with her on this shopping expedition.

"My mom said she thought I'd have more fun shopping with you for my birthday present, so she gave me her credit card and told me to 'be reasonable,'" Jenny said as we entered the clothing store.

I tried to smile at Jenny's remark, but I could tell my effort left something to be desired. I could feel my facial muscles tightening with forced cheerfulness as I imagined what "reasonable" meant. *You'll probably only buy three new outfits instead of five,* I thought, and each one complete with shoes and accessories.

Before I could stop it, the green-eyed monster was rearing its ugly head.

Jenny and I had been best friends since the sixth grade. Over the years, we'd done everything together —gotten our hair cut short and hated it, discovered guys, and complained about school.

At first it never bothered me that Jenny's family was much better off than mine. Now that we were in high school, though, I began noticing the things Jenny had that I didn't—a bulging wardrobe, her own car, membership in a fitness club. It seemed the list could go on forever. More and more I was envious of her life-style and the things she had. Sure, I'd pray halfheartedly that God would take away those feelings, but I think what I really wanted Him to do was to give me all the things Jenny had.

I couldn't help comparing this shopping extravaganza with birthdays in my family. Even though we weren't poor, four children in the family meant budgeting—even for birthdays. We had a good time, but my parents put a $20 spending limit on presents.

I remembered my last birthday. In our family, it's a tradition that the one who's celebrating a birthday gets to pick the menu and invite one special person to the celebration. I invited Jenny, of course, and ordered my favorite meal complete with chocolate cake for dessert. It was fun, but nothing like this credit card shopping spree.

I was brought back to the present when Jenny held up a white sweater and matching skirt. "Do you like this?" she asked.

"It is gorgeous," I said. Jenny nodded and continued looking while I moved from rack to rack, touching the beautiful clothes. "I'm going to try this on," Jenny headed for the dressing room. After a few minutes, she reappeared in the outfit she'd just shown me. She looked beautiful.

I sighed. While part of me wanted to tell her how good she looked, another part of me snatched the words back before they were uttered. Jenny was in such good shape that she'd look good in a potato sack. Sometimes I doubted my judgment in choosing a best friend who was so pretty. Lord, why can't I be the one with the rich parents and the great looks?

"Well, Teresa, what do you think?"—a question Jenny had asked me more than once. "Do you like it?"

The outfit looked great on her, but the green-eyed monster struck again. "Not really," I lied. "I think you need something with more color."

"You think so?" Jenny said doubtfully. "I don't know."

"Just trust me. We'll find something better," I told her, pushing her back into the dressing room. "You just can't buy the first thing you see." I would have said anything to get Jenny out of this store and away from that outfit. As we left, Jenny gave the sweater one last look.

Just down the mall, we passed a frozen yogurt place. "My treat," Jenny said, pulling out her wallet. "The Taylors stayed out late Saturday night, so I've got a few dollars to spare."

I never could resist chocolate yogurt so we got our cones and sat down at a table. As Jenny chattered away about a million things, I thought about the feelings I'd had toward my best friend lately. Those feelings weren't very kind.

As I sat there, I began to see Jenny in a new light. I saw how attractive Jenny was—not just treating me to yogurt, but in all areas of her life. Even though she was the one who belonged to the fitness club, she took me every chance she got. She also let me drive her car and borrow her clothes.

I also realized this wouldn't be a shopping extravaganza. Jenny would go home with only one gift. I'd let envy take over my vision until it distorted the picture I had of my best friend.

With that thought, the green-eyed monster seemed to shrink in size.

After we finished our cones, we headed for the next clothing store. "Look at that red sweater," Jenny said as we passed the window. "It would be perfect for you Teresa with your dark hair. How are you doing saving your baby-sitting money? Maybe you'll have enough soon to buy something like that?"

A few minutes ago, all I would have heard was the part about saving my baby-sitting money. I would have resented the fact that all Jenny had to do was ask her parents for the sweater and they'd buy it for her. This time, though, I heard more. I heard my best friend complimenting me and saying how good I'd look. I heard the voice of someone who loved and cared for me for who I was. I needed to extend that same courtesy to her.

I'd let envy and jealousy take hold in my life and I almost let them ruin a wonderful friendship. I knew now that it wasn't that God hadn't heard my prayers to take away those feelings. He just wanted me to see the ugly reality of how it looked when the green-eyed monster took over. Now that I'd seen it, I didn't want to see it again.

"You know, Jen, I've been thinking," I said, linking my arm with her and pulling her back to the first store, "that white skirt and sweater really was beautiful on you. . . ."

wwjd power statement

The world we live in measures people by what they look like and how much they own, so it's not unusual to feel jealous when someone else has more than we do. The good news is that Jesus places value on people because they are made in God's image and on the qualities that only He can see—the qualities of the heart.

scripture

Do not want anything that belongs to someone else.

Exodus 20:17 CEV

Down in My Heart

By Teresa Cleary

Rachel Ellis read the paragraph from her history book for the third time, but she knew the information wasn't sinking in. The loud music from her brother's room next door was breaking her concentration.

My friends have older brothers who crank up their D.C. Talk tapes, she thought, *but not me.* I have to contend with a five-year-old who likes to listen to his *Kids' Praise!* tapes at full volume.

Rachel pushed back her chair and headed for Danny's room. As she opened the door she was met with the chorus of "Jesus Loves Me." Danny was singing along at the top of his lungs while he pushed his Matchbox race car around obstacles he'd set up all over the floor.

"Hey you! Al Unser Jr.!" Rachel yelled. "There are people in this house who are trying to study."

Danny hopped up and turned down the child's tape player that sat on his dresser. "Sorry Rach," he said. "I like it that way."

"Well, I've got a test tomorrow," Rachel told him, "and I can't concentrate with your music so loud. Can you keep it down to a dull roar?"

Danny nodded.

Rachel returned to her history book and continued reading. A half-hour later she realized that Danny's loud music hadn't been the only thing breaking her concentration. She'd finished the entire chapter, and she couldn't remember a thing she'd read. Her mind was already full—of everything but history.

Rachel couldn't remember when her life had been this busy. There was school, homework, and soccer practice. She had student senate meetings to run, her work on the decorating committee for the spring dance, and the youth group retreat to help plan. None of this left much time for helping out at home and spending time with her friends, but she tried to fit that in anyway. It seemed like every minute of her day was accounted for before she even got out of bed.

Rachel sighed and closed her eyes to give them a rest. She was already tired, and she hadn't even scratched the surface of what she needed to cover for the test. *Lord,* she prayed, knowing full well this was one of those "hour of desperation" prayers, *help me do okay on my history test tomorrow.*

Rachel knew God had heard her prayer, but she had to admit she doubted its effectiveness. After all, she really hadn't done her part in preparing for this test. What did she expect? A miracle grade? Rachel saw that as her list of school activities lengthened, her time for Bible reading and prayer shortened. Too often her prayers were reduced to ones like her desperate plea for a good grade on her history test.

She heard Danny's door open. The strains of "I've got the joy, joy, joy, joy, down in my heart" floated down the hallway along with Danny's joyful accompaniment.

Where's your joy, Rachel? the Lord seemed to whisper.

Rachel sat there. *I don't know,* she answered truthfully.

She turned back to her history book, but the thought kept interrupting. *Where did my joy go,* she wondered, *and how do I get it back?* When she finally finished studying and turned off her light that night, neither of her questions had been answered.

The next morning Rachel hit the floor at a run. After a quick shower and a cup of juice, she raced upstairs to look over her history notes. She was so absorbed in her reading that she almost didn't hear her mom call that the bus was coming down the street.

At school, her first two classes sailed by, and then it was time for her history test. When it was over, Rachel wasn't sure if she'd passed. *Where's your joy, Rachel?* she heard in her ear as she headed for fourth bell. *I think I lost what little I had in history class, Lord,* Rachel answered.

Throughout the rest of the day, Rachel heard God's whispered question over and over. She heard it as she moped when the dance committee vetoed her idea for using springtime flowers and voted for a trendy black-and-white theme for the decorations instead. She heard it at soccer practice when she felt like a failure because she couldn't seem to block any of the goals kicked her way. She heard it as she walked in the front door at home and was greeted by the smell of cooked cabbage—her dad's favorite dish, but one she loathed. *Where's your joy, Rachel?*

As she headed for her room, her mom's voice called behind her, "Rachel, check Danny for me. He was sent home from school with a fever. I want to know how he's feeling now."

"Sure, Mom." Rachel opened her brother's door.

"Hi, Rach," Danny said. "did you come to visit me?"

"Sure did, buddy." Rachel walked over to Danny's tape player and turned it down. *Doesn't this kid own any other tapes?* she wondered as the familiar Kids' Praise! songs played on. "Mom says you're not feeling well."

Danny shook his head. "My head hurts, and sometimes I feel like I might throw up. But not now," he reassured his sister.

Rachel felt Danny's forehead and hand. He had a fever all right.

"Will you find my bear for me, Rachel?"

As Rachel searched the closet, she heard Danny begin to sing softly with his tape. "I've got the joy, joy, joy, joy, down in my heart. Where? Down in my heart. . . ."

"I found him, Danny," Rachel said as she pulled her brother's battered teddy bear from the bottom of the closet. She tucked the covers around the two of them and gave her brother a quick kiss on the forehead. She knew he'd be asleep within minutes.

Rachel went downstairs to update her mom and then headed for her room. *Where's your joy, Rachel?* she heard for the final time as she sat on her bed. She knew now she had an answer.

As she watched Danny she realized that even though he was sick, his joy just seemed to spill out of him. Hers though depended solely on the circumstances in her life. Having too much to do, being outvoted by the dance committee, knowing she was going to eat cabbage for dinner—all those had made for a pretty rotten day. Yet when things were going well, she was happy. In fact, it was easy to praise God when things were good. When they weren't—now that was a different matter.

Rachel knew she had a choice to make—one she'd have to make over and over. She could either choose to be joyful, to look on life's bright side, or she could go through life with a perpetual cloud over her head.

Rachel slipped out of her door and into Danny's room. Her brother didn't even stir as she took the tape from his player and brought it into her own room. She quickly found the song she wanted and began to sing along, getting louder as the song progressed. "I've got the joy, joy, joy, joy, down in my heart. Where? Down in my heart. . . ."

w w j d   p o w e r   s t a t e m e n t

Joy is different than happiness. You may feel happy one day and down the next. Joy is more than just a state of being. It comes from the knowledge that God loves us, is in control of our lives, and genuinely wants the very best for us.

s c r i p t u r e

You make our hearts glad
because we trust you, the only God.

PSALM 33:21 CEV

Mental Giant

By Alan Cliburn

I was sitting in a far corner of the library when Sean Collins came through the door with a big stack of books. Didn't surprise me a bit. Sean was smart; a lot smarter than I am anyway.

"Is this one right?" Ben Culver whispered, sticking his math assignment in my face. "Is it right, Randy?"

I glanced at the paper. "Yeah, that's right. Try another one."

"Did I tell you I passed that math test we had the other day?" he said excitedly. "I got a C!"

"You told me. That's great."

"It's only because you're tutoring me," he went on.

I shook my head and grinned at the same time as Ben tackled the next problem. Tutoring somebody with his limited ability was not the easiest thing in the world, but I could finally see some improvement. More important, he could see improvement as well.

I glanced up just as Sean Collins looked my way. He nodded, I waved. We weren't close friends or anything, but we did have a couple of classes together. Suddenly all that had changed. During a discussion in our science class several months earlier, Sean made some comments which indicated that he disdained anything of a spiritual nature.

I kept my mouth closed in class, because I knew my limitations as a debater. Actually I didn't want to debate Sean; I just wanted to tell him that as a Christian I believed the Bible.

It took a while to work up the nerve to do it, but finally I just walked over to him one day while he was sitting alone in the quad.

"Hi, Sean," I began, mouth dry and heart pounding.

"Hi, Randy. What's on your mind?"

He was pretty direct, so I figured I should be, too. "I heard what you said the other day in science," I continued. "You know, about the Bible."

"It's full of fairy tales," he said, shrugging. "Totally impossible to believe or take seriously. According to the latest research—"

"I believe it," I interrupted.

"What do you mean?" he wanted to know.

"I mean that I believe man was created in the image of God and that because of man's sin, Jesus Christ came to provide salvation for those who believe in Him. I've seen the changes He can make in a person's life."

"Religious experiences are strictly psychological," Sean replied simply, not looking a bit impressed. "Still, if it makes you happy, go right on believing anything you want, Randy. Excuse me, I have to see Mr. Ritter about a special project I'm working on for college credit."

I hadn't given up after my slightly less than successful experience with Sean Collins. Regardless of what he thought, he still needed Christ. At the same time, I figured somebody smarter than me would have to do the job. Somebody like Dan Scribner from church, a brain if there ever was one.

"Sure, I'll talk to Collins," he had agreed. "I personally think it takes a whole lot more faith not to believe in God," Dan answered. "Take the size of the earth. If it were smaller, we couldn't breathe."

I frowned. "Why not?"

"Because there wouldn't be enough gravity to hold the atmosphere in place. And of course if it was much larger, the gravity pull would be so strong that we couldn't move."

"I never thought of that," I admitted.

"Even the position of the earth in relationship to the sun is pretty significant," Dan went on. "If we were closer it would be too hot to survive, and if we were farther away than we are now, we'd freeze. Everything points to a Supreme Being Who put it all in motion and keeps it going."

It made sense to me, and of course I couldn't wait to hear how Sean reacted in the face of all that knowledge.

"Did you talk to him?" I asked the next time I saw Dan.

"I talked, all right," he said, "but I don't think he really listened. Oh, he admitted that everything I told him was accurate, but the most he would agree to was that there could be a God. He's an agnostic, not an atheist."

"Look, Ben, it's getting late," I told him, glancing at my watch, "you about ready to go home?"

"Uh huh," he replied. "only one more to go. I think I'll need some help, though.

I stayed, even if there were other things I had to get done. By the time I ate dinner, it was time to go to youth group. I did as much of my own schoolwork as I could when I got home, but it was far from finished.

I planned to catch up with my assignments during lunch, but that didn't help during fourth period science. Mr. Tillman hardly ever quizzed the class orally, but suddenly he was calling my name and asking me a question.

"I don't know," I admitted.

"Did you do last night's reading?" he asked.

"Not all of it," I told him, red-faced. "Didn't have time."

Much to my surprise, Sean fell into step with me after class. "Mind if I visit your church this week?" he asked.

"Uh, sure," I agreed, still in shock. Maybe Dan had gotten through to him, after all!

"And it has nothing to do with Scribner and his scientific evidence," Sean went on, as if reading my mind. "You like tutoring kids like Ben Culver?" Sean continued.

I shrugged. "He just needs a little extra help, that's all."

"Yeah, but if you hadn't been with him yesterday in the library, you could've been doing your own work," Sean explained. "I see you with him nearly every day."

"It's finally starting to pay off, too," I told Sean. "He passed a math test earlier this week."

"So what? What do you get out to it?" Sean wanted to know. "You don't even get credit for helping him."

"I don't know, depends on what kind of credit you're talking about. Do you want me to pick you up Sunday?"

"No, I'll make it on my own," he decided. "Listen, Randy, don't get the idea that I'm getting religious or anything. I'm just—well, curious, I guess. Dan was right about one thing; it's intellectually dishonest to reject a philosophy without knowing something about it."

"See you Sunday," I said, heading for my locker. Curious, huh? Well, I didn't care why Sean Collins was coming, as long as he came.

w w j d   p o w e r   s t a t e m e n t

It is important to be able to try to answer the questions others have about God and being a Christian. But God's word says they will know we are Christians by the way we love one another.

s c r i p t u r e

I want you woven into a tapestry of love,
in touch with everything there is to know of God.
Then you will have minds confident and at rest,
focused on Christ, God's great mystery. All the
richest treasures of wisdom and knowledge are
embedded in that mystery and nowhere else.

COLOSSIANS 2:2-3

Scott's Dream Job

By Clint Baxter

I thought about it off and on all afternoon. Yes, there were clients to phone and appointments to keep, but in the back of my mind I could still see that sixteen-year-old son of mine stretched out in the hammock in our backyard, sipping lemonade and listening to what passed for music blaring from his CD player.

It was rare for me to return home during the day, but on this occasion I had forgotten a contract I needed. I took my lunch hour to go home and get it.

That's when I had spotted Scott stretched out in the back yard. First I heard the "music" and went to the window to investigate.

It was Margo's volunteer day at church; not that she would've been listening to that noise anyway, of course.

I glanced at my watch. It was still early. In any case I couldn't have left without satisfying my curiosity and appeasing the probable wrath of the neighbors at the same time.

I pointed to the CD player. "Keep it low, huh? Not everybody shares your taste in music."

He shrugged and took another sip of lemonade. "Did you get off early or what?"

"I had to pick up something," I replied. "Scott, I thought you were working."

"Hey, I am working," he informed me. "Can't you see the sweat rolling off my brow?"

"Very funny. What happened to all those yard jobs you had lined up?"

"Everything's on schedule," he said, "trust me."

"Just so we understand each other," I replied, "about camp, I mean."

"I know, I know. I have to earn my own money or I don't go," he began in a bored monotone. "And no last minute attempts to borrow it from Mom or Grandma. No problem. In fact right at this very minute I'm probably making between five dollars and ten dollars an hour!"

"Somebody's paying you to warm a hammock?"

"Not exactly. It's kind of a long story. Got a minute?"

I checked my watch. "Not now, Tell me later."

"Will do."

By the time I reentered the house he had already closed his eyes and turned up the volume on the CD player. At least it wasn't as loud as before.

Scott was a good kid. Margo and I had raised him in the church and he didn't give us much trouble. He had accepted Christ at an early age and was active in the youth group. Going to camp was important to him.

Margo was home when I got there on this particular day, but Scott wasn't.

"He was gone before I got back from church," she said. "Why?"

I quickly told her what I had found when I returned home at noon.

"He loves that hammock," she informed me in a motherly way. "He spends a lot of time out there."

"So when does he work?" I asked. "And what did he mean about making money while he was lying around?"

"I have no idea," Margo admitted. "But he's on the phone quite a bit, and I've seen him talking to some of the other boys in the neighborhood more than usual."

I frowned. There were no other boys Scott's age in our neighborhood. "Like who?"

"Well, there's Danny Wilcox down the block and Paul Winters across the street and. . . ."

"Those are just kids," I interrupted. "They couldn't be more than ten or eleven."

"I believe Danny just turned twelve," Margo said. "Yes, I'm sure of it. He is small for his age, though."

Scott came home just in time for supper. I was waiting for him.

"Lined up three more lawn jobs today," he began before I could ask. "It really helps if the people know you."

"Where are you getting your leads?" I wanted to know.

"I'm using the church directory," he explained.

"Scott, there's something I still don't understand," I told him.

Margo put a platter of chicken on the table and sat down. "Will you pray, Honey?"

We asked the Lord's blessing on our dinner, but I still had to have some answers, "How can you make money when you're lying in the hammock in the back yard sipping lemonade?"

"Simple," he replied. "Just because I line up the lawns that need mowing doesn't mean I actually have to do the work myself. Pass the chicken, please."

I handed him the platter. "If you aren't doing the work, who is?"

"I have a whole bunch of kids working for me," he explained. "See, I got to thinking: if I do the work myself, I can only do one yard at a time. If I have kids doing the work, I can handle more than one at a time. In fact, I can do half a dozen yards at the same time. On paper I've made more than enough for camp already. Now I'm saving for a car."

"What about these kids," I asked. "You have to pay them something, don't you?"

"Sure, but they work for about half of what I'm charging the customer," Scott replied. "The other half comes to me. For example, if I charge ten dollars per yard, which is pretty cheap, I get $5.00 and the kid gets $5.00. If I have four kids mowing four lawns at the same time, I'm making twenty bucks for lying in the hammock!"

"And you think these kids can do the work?"

"I only hire kids who have their own lawnmowers," he assured me. "And all the jobs are within a few blocks."

I shook my head. It sounded almost too easy. "And you haven't had any complaints?"

"Not yet. Of course, it would be kind of impossible to get complaints at this point."

I frowned. "Why?"

"My service is kind of special," he told me, wolfing down mashed potatoes smothered in gravy.

"I only look after a yard while the owner is on vacation. I expect my first customers back from vacation next week. Then I'll collect."

"Well, I'll have to admit it sounds pretty good," I answered. "Wouldn't hurt to check up on your boys, though. After all, you're the one responsible if they do sloppy work."

He shrugged. "Couldn't hurt, I guess."

So, we all went that night after supper. I had to admit that Scott was very well organized and had an alphabetical list of all his clients. The name of the worker assigned to a particular job was written right on the work order.

"Over on the right, Dad," Scott said as we drove down Tremont. "6732. It's that house with the fence."

"Helen Applegate lives here," Margo said.

"Right," Scott agreed. He glanced at his list. "Danny Wilcox is taking care of her place."

I parked the car and we took a fast look at the yard. Her lawn had been mowed and watered. "Not bad," I admitted.

"Doesn't surprise me a bit," Scott replied.

"Helen wouldn't like all those weeds in her flower bed, though," Margo informed her son, pointing.

"I'll make a note of that," Scott answered, writing it down on the order. "Pull weeds. I thought I told him."

Unfortunately, most of the other yards were in pretty sad shape.

"I can't believe it!" Scott exclaimed when we stopped at a particularly bad one. "This whole yard will have to be done again! If Paul thinks I'm paying him for a crummy job like this. . . ."

"Wait a minute, son," I interrupted. "He'll have to be paid. It's obvious that he tried; he just couldn't handle it. He's a little young to mow a yard this size anyway."

"But there goes my profit," Scott complained. "And if I have to do the yards over myself, I won't have time to line up other jobs!"

"Relax, " I told him. "You can do it. Camp is still six weeks away. Maybe keep Danny, since he's a little older and more dependable, and let the others go."

"Or maybe I'll just forget about camp," Scott began.

"That's up to you," I said.

Of course Scott went to camp and paid for everything himself, with money to spare. All his workers—including the lousy ones—were paid off, too, before he pocketed even a penny for himself. He didn't spend a lot of time in the hammock after that first week, but that didn't seem to bother him, either.

"If you want anything done right," he told me, "do it yourself." Okay, so he wasn't original. I was proud of him anyway. He had learned as much as he had earned that summer.

w w j d   p o w e r   s t a t e m e n t

Laziness is easy, it just doesn't get you anywhere. Anything worth doing—having a job, building relationships, or maintaining your Christian walk—is worth doing well and with substantial effort.

s c r i p t u r e

No matter how much you want, laziness won't help a bit, but hard work will reward you more than enough.

PROVERBS 13:4 CEV

Me? A Ten? No Way!

By Cindy Wainwright

So there we were, stuck in the church parking lot! "Why'd they have to schedule a meeting right after church?" I wanted to know. "It's such totally dumb timing!"

Denise Whitney and Carla Alexander had been waiting with me, but they were so busy yammering away about Sunday school and the new youth pastor that they didn't even hear me.

"What'd you say, Alyson?" Denise asked suddenly.

Well, what do you know! I thought. *They knew I existed, after all.* I checked my hair in the window of Mr. Peterson's Porsche. *Wow, what a car! I'd love one like it someday!*

"I said, why'd they have to schedule a meeting right after church?" I repeated.

"Weren't you listening? They're voting on whether or not to call Tom Driscoll as our new youth pastor," Carla explained.

"They'd better keep him!" Denise added. "He's cute! And he knows how to talk to us too."

"Like this morning," Carla went on.

I shrugged. Big deal. It was a lesson on the Ten Commandments. So what? I yawned.

"You don't look impressed, Alyson," Denise said. Boy, was she perceptive! "You like Tom, don't you?"

"He's okay," I admitted. "But couldn't he have picked a topic more current?"

"But didn't you hear what he said?" Carla replied. "He said the Ten Commandments are relevant for today!"

"And he really made them come to life, at least for me," Denise chimed in.

"But they're Old Testament!" I explained. "This is supposed to be a New Testament church! Where'd you get those shoes, Carla? I wish I had some!"

"That little shoe store in the mall," she said. "Darnell's. I'll admit I hadn't really given the Ten Commandments much thought in a long time, but the way Tom talked about them today—"

"He put it in a whole new light for me," Denise interrupted.

"But they're so obvious," I answered, admiring Denise's watch. I needed a new one. "I mean I'm not going to go around killing people or stealing or doing any of that stuff!"

"How about honoring your parents?" Carla asked. "That's a hard one for me."

"No problem," I told her. "We get along fine. Anyway, that's in the New Testament, too. I've heard 'Children, obey your parents' for as long as I can remember."

"The one about having other gods before you really got to me," Denise said "When Tom was saying a god could be anything that takes our eyes off the Lord or gets in the way of our serving Him—like hobbies or watching TV—I realized just how much time I spend on my gymnastics."

I frowned. "You aren't giving up gymnastics, are you? I wish I was half as good as you are!" She really was good too. Olympics potential, the coach said.

"Well, no, not give it up," Denise decided. "But lately it's like all I do. I need to keep it under control, so it's not the most important thing in my life."

"Don't any of the Ten Commandments give you trouble, Alyson?" Carla questioned.

I thought about it for a second. "No, not even one. Why don't we walk across the street to Starbucks?"

"Good idea," Denise agreed. "Got any money?"

I checked my purse. "Only some change. How about you guys?"

"I put it all in the offering," Carla said.

"Fifty cents," Denise announced. "Doesn't matter, the meeting should be out any second."

"I wish I had money," I told them. "Lots of it! Like this man at my dad's work who won a million dollars in a sweepstakes! I am so sick of being too young to get a job and not having money! The girl who lives next door to me has a job at the Taco Shack, and she's bringing home good money every week! I'd kill for this one outfit she bought a couple of weeks ago—"

I stopped talking because Carla and Denise were looking at each other and laughing. If you ask me, it was pretty rude. I got the definite impression that they were laughing at me too.

"What's so funny?" I demanded.

"You really don't think one of the Ten Commandments applied to you?" Carla asked, still snickering.

"Think really hard," Denise added, giggling.

"No!" I replied, more than a little bugged, but curious too. "Which one?"

"Well, it comes right after 'Do not bear false witness against your neighbor,'" Carla answered.

"In fact, it's the last one," Denise said. "You know, number Ten."

"The last one," I repeated, thinking. Then I frowned. "You mean the one about coveting? That's ridiculous! I wouldn't covet! You don't know what you're talking about!" I glanced toward the church. "Oh good! The meeting's over. I can't wait to get home. We have new neighbors moving in across the street, and I want to see what kind of stuff they have!"

Denise and Carla started cracking up again, like I had said something funny. No kidding, those two are weird!

w w j d   p o w e r   s t a t e m e n t

Jesus spoke more about the love of money and its danger than almost anything else. He warned against the power that money and possessions would have in our lives. Seeing the world as He sees it means having the proper perspective on material possessions and eliminating their power over us.

s c r i p t u r e

If you decide for God, living a life of God-worship, it follows that you don't fuss about what's on the table at mealtimes or whether the clothes in your closet are in fashion. There is far more to your life than the food you put in your stomach, more to your outer appearance than the clothes you hang on your body.

MATTHEW 6:25

Tough Break

By Walt Carter

The whole class sat quietly while Mr. Hendricks read the list. I'll have to admit it was kind of exciting, wondering who my partner for the project would be.

"The next team," Mr. Hendricks said, "is Andrew Cavanaugh—"

I froze as he called my name, and Lori Whelan's eyes met mine. Was that a hopeful look in those blue eyes?

"—and Reese Butler," Mr. Hendricks finished.

Reese Butler! My throat was suddenly dry and a big heavy knot was forming inside my stomach. Bruce Grant, sitting behind me, snickered and whispered, "Better luck next time, buddy!"

Out of the whole class, Reese was the only person I didn't want as a partner. Of course no one else would have wanted him either, so I guess Mr. Hendricks had been stuck. And now I was too!

What's wrong with Reese? I guess the best way to describe him would be "slow" and that's putting it mildly!

"You're in big trouble," Bruce told me after school.

I shook my head. "Yeah, I guess." I couldn't figure out why Mr. Hendricks made such a big deal about his choice being final on this assignment until he teamed me up with Reese. And he also knows that I'm a Christian. It wouldn't look very good if I tried to get out of working with Reese."

Bruce made a face. "That religion stuff sure isn't helping you now. See you tomorrow, Andrew."

Reese answered the door when I got to his house that night and turned away without even asking me in. I felt like going home.

"Hello, Reese," I began, extending my hand as I crossed the room.

"Hello," he replied, ignoring my hand and plopping down on the couch.

"About our project," I said. "It's on friction, you know."

He just sat there ignoring me and playing with a model car.

Instead I smiled. "That's a nice car, Reese. Did you make it?"

He nodded, "Would you like to see all my cars, Andrew?"

"Well, I—"

"Come on!" he said, jumping up and starting for the hall. That was it for the night!

While eating lunch with Bruce the next day, I invited him to church on Sunday night.

"I told you I was spending the afternoon at Lori Whelan's," he informed me. "She is my project partner. I could be there for hours."

"Yeah, but Lori goes to church on Sunday nights," I said. "Why don't you—"

"You have about as much chance of getting me to church as you have of getting a passing grade on your science project!"

Finally, Mr. Hendricks began to assign days for presenting our projects. I was hoping for one of the late dates.

"Starting off our presentations this Friday will be Andrew Cavanaugh and Reese Butler." Despite all the time I had spent with Reese, he wasn't ready to define friction, much less demonstrate it in front of the class. And it was a joint project. He had to do his share or both our grades would suffer.

"I saw your face when Hendricks set Friday for your project," Bruce said. "You'll bomb out—right?"

There was something almost arrogant in Bruce's attitude, and it bugged me. "You may be in for a few surprises," I replied. "How are you and Lori coming along?"

"Okay on the project, but otherwise lousy," Bruce said. "She invites me to church almost as much as you do."

That sounded like Lori, all right. "So why not come?"

He shrugged. "Maybe I will sometime. There's too much I don't understand about it, though."

"Like what?"

"Well, you believe that God loves you and wants to help you, and then you get stuck with Reese for your project," Bruce began. "If God really cared about you, why didn't He give you the best partner?"

"I don't know why I was teamed up with Reese," I admitted, "but I trust that God does."

I had been praying about Reese and our project all along, but before I went to his house that night, I prayed harder and longer than I ever had.

He was in his room when I got there, sitting on the floor, playing with those model cars. I almost turned around and walked out, but I couldn't. Somehow there was more at stake than just my science grade."

I'm trying to get them to go faster," Reese explained. "Why do some of them slow down so soon?"

"Reese, we have to get started on—" I began. Suddenly I stopped. "What did you say?"

The rest of the week was unreal. Once Reese understood that it was friction that slowed his precious cars down, and that the weight of each individual car was involved—plus the surface they were riding on—our project really got underway.

We did a huge assortment of experiments in class on Friday—every one involving model cars—and Reese handled each experiment perfectly! I did most of the talking, and held my breath when Mr. Hendricks directed a fairly complicated question at Reese right before we finished. Reese thought about it for a minute and answered the question slowly but accurately. The class applauded and Mr. Hendricks nodded approval.

Kids crowded around both Reese and me after class to congratulate us, but eventually they had to get to their next period. So Bruce and I walked alone to the gym.

"I have to hand it to you," Bruce said, shaking his head. "You pulled it off. I never thought it was possible."

"Thanks," I replied. "Bruce, remember when you said I had as much chance of getting you to church as I had of getting a passing grade on the project?"

He nodded.

"Well, Reese and I got a B on our project. Know what that means?"

He smiled. "I'm going to church with you this Sunday night?"

"Right."

w w j d   p o w e r   s t a t e m e n t

Patience is one of the most visible fruits of God's Holy Spirit at work in our lives; one that's clearly obvious to those who are watching.

s c r i p t u r e

So, chosen by God for this new life of love, dress in the wardrobe God picked out for you: compassion, kindness, humility, quiet strength, discipline. Be even-tempered, content with second place, quick to forgive an offense. Forgive as quickly and completely as the Master forgave you. And regardless of what else you put on, wear love. It's your basic, all-purpose garment. Never be without it.

COLOSSIANS 3:12-13

Just Push Enter

By Marlys G. Stapelbroek

It was your basic Monday morning. The alarm clock screamed; I thumped the snooze delay. The alarm clock screamed; I thumped—

"Jessica Lynn," Mom's voice echoed up the stairs. "It's 6:30!"

Six-thirty? Mom didn't usually hassle me until seven. Then I remembered my science report. It was due sixth period so I needed to be at school when the computer lab opened at 7:15.

By the time I arrived, the world was coming into focus. I only had to dial my locker combination twice before it swung open. I was rummaging on the top shelf for my folder, when I heard voices. Weird, since one of them belonged to Monica. We used to play together when we were kids, but now she's into stuff that makes me nervous, like hitchhiking to the mall and crashing her older brother's parties.

I couldn't see why she'd be looking for me. Then I realized she and her friends had stopped at the locker next to mine. Were Monica and her friends looking for Andrea Walker? That was weird. Andrea's really shy, and she knows some weird Zulu language because her dad used to work at this medical clinic in Africa.

I was pulling out my folder, wondering what they were up to, when I noticed Monica slipping a note into the vent at the top of Andrea's locker. There was a flap of that white first-aid tape on the paper, and Monica stuck the other end on the outside of the locker so the note hung inside the door.

I frowned. "What are you doing?"

Monica jumped like she hadn't noticed me. Then she smiled. "Oh, Jessica," she murmured, "I had a slumber party—" She glanced at the other girls, letting me know they were the lucky ones she'd invited. "We thought of the best joke. We wrote this note to Andrea about how pretty she is, and will she please come to the football game Friday night. And then we signed it—" Monica giggled. "We signed it, 'Love, Eric.'"

Eric Samuels. He'd transferred to our school a couple of months ago and already half the girls had a crush on him. Andrea probably did too, which meant that when she read it, Andrea would go to the game and hang around Eric, waiting for him to say something. When he didn't, she'd be crushed.

The pain in my stomach tightened into a hard knot. Talk about mean! When I looked at Monica, she and her friends were huddled together giggling. Banging my locker closed, I hurried to the computer lab. I was glad I hadn't been at her slumber party and glad I wasn't in her little clique. Really glad. And sorry for Andrea.

I slipped into the computer room and took the first empty seat. Calling up my file, I got out my notes and started typing. By 7:50 I was done. "Just enough time to print it out," I muttered, rolling a piece of paper into the printer beside me. I pressed "P" and the screen filled with a list of questions.

Number of copies? I shrugged. One should do it. Hybrid Seeds in American Agriculture wasn't the kind of reading material you handed out to your friends.

Starting page? Duh. I pressed the one. Ending page? I groaned. How did I know what page it ended on? I looked around for Mr. Patterson, but he was busy across the room. The boy next to me looked up.

"Having trouble?" he asked.

I nodded. "The print program keeps asking me dumb questions."

"Just press 'Enter.'"

"But the answer isn't 'Enter.' It's supposed to be a page number."

He shook his head. "'Enter' tells the computer to skip that question."

I must have looked skeptical because he shrugged and said, "It's your detention." Meaning, if I didn't get it printed out in time and was tardy, I'd be the one sitting in detention after school.

"Good point," I muttered, pushing "Enter" for the six questions still on the screen. The computer whirred, hummed, and then the printer started its thap, thap, thap. Picking up a clean sheet of paper, I watched it type the last line on page one. . . .

I caught the first page as it rolled out of the printer and turned to set it on my folder—Thap, thap—thap, thap. . . .

I spun back and stared at the printer. It was clacking away, mindlessly printing without any paper.

"Stop!" I hissed as Mr. Patterson hurried up.

"What's the problem?" he asked calmly.

I pointed to the printer. "It didn't wait for me to put in the next sheet of paper." With a quick nod, he tapped a few keys, and a moment later the printer stopped. "Thanks," I muttered, "but why didn't it wait for me?"

"Did you ask it to?"

I thought he was joking, but when he didn't smile, I shook my head. "I didn't know I had to."

Leaning over the keyboard, he started the print program again. The list of questions flashed on the screen and he pointed to the fourth line.

Pause between pages?

I gulped. "You mean I can't just push 'Enter' and skip all those questions?"

He gave me his patient smile. "The system has to have an answer for each question before it can start, so the programmer built in a default response. If you don't actively tell the computer what you want, it assumes you agree with that default position. If you want to roll in individual sheets, you have to tell it. Why don't you give it another try at lunch," Mr. Patterson offered.

Hurrying down the hall, I turned the corner. As I walked up to my locker, I noticed the white square of tape stuck to Andrea's door. That tape was like a magnet. I couldn't take my eyes off it.

And then Mr. Patterson's words echoed in my head. "If you don't actively tell the computer what you want, it assumes you agree with that default position."

Staring at that tape, I got this funny idea that life isn't all that different from a computer program. I would never do something mean like write a fake note to someone, but I hadn't said that to Monica. I hadn't told her that leaving that note was wrong. I hadn't even tried to stop them. By avoiding the whole thing, I'd let Monica and her friends assume I agreed with them.

But I didn't and suddenly, I didn't want anyone thinking I did. I shoved my books in my locker, then picked at the corner of tape until it finally came up. By the time I'd tugged the note out of the vent, Monica and her friends had me surrounded.

"What are you doing?" she demanded.

I ripped the note into little pieces. "Hurting someone else to get a laugh is really mean." Monica glared at me, but a couple of the other girls looked away. Then one of them pointed down the hall.

"Here she comes!" Instantly, they disappeared into the stream of kids moving through the hall. A second later, Andrea saw me. "You're here early today," she said softly, twirling the dial on her locker. The door swung open and she smiled.

"Yeah, early," I echoed, smiling back. Which is when I figured out that life is too important to just push "Enter."

w w j d p o w e r s t a t e m e n t

It takes a lot of courage to do or say what you know is right when it goes against the crowd. But God is honored and will honor you for choosing to be true to your convictions and to Him.

133

s c r i p t u r e

If you do the right thing, honesty will be your guide. But if you are crooked, you will be trapped by your own dishonesty.

PROVERBS 11:3 CEV

Blessing in Disguise

By Alan Cliburn

I hadn't expected it to be easy, but living with Uncle Dan and his family was a lot worse than I had anticipated. There were plenty of times when I felt like picking up the phone and calling my parents. One phone call and I could be on my way to New York.

But I wouldn't let myself make that call. It had been my decision to stay in Springfield and finish high school and I usually stuck with the decisions I made.

"Are you sure you won't go with us?" Mom had asked when Dad's transfer came through last fall.

"I'm a senior, Mom," I reminded her. "I'd like to graduate with my class."

"Makes sense to me," Dad said. "I'd do the same thing. And I'm sure Dan will let him stay there."

That had stopped me for a second. "Uncle Dan?" I repeated, frowning. "I thought maybe I could stay with Patrick Gilmore or one of my other friends."

"No," Dad replied firmly. "If you stay here at all, it'll have to be with my brother. It's only right. Besides, you and Kevin can get better acquainted."

I had forced a smile, but it was weak. Kevin was a year older, four inches taller, fifty pounds heavier, and mean. We had never gotten along, not even as kids. But if I didn't stay with Uncle Dan and Aunt Caroline—and Kevin—I'd have to go to New York. So I reluctantly agreed.

That's how I wound up sharing a room with a cousin who hated me, Jesus, and anything remotely connected to Christianity. I knew Uncle Dan's family wasn't religious, but that was putting it mildly. My parents weren't Christians either, but they didn't discourage me about my faith.

"Well, well, here comes the Jesus freak," Kevin said when I got home from church on Sunday. "And I do mean freak!"

"That's enough, Kevin. But do you have to go to that church every Sunday, Jason?" Uncle Dan asked

"I don't go because I have to," I explained. "I go because I want to. I wish you would go with me sometime."

"Are you saying we aren't good enough the way we are?" Aunt Caroline asked, sounding a little insulted.

"It's not a matter of being 'good enough,'" I began.

"Because I know an awful lot of church people who are no better than we are," Aunt Caroline went on. "And some are much worse."

"Yeah, there's this handyman at work who's all the time quoting verses out of the Bible," Kevin said. "But man, when he hits his finger with a hammer, you should hear him! He can outswear anybody I ever heard!"

"We'll be ready to eat as soon as you wash up, Jason," Aunt Caroline said, changing the subject.

Kevin was a pretty foul-mouthed guy anyway, but he went out of his way to swear when I was around. He'd tell me the filthiest jokes he knew, even though I told him I didn't want to hear them. Depending on his

136

mood, he'd physically restrain me from leaving the room if he was in the middle of a really bad story.

"Don't be rude, Jason," he'd snarl, shoving me against a wall. "Now I'll have to start all over!"

I was careful not to complain to Mom and Dad when I wrote them. Since they weren't Christians I knew they wouldn't understand.

"We miss you, Jason," Mom usually added at the end of her letters. "Let us know if you want to join us."

"It is tempting," I told my friend Patrick. "There are some nights when I don't think I can stand it another second in my uncle's house."

"You mean you'd leave in the middle of your senior year?" Patrick asked, frowning.

"It's not that I want to leave," I explained, "but you just don't know what living with Kevin is like."

"I think you're doing okay," Patrick replied. "Better than okay, in fact."

That surprised me a little bit, because I had kept Patrick informed of exactly what was going on in my life and somehow expected him to be a little more sympathetic. "You really think living with that heathen cousin of mine is okay?" I demanded.

"All I know is that you used to miss church and Sunday school occasionally," he began. "Now you're there every week. And not just on Sundays either. I don't think you've missed a single Bible study or anything."

"No, of course not," I replied. "I get out of the house whenever possible."

"It's more than just getting out of the house," Patrick corrected. "Otherwise you'd go to the library instead of going to church. The library's a lot closer to your uncle's house."

"Yeah, but after being around Kevin, I need to be with my Christian friends," I said.

"Are you still having your devotions every night?" Patrick wanted to know.

I nodded. "Sure. Why?"

"Because when you were living at home you used to forget," Patrick reminded me. "How's your prayer life?"

"Never better," I admitted. "If I didn't have God to talk to, I think I'd go out of my mind. You know, it's funny, but when Kevin starts telling one of those dirty jokes of his, I start praying. It really works, too, because I haven't even heard him the last few times."

"I'm not surprised," Patrick told me. "This explains a lot of things."

I frowned. "Like what?"

"I couldn't figure out why you seemed to be growing as a Christian," Patrick answered. "After all the stuff you've been going through, I kind of expected you to get away from the Lord, but just the opposite has happened. And I'm not the only one who's noticed, either."

I shrugged. "Well, maybe so; I really hadn't thought about it. Of course I rely on God a lot more, but that's because I have to."

"You're just like Paul!" Patrick exclaimed suddenly. "Remember how his faith seemed to grow while he was in prison and suffering so much persecution? And not just Paul, either. Persecution and Christian growth seem to go together!"

I decided then that I would stick it out at Uncle Dan's house until June, no matter what. Either God could supply all my needs or He couldn't, and I had ample evidence that He could.

During those next few months I would pray like never before; but not only for myself, as I had been doing. I decided to pray for Uncle Dan and Aunt Caroline and Kevin—especially Kevin. He needed Jesus more than anybody else I knew.

It seemed like a lost cause, at times, but that Philippian jailer probably seemed like a lost cause, too, in Paul's day. God worked it out then; He could work it out now.

w w j d   p o w e r   s t a t e m e n t

It's easy to go through the motions of being a Christian. It's when we are up against some resistance though that our faith is strengthened. Dealing with persecution is rough, but it does teach us to rely on God, just like Jesus did.

s c r i p t u r e

You're blessed when your commitment to God provokes persecution. The persecution drives you even deeper into God's kingdom.

MATTHEW 5:10

The Professor

By Clint Baxter

Talk about dumb ideas! Our new youth director was full of 'em. I mean, if there was anybody in the whole youth group I couldn't stand, it was Craig Rimstead. So naturally we were assigned to the same prayer team.

To tell you the truth, I would've dropped out if my dad had let me.

"Do I have to go?" I asked that first Tuesday.

"Have to?" Dad repeated, frowning. "Isn't this the night you're starting prayer teams?"

"Uh huh." Prayer teams! I didn't even like the sound of it.

"Then I suggest you show a little more enthusiasm, Scott," Dad told me. "Prayer is a privilege."

"Look, Dad, I don't have anything against prayer," I began.

"Good," he said. "Get your jacket and I'll drop you off on my way to the post office."

There was no use arguing with my dad; I had learned that a million years ago. Most of the time I didn't mind too much—at least I had a father who cared enough to be strict—but this was different. If I didn't want to be on the same "prayer team" with Craig Rimstead, that should be the end of it.

It wasn't just Craig, though. I didn't like the whole idea of praying in a group. To me prayer was a very private thing and what I said to God was nobody else's business. I liked that verse about going into a closet and praying, but I guess Jim Collins had never read Matthew 6:6.

"The importance of prayer is grossly underrated by most Christians," Jim began the night he brought up the subject of prayer teams. "There's a lot more to it than rattling off a few memorized words before you eat or thanking God for getting you through the day as you doze off at night."

I couldn't argue with that. So what's your point? I wanted to know.

"At my last church we tried something which was quite successful," he continued. "It's based on Matthew 18:19 and 20. Tonight each of you will be assigned to a team of three and these teams will meet once a week for prayer. Naturally you can meet more often if you wish."

There was stunned silence. We all just sort of looked at each other. Admittedly there were a few people in the group I wouldn't have minded praying with. Cindy Daniels looked like a perfect prayer partner.

"When you came in this evening, you wrote your name on a slip of paper," Jim went on. "All those names are in this fish bowl and I'm going to pull out three at a time. Our first prayer session will be Tuesday night at 7:30."

He started reading the names. I just sat there and listened, hoping I'd be on the same team with somebody I liked.

"Josh Atwell, Jan Salter, and Cindy Daniels," Jim read.

Well, that takes care of Cindy, I thought, disappointed.

"Scott Reller," Jim read, pulling my name out of the fish bowl. "Bryce Colter," he continued. That was okay with me. Bryce was a friend. "And Craig Rimstead."

I nearly groaned. Not Craig! Anybody but Craig! Well, I'm just not showing up Tuesday night, I decided.

But of course I did. Bryce didn't come, so it was just Craig and me. *Well, one time won't hurt,* I thought.

"I believe I have located an excellent place for our team," Craig began in that sickening voice of his. No kidding, he always sounded like he was making a report when he talked. Some of the kids at school called him "The Professor," among other things. He wasn't very popular.

"I really don't know you very well, Scott," Craig went on, "so I'm glad we're on the same team. Maybe we should get acquainted before we start praying together. I think we should know when our fellow team members accepted Christ and a little about their families."

"Yeah, okay," I agreed halfheartedly. "I became a Christian when I was twelve. My parents are both Christians. Your turn."

"My father died when I was four," Craig began. "My mother had never worked before, but after that she got a job at the library so she could support my sister and me. I accepted Christ when I was six. Do you have any prayer requests, Scott?"

Just one, I thought. "Uh, no," I replied. "None that I can think of right now anyway."

"I know it's difficult because we don't know each other very well," he said, "but it's really quite essential that we learn to open up to each other during this prayer time each week. As it says in Galatians 6:2, we're to share our problems with our fellow believers."

My main problem is being here, I felt like telling him. "Well, I guess I could be doing better in school," I decided.

"Good," Craig answered, writing it down on a little pad. "I'm keeping track of our prayer requests. By the way, I wish you'd pray for a neighbor of mine. He really needs the Lord, but I can't seem to reach him."

"Yeah, okay," I agreed. "What's his name?"

"Danny Slagle."

I frowned. "Danny Slagle? You mean from school?"

"Yes. Do you know him?"

"Who doesn't! We've been friends for a long time. Well, sort of friends. He's about the last guy I'd expect to come to church, though."

"Will you pray first?" Craig asked.

I swallowed. "Well, okay. I'm not real big on praying out loud, though."

My prayer that first night was about the shortest on record. Oh, I prayed for Danny and asked God to help me get better grades, but the whole thing was over in about a minute.

Craig, on the other hand, went on and on and on. I thought he was going to pray all night. Sure, some of the things he said were good, but he could've kept it a lot shorter as far as I was concerned.

"I'm going to pray for you every day, Scott," he told me before we left that first night. "I hope you'll pray for me, too. I need help with my priorities. I spend so much time studying that I don't always have time for people."

I can believe that, I thought while I was waiting for Dad to pick me up. But at the same time, I kind of liked the fact that Craig had been honest enough to admit something like that. But he still prayed too long.

The first couple of weeks Dad had to prod me a little, but after that I started going because I wanted to. Not only was Craig my prayer partner, he also had agreed to help me with English and Algebra.

Praying with Craig every Tuesday night made me realize that he was okay underneath all that intellectual exterior. I mean he had feelings and needs and wants just like anybody else. Before long I was willing to share some fairly personal stuff with him.

I thought I knew how to pray before Jim started the prayer teams, but my prayer life really improved when I had someone to pray with on a regular basis. I also learned that prayer is a lot more than just asking for stuff. It made a big difference, that's for sure, and not just on Tuesday nights either, but even when I prayed alone in my bedroom.

And we began to see some results, too. Danny Slagle didn't suddenly show up at church and march down the aisle to receive Christ or anything, but he did agree to go to a sports night with me. And he had a good time too, even if he wouldn't admit it.

But the biggest changes that occurred happened within the youth group itself. A lot of kids—like Bryce, for example—had decided that prayer teams were dumb and so they just didn't show up on

Tuesday nights. But those of us who were faithful each week really began to grow. I wouldn't have believed it if it hadn't happened to me, but praying together on a regular basis can make all the difference in the world.

And if you don't believe me, just ask my good buddy Craig Rimstead!

w w j d   p o w e r   s t a t e m e n t

God wants us to bring every concern of our lives, big and small, to Him in prayer. He cares about each and every concern because He cares so much for us. Prayer doesn't always bring about the changes we want in our lives; but it does change us.

s c r i p t u r e

Pray all the time; thank God no matter what happens. This is the way God wants you who belong to Christ Jesus to live.

1 THESSALONIANS 5:17

The Queen

By Misti Chapman

"Hey, Jay just drove past the house again!" I shouted.

"Not so loud," my sister "Queen Gloria" commanded from her throne—otherwise known as the couch—where she was polishing her fingernails.

"But Jay—"

"As I've said before," Queen Gloria proclaimed, "Jay Watson doesn't interest me in the least, and just because he has been smitten by my great beauty in no way obligates me to grant his request for an audience, much less a date."

"I think I'm gonna be sick," I said, making a face. "And how do you know he even wants a date with you?"

"I suppose he's driving by to catch a glimpse of you?"

"No, of course not," I admitted. "But there is another girl who lives here."

"That's it!" Queen Gloria exclaimed. "He's one of Megan's!" She laughed uproariously at the idea.

"It would serve you right if he was," I told her as I stomped out of the room.

A moment later I came upon Megan, dressed in jeans and an old shirt, absorbed in her latest oil painting. I studied her, and the canvas. She was talented, there was no doubt about that, and not bad looking when she took the time to get herself fixed up. But she wasn't in Gloria's league.

While Megan was painting each afternoon, Gloria would perch on the couch and do her nails or read fashion magazines. She always sat in the same place, which just happened to be in front of the picture window. I started calling her "Queen Gloria" because of the regal way she sat.

It had begun when Jay Watson started coming to our church. He was a year older than Gloria and they had gone to junior high together. But he hadn't paid attention to her, despite the fact that she had a huge crush on him. Admittedly, Gloria didn't look her best in seventh grade. She had braces, pimples, and skinny legs.

But something happened during that year when Jay went to high school and Gloria finished junior high. Almost overnight she blossomed and became beautiful.

Right away boys started asking her for dates, but my parents wouldn't let her go out with anybody until she was fifteen, and then it was only with boys from the youth group.

Jay Watson was a member of the youth group, so that wasn't why Gloria pretended she wasn't interested. And he was a good looking guy, which was Gloria's specialty. No, it all went back to the way he had treated her in junior high. To make it even more insulting, he didn't remember her!

It was obvious from the beginning that Jay wanted to talk to Gloria. I was standing right there next to her that first night at youth group when he walked up to her. She had recognized him instantly, of course, and told Megan and me who he was.

Megan was on the refreshments committee and left for the kitchen before the meeting was over. I was in charge of putting away the chairs, but hadn't really started my job when Jay made his move.

"I'm Jay Watson and I—"

"Welcome to the group, Jay," Gloria interrupted coldly. "So nice to meet you. Now, if you'll excuse me—"

"Hey, wait a minute," Jay called after her, frowning. But it was too late, and Gloria was soon surrounded by her many admirers, not giving Jay a chance to say another word. If it had been me, I would've forgotten about her, no matter how pretty she was.

Not Jay. Before long he started driving past the house. Just once or twice a day in the beginning. Gloria pretended to be annoyed, but I knew better. She wasn't fixing herself up for me, after all.

One day he stopped in front of the house and got out of the car. Gloria was holding court in the living room, as usual, and she nearly went berserk when her mirror reflected the image of Jay Watson walking up the driveway.

"The nerve of him, not even calling first!" she exclaimed. "Well, if he thinks I'm available on such short notice. . . ."

The doorbell rang.

"Tell him I'm busy!" she ordered softly, heading for the staircase.

"Tell him yourself," I replied, disappearing into the kitchen.

"Kyle! Come back here!"

But I refused to obey. I was curious about how Queen Gloria would handle the situation, and there was no excuse for her not to open the door.

The bell rang again.

"Will somebody get that?" Megan called from upstairs.

She, Gloria, and I were the only ones home, so a moment later I heard the front door open. I sneaked into the dining room so I wouldn't miss a word.

"Hello, Jay," Gloria began.

"Well, hi! Do you live here too?"

"Too?" Gloria repeated. "Yes, I do. Who were you expecting?"

"Megan, of course."

That was too much for me, so I emerged from my hiding place. "Hi, Jay."

"Hi, Kyle. I'm finding out things about this family I didn't know before."

"Like what?" I asked.

"Well, I knew that you and Megan were related, but I didn't know Gloria was your sister too." He turned to Gloria and smiled. "I got your name right, didn't I?"

Gloria nodded blankly, almost as if in a trance. "Uh, I'll see what's keeping Megan. Excuse me." She ran up the stairs.

Jay looked after her. "That girl is always on the move!"

I frowned. "Were you serious—about not knowing Gloria lived here, I mean?"

"Sure. Why?"

"Because you drive past here all the time and Gloria usually sits in the front window."

Jay blushed. "You've seen me driving by, huh? I hoped nobody would notice, except Megan. But I didn't know who that was in the window. All I ever saw was the back of her head."

I could barely keep from laughing, but there were a few more things I had to get straight. "That first night at youth group you walked right up to Gloria," I began.

"Yeah," Jay agreed. "That second time too. I wanted to find out what had happened to the girl who was sitting next to her, but Gloria flew off without telling me. Finally I found out that it was Megan and she was fixing the refreshments. I got her address and phone number."

"You like Megan?"

"Sure. We talk on the phone a lot, and sometimes she waves to me from the upstairs window when I drive past!"

"Sorry to keep you waiting, Jay," Megan said as she descended the staircase looking prettier than I had seen her before.

I was standing at the picture window, watching them drive off together, when Gloria appeared at the top of the stairs. "Are they gone?"

"Yes."

"I always thought Megan had better taste than that."

I could've said something—a lot, in fact—but I didn't. Megan had gone off with Jay, and she was his first choice. That was quite enough for a queen to accept all in one day.

w w j d   p o w e r   s t a t e m e n t

A safe way to measure your own value is to see yourself as God sees you—no more but no less.

s c r i p t u r e

The stuck-up fall flat on their faces,
but down-to-earth people stand firm.

PROVERBS 11:2

Roi Lkc and Love

By Marlys G. Stapelbroek

I was pocketing the money from raking Mrs. Taylor's leaves when Mom called over the fence. "Wes? Mrs. Evan's new neighbors need a baby-sitter this afternoon. Are you interested?"

I was definitely interested in the money. I'd be sixteen next spring. When Randy Ericson graduated, I wanted to buy his '65 Mustang. But baby-sitting meant diapers. I wrinkled my nose.

"Rick gets out of school at three," Mom added.

"School?" So no diapers.

"And Mrs. Bradshaw pays $3.50 an hour."

"Three fifty?" Three was the going rate. I bicycled right over to the Bradshaws.

When I introduced myself, Mrs. Bradshaw gave me a huge smile. "What a Godsend," she said.

"Me?"

"Not many boys want to baby-sit," she explained, "but since my divorce, Rick needs male companionship." She sighed. "Each year it gets harder to find someone older."

I frowned. "Older than who?"

"Rick. He accepts authority better from someone older."

"Sure," I agreed, wondering what she was talking about. Of course, I was older.

Then I saw Rick. He looked about thirteen and almost my height, but his face was flat and his eyes slanted.

"Rick has Down's Syndrome," Mrs. Bradshaw explained quietly.

I swallowed. I wasn't even sure how to talk to someone like Rick. How was I going to baby-sit him?

I guess Mrs. Bradshaw understood because she murmured, "Rick needs the attention you'd give a child, but he craves the respect you'd show your friends."

I was still thinking about that when Rick held up the silver engine from a toy train toward me. "Engine," he announced.

Mrs. Bradshaw gave him a hug. "Why don't you and Wes set up your trains?"

Nodding, Rick laughed as cows spilled out of a green cattle car. He was unwrapping a red caboose when I realized Mrs. Bradshaw had left.

The train table was in the basement. Spreading out the track, we started hooking it up.

"Don't make the curves too tight," I warned. Rick's stubborn frown reminded me of his mom's advice, and I added, "If the curves are too tight, the train will tip over." His quick nod made me feel good, and a moment later he was looking for straight pieces, too.

After we finished the track, Rick emptied a box of toy buildings on the table. I sorted them into piles. "Houses, the school, a church—"

"God house," Rick corrected me, setting the white building in the middle of the table.

"God house," I agreed. It made as much sense as church.

The train was cruising through the model town when Mrs. Bradshaw returned. "It's time for Wes to leave," she told Rick, shaking her head at his protest. "I'm going to see if he can come again next week."

"Come next week," he told me, holding out his hand. I felt odd shaking it. He seemed like such a little kid.

Upstairs, Mrs. Bradshaw opened her purse. "I've never seen him take to someone so quickly. When I start work next Monday, I'll need a sitter after school." She handed me $7.00. "Would you be willing to come each day for a couple hours?"

Two hours a day, five days a week? At $35 a week? That wouldn't be enough to buy Randy's Mustang in June, but maybe I could make up the difference on weekends.

"Okay," I told her, pushing the money into my pocket. Playing trains after school wouldn't be so bad.

But Monday when Rick got off the school bus, he looked mad. Stomping into the kitchen, he threw a notebook page on the floor. "Can't make 'k,'" he shouted.

Picking up the paper, I studied the large, shaky letters. R-I-C, R-I-C. Again and again he'd tried making a "k," but the lines wouldn't meet in the middle.

"We could practice," I offered.

Snatching the paper out of my hand, he ran upstairs and slammed the door. I almost went after him, except I wouldn't chase a sulking friend.

Then I remembered the soccer ball downstairs. A few minutes later I was kicking it against the garage door. Smack, smack, smack. I was sure the rhythmic sound would break through Rick's sulk.

When I finally saw him in the kitchen doorway, I waved. "Come on," I called, gently kicking the ball toward him. With a shy grin, he ran down the steps and kicked it back.

We didn't work on his "k" that day or even the next, but eventually he let me help. It took a couple weeks, but when he finally showed his mom, Mrs. Bradshaw cried.

"I'm sorry," she sniffed, "but he's been trying to get 'k' for so long." I nodded, glad I'd helped make things click.

Over the weeks, we fell into a routine—soccer or the park on nice days, trains and coloring when it rained.

The first week of November, we had our first snow. I was trudging through dirty slush when I saw the sign in Lawson's Hardware Store. Hiring part-time for Christmas.

Pulling open the door, I found Mr. Lawson and asked for an application. "I only need one clerk," he explained. "It's just through Christmas and I pay minimum wage."

Minimum wage? That was over $5 an hour. "No problem," I told him, then headed for the Bradshaws.

I fixed Rick a peanut butter and jelly sandwich, then sat across from him at the kitchen table with my application. Name, address, and social security number were easy. Experience was harder, but I knew a lot about hardware from my odd jobs.

The real problem was Mr. Lawson's scribbled note at the bottom. Hours available. I couldn't work during school, and if I was with Rick afternoons, I needed evenings for homework. Mr. Lawson would never hire me if I could only work weekends.

I thought for a long time, but there was only one answer: I had to quit baby-sitting. Just through Christmas. Two months at the hardware store would give me a real shot at buying that Mustang. Mrs. Bradshaw would understand. And Rick—

He was coloring, drawing big letters.

"What are you doing?" I asked, puzzled.

He pointed to my application. "What you do."

Copying me. That's how he'd learned to make a "k" and head a soccer ball. But he'd written Roi Lkc.

"What are you writing?"

He sat up proudly. "My best words."

"Can you read them?" I asked, not wanting him to know I couldn't.

He pointed to Roi. "Trains and—" his finger slid over to Lkc "—God."

Trains and then God. I smiled, wondering how God felt about coming in second to a toy train. My smile faded. How would Rick feel about coming in second to a '65 Mustang? How could I throw away the trust and friendship we had for minimum wage?

Sighing, I picked up my pen and filled in my hours available—weekends. As I finished, Rick pointed to it.

"Your best word?"

I shook my head. "Not really." But what was my best word? How did I know God should come first and that Rick was miles ahead of an old Mustang?

Smiling, I realized there was one thing that put everything else in the right order. Reaching for one of Rick's crayons, I wrote in big red letters: Love.

w w j d   p o w e r   s t a t e m e n t

Jesus always put people first. When there is a choice between better and best, you can always know that God wants you to choose to behave out of love for another person.

s c r i p t u r e

Self-sacrifice is the way, my way, to finding yourself, your true self. What kind of deal is it to get everything you want but lose yourself? What could you ever trade your soul for?

MATTHEW 16:26

Trusting

By Julie Durham

"Dad, can't we please stay up just a little while longer?" Michelle and Michael begged, their eyes full of pleading. "Please."

Uncle Doug smiled slightly but then he shook his head. "No, kids, for the last time, go to bed."

They pouted a little as they came and gave me and mom and dad hugs goodnight. "Hey, aren't you forgetting someone?" Doug asked as they started to drag out of the room. Still pouting, they gave him a hug and kiss and shuffled off to bed.

"They've grown so much, Doug." Mom said softly. "How do you do it?"

We hadn't really seen Michelle and Michael since they were only a year and two years old. At that time, Uncle Doug and Aunt Katie had moved to California. Since we live in New Hampshire, we didn't get together with them very often. After Aunt Katie died from cancer, Uncle Doug stayed out West for about a year. Then he decided to come back.

I was excited that Uncle Doug was back. He'd always been my favorite adult. I remember when he and Aunt Katie first had Michelle and Michael, I spent lots of time at their house. When I was afraid to talk to my parents about something, or they didn't seem to have time, I could always count on Uncle Doug and Aunt Katie to listen. Although we were heart-broken when Aunt Katie died, I was glad that Uncle Doug was coming home.

I'd hit it off with eight year old Michelle and nine year old Michael right away, even though I'm seventeen.

It wasn't that late. I didn't understand why Uncle Doug didn't let them stay up later—especially since it was their first night with us. But I soon forgot about it.

Since Uncle Doug only lives a couple of blocks from our house, Mom would watch the kids after school until Uncle Doug got home and I'd often go over on weekends to take them to the park or spend time with them. One day, I took some licorice with me to share with them. I was kind of surprised when Michelle grabbed hers and stuffed it into her pocket. Then she ran into the other room.

Michael started to tell me something, but Uncle Doug came into the room and I offered him a piece. He looked at me like he was trying to decide whether or not to say something.

"Julie, did you give a piece to Michelle?"

"Yeah, I did."

Uncle Doug sprinted through the other room and out into the back yard, with me and Michael close behind. He found Michelle hiding behind a bush.

"Okay, hand it over."

"What?" Michelle said looking innocent.

"You know what." He answered sternly. "Now."

Michelle scowled as she passed over the gummy, half-chewed licorice.

"You're mean," she announced, and began to cry. I didn't know what to do. From the baby-sitting I'd done, I knew never to butt in when parents were having a problem with their kids, but this was my cousin. And Uncle Doug was being awfully mean. What was the big deal about a lousy piece of licorice? Michelle looked at me and hurtled herself into my arms, sobbing like her heart was breaking.

Uncle Doug touched my shoulder. "Julie, I think you'd better go home for right now," he sighed. "I need to talk with the kids for a while."

"I was going to take them to the park . . . ," I started to explain.

"Thanks, but not today," Uncle Doug told me. I unwrapped my arms from Michelle and began walking away. "No, no, no. . . ." she screamed hysterically. I hesitantly looked back, but Uncle Doug had a hold of her hand and was leading her into the house.

Uncle Doug and the kids didn't come over that night, like normal. And I was afraid the kids were being punished because I took them licorice. I felt awful. All afternoon I thought about them and about Uncle Doug. He sure had changed. He seemed so strict—more than strict, he seemed mean.

I was moping about it all afternoon. Then Tony called. Tony Graziano. Dark skin, jet black hair, long black lashes, and clear blue eyes. Lately, Tony's been hanging around me at school. I don't know that he's a Christian. But as I told my best friend Pam when she mentioned something, I don't know for sure that he's not a Christian either.

Pam had frowned at me, "I think you have a good idea that he's not." I know the Scripture about being unequally yoked and everything. But it's not like I was planning to marry the guy. Who knows, maybe being around me will help him see that Christians aren't so bad. Maybe he'll even become one.

Tony and I talked for forty-five minutes before Mom made me get off the phone. Right before he hung up, he asked me to go to a picnic the next morning. "Sorry, I can't. Church." I told him. "I'd love a rain check though."

He didn't give me a hard time at all. That's one thing I liked about Tony. He's nice. Even nicer than all the Christian guys I knew—and a lot cuter than most. I mean, I figured that surely God doesn't want me to go out with a Christian guy when I can go out with a non-Christian guy who's nicer. After all, I'd been raised to believe that God wants the best for me. Tony doesn't drink or smoke or do drugs or even swear. And he's as moral as any Christian guy I know. And just like Tony didn't try to get me to skip church, I know he'd never resent my going to church, even if he doesn't go himself.

"How about next Saturday?" Tony asked.

"It's a date . . . er, an appointment," I answered with a smile and a bit of a blush—good thing he couldn't see me.

As I hung up the phone, Mom frowned. I knew she'd have fits about my plans to go out with Tony Saturday. I'd worry about that later in the week.

It was hard to sit through church Sunday— partially because I kept thinking, *I could be with Tony right now.*

And partially because the pastor was talking about obeying God—even when we didn't agree or understand. I quickly tuned him out and concentrated on Tony. I did feel another little flinch of guilt when we sang the closing hymn, *Trust and Obey*, but by the time we got home, I'd shrugged it off.

After supper on Monday, Mom handed me Michael's jeans and asked me to run them over to Uncle Doug's house. He'd ripped them at school and mom had patched them.

When Uncle Doug opened the door, he gave me a warm smile, "Julie! I just put the kids to bed, but come on in and have a Coke. It seems like forever since I've really talked with you."

We ended up sitting on the front porch swing, making small talk for a while. I told Uncle Doug a little bit about school, but I didn't mention Tony. I didn't want another lecture. Then Uncle Doug started talking about the kids.

"Julie, I know sometimes I must seem mean to you. Like Saturday. I didn't have a chance to explain, but Michelle's allergic to licorice. We've had a few scary times with her when she's eaten it.

"I know there are other times when I may seem too strict. Like making the kids go to bed early. I know when you were little your parents let you stay up. But you had a different temperament. You've always been a little bit of a night owl. Michelle and Michael aren't. If they're up past 8:30, they're at each others throats all the next day.

"Sometimes it's hard when I know other people think I'm being too strict or mean, but I do have a reason for every regulation I place on the kids."

I didn't know what to say, so I didn't say anything. He pushed the swing with his foot and continued.

"You've experienced it many times in your own life. Your parents tell you something and you don't understand their reasoning. But when your parents come down hard on you, it's because they love you and want to protect you. They know you don't always understand. And that hurts them almost as much as it makes you angry . . . parents hate it when their children just think they're being mean. But it's smart to obey them. Even when you don't understand."

Suddenly I remembered vague words I'd only half heard the pastor preach Sunday "When God gives a command it's usually for two reasons—because He wants to protect you and because He wants to provide for you—His way. When we disobey Him, we step out from under His umbrella of protection. And when we try to provide for ourselves instead of letting Him do it, we might miss the provision He had for us all along."

Sitting on Uncle Doug's front porch, enjoying the warmth of the early spring, I suddenly began to see God's command about not being unequally yoked in a new light. Maybe God was trying to protect me. And maybe if I stayed so set on Tony, I'd end up missing the provision that God has for me.

I knew I needed to do some thinking. Alone. As I walked down the street, the words floated back through my mind, "Trust and obey, for there's no other way to be happy in Jesus, but to trust and obey."

Mingling with the "enemy"—someone who wasn't on God's side of the battle—wasn't the only command

I'd broken lately. I needed to sit down with God and do some heavy-duty apologizing. But first, as I walked into the house, I walked straight to the phone. "Hello, Tony? I'm sorry, but about Saturday. . . ."

w w j d   p o w e r   s t a t e m e n t

God's commands for our lives are for one of two reasons: to protect us or to provide for us. When those limits seem restricting, remember that God is acting out of His love for us.

s c r i p t u r e

This is your Father you are dealing with, and he knows better than you what you need. With a God like this loving you, you can pray very simply.

MATTHEW 6:8

The New Neighbors

By Alan Cliburn

A big white moving van was parked in the Brewster's driveway when I got home from school that Wednesday. *So it really is true, after all,* I thought.

The Brewster's house had been empty for a while and we'd been hearing rumors that the family that was moving in didn't really belong in our neighborhood, if you know what I mean.

Of course just because that moving van was there didn't tell us anything about the new owners, I thought, standing on the front porch and watching the movers carry in a red couch. I could see they liked bright colors. But lots of people do; that didn't mean anything.

Before long a big car pulled up in front of the Brewster's house and my worst fears were realized. A whole family of them got out! There was a mother and father and three kids, including a guy about my age.

"Look at that fancy car," Dad said Saturday morning as he stood at the picture window. "Doesn't surprise me a bit!"

"Fred, it's no bigger than our car," Mom answered. "I'm going over to meet them this morning. Who's coming with me?"

"I-uh-I have chores to do," Dad replied quickly, heading for the garage.

"How about you, Kent?" Mom asked, looking at me.

I swallowed. It was bad enough having them in the neighborhood; did I actually have to go over there?

"I'm sure the boy will be attending your school," Mom went on. "He might already be enrolled, in fact."

"If nothing else, you can invite him to church," Mom said.

"Church?" I repeated, frowning. "You want me to invite him to our church? I thought they had their own churches!"

"Well, it's true that some churches do seem to be made up of members of one race," Mom admitted, "but all races are welcome at our church. Isn't Joe Wong in the youth choir?"

"Well, yeah," I agreed. Somehow that seemed different. Besides, Joe didn't live on my block.

Mom continued. "We know nothing of this family's religious background; we only know that their skin is a different color than ours."

Isn't that enough? I thought. But I shrugged. "Okay, I'll go. Let me put on a different shirt."

"Come right in!" the woman said after Mom introduced herself and me. "I'm Roxie Harris."

She was friendly and so was her husband, but that didn't mean anything. Anybody can act friendly, after all. The girls were kind of cute, I guess; probably about seven and ten, although it's hard to tell.

"And this is Chris," Mr. Harris announced as a tall, lanky guy about my age came into the room. He looked a little embarrassed.

"I'm Kent," I said, shaking hands with him. "Wanna come over and shoot some baskets later?" I heard myself ask.

"Yeah, that'd be great," he answered.

Chris was pretty good at basketball, which wasn't surprising, if you know what I mean. Actually we were pretty evenly matched, which made it fun. Chris wasn't loud or dirty talking or anything either, which caught me off guard. I guess you can't believe everything you hear.

"Would you like to go to church with me tomorrow?" I asked him before he went home. "We have a pretty good youth group."

"Is it okay?" he wanted to know.

"Sure, anybody can go to our church," I said before I realized how that sounded. "I mean, it doesn't matter what your church background is."

He smiled. "I knew what you meant. Yeah, I'd like to go."

And he went. I wasn't too sure how the other kids would treat him—some Christians are really prejudiced, if you can imagine such a thing—but nobody made any snide remarks; none that I heard anyway.

I thought Chris would only go that one time, but he really liked it and wanted to go back. In fact, his whole family went a couple of weeks later. Dad smiled and shook hands with Mr. Harris and all that, but I could tell it was killing him.

"We're thinking about joining your church," Chris told me one afternoon as we were walking home from school. "Have you heard any negative comments about our being there?"

"What do you mean?" I asked, feigning innocence.

He gave me a look. "You know what I mean! We're the only family of our race attending your church. Do you think it'll create any problems if we join?"

"It shouldn't," I replied. "I mean, the important thing at our church is a personal relationship with Jesus, not the color of someone's skin."

"Well, we are Christians," Chris assured me. "I accepted Jesus when I was nine."

I was sitting right up front the Sunday morning the Harris family joined our church. I knew there were some people, like my father, who weren't thrilled, but nobody said anything and Pastor Willis welcomed them warmly into our fellowship.

I wasn't home the day of the accident, but later Mom told me that Dad had fallen off the ladder while pruning some trees and gashed his arm really bad. It was Mr. Harris who drove Dad to the emergency room.

There's more. Despite Mr. Harris' fast work, Dad lost too much blood and needed a transfusion. Turned out he has some rare blood type and they couldn't find a donor. Mr. Harris volunteered to be tested and wound up giving Dad some of his blood!

"Well, we were brothers in Christ before," Mr. Harris told Dad one evening when the whole family was over for dinner. "Now we're blood brothers!"

"You probably saved my life," Dad said. "God brought your family into our neighborhood for a reason."

"We like it here," Mrs. Harris replied. "Thanks to you, we feel we really belong."

"If you guys are gonna get mushy about it, can Chris and I be excused?" I asked.

They laughed. "We're having dessert later," Mom reminded me.

"We'll be right outside," I promised.

Chris and I just sat on the front porch without saying anything for a while.

"I really am glad we moved here. I didn't want to at first. It was kind of scary moving into a minority neighborhood—you hear all kinds of stuff—but this is home now. Thanks for everything, Kent."

"That's okay," I told him. "For a white guy, you aren't so bad."

w w j d   p o w e r   s t a t e m e n t

Jesus sees us all the same. Remember that the person who may look different from you on the outside, is like you on the inside. He or she has the same hopes and fears, joy and hurt. It honors God when you choose not to make judgments about others based on their race.

s c r i p t u r e

Do as God does. After all, you are his dear children.
Let love be your guide. Christ loved us and
offered his life as a sacrifice that pleases God.

EPHESIANS 5:1-2 CEV

Emilio

By Dennis C. Gerig

Emilio stood at the end of the counter, polishing it for all he was worth. There wasn't a customer in the place and Mr. Reynolds had gone to the bank, but there he stood, working!

The other guys and I sat in a front booth, drinking free Cokes and talking about Emilio. They didn't like him much.

"What's he doing anyway?" Adam hissed. "Trying to make us look bad?"

Justin shrugged. "To who? There's nobody here but us. He'd be taking a break if he had any sense at all."

"So who says he has any sense?" Adam snickered.

Emilio glanced up self-consciously at the sound of Adam's snicker.

"Hey, there's the boss' car!" Adam exclaimed suddenly, pointing out the window. By the time Mr. Reynolds entered the restaurant a minute later we were all working. He glanced around and nodded approval.

It was a fast food restaurant with a dining room section for people who wanted to eat there, so the four of us were kept busy once the customers started coming in. Emilio really was a good worker, but that didn't matter to Adam and Justin. They hadn't even given him a chance.

Emilio had tried to fit in, being friendly and all that, but when he didn't get any encouragement he soon stopped trying, concentrating on his work. I felt sorry for him, but I couldn't do anything, not with Adam and Justin watching. They were friends of mine, after all.

"I need somebody to work tonight," Mr. Reynolds said one afternoon. "One of the girls on the night shift is sick. How about you, Scott?"

"No, I can't," I replied. "I have an appointment."

"Anybody interested in working tonight?" Mr. Reynolds asked.

"Not me," Adam decided.

"We got tickets to the ball game," Justin explained.

"I'll work," Emilio volunteered. "I don't mind."

Adam and Justin gave each other a disgusted look.

I would've worked that night, but I was taking a class at church, taught by the pastor. It was a class on witnessing, with a lot of on-the-job training. We usually went out in teams of three, with one experienced person as the leader and the other two as trainees. I was in the trainee stage.

"Most people are scared of witnessing and visiting people in their homes because they haven't done it before and are afraid of the unknown," Pastor Miller had explained the first week. "This course is designed to help you get over that fear."

It was a lot easier than I expected it to be. Most of our contacts were people who had visited the church, so they were usually glad to see us. After we invited them to come back to church and explained the various activities available, our leader shared the Gospel. Several people came to Christ as a result.

I kept hoping I'd learn how to share my faith well enough to tell Adam and Justin about the Lord, but considering the way they acted when I invited them to a youth group sports night I decided to wait a while. They just didn't seem at all interested.

"I thought of a way to get rid of Emilio," Adam whispered after Mr. Reynolds left for the bank and Emilio headed for the storeroom.

"How?" Justin questioned.

I didn't say anything.

"It's his turn to fill the salt and pepper shakers," Adam explained. "What if he puts sugar in the salt shakers?"

"All right!" Justin hissed.

I wanted to object, but I didn't. It wouldn't have done any good, after all.

Naturally there were lots of complaints from customers who were less than thrilled with sweet French fries.

"Who is responsible for this?" Mr. Reynolds demanded after the lunch crowd had thinned out.

"Emilio filled the shakers today," Adam announced.

"Yeah, I saw him," Justin chimed in.

"With salt," Emilio said, "not with sugar!"

"Take care of it," Mr. Reynolds told him. "Check every shaker."

"Yes, sir," Emilio agreed.

After that they played dirty tricks on Emilio whenever they could, like putting mustard in his change drawer.

"What is going on around here?" Mr. Reynolds wanted to know. I could tell he was really upset.

"My drawer was okay earlier," Emilio insisted.

"What do you know about this, Scott?" Mr. Reynolds asked.

"Me?" I replied. "I didn't see a thing!" It was true, but I probably wouldn't have told him even if I had seen Adam or Justin in action.

Eventually he quit, even though Mr. Reynolds tried to get him to stay on. "Accidents happen," he told Emilio.

Emilio shook his head. "There have been no accidents."

Adam and Justin thought it was great and spent most of their spare time congratulating each other. They liked the girl Mr. Reynolds hired to take Emilio's place, so everything ran pretty smoothly.

We were having good results in our witnessing class at church. "With all the teams we have now," the pastor said one night, "we have more than enough to handle the church visitors. So we're going to ask the more experienced teams to try going into a neighborhood and talking to whomever will let you in. Your assignments are on the table. Pray together and then be on your way."

My team was sent across town to an older section. I was really nervous, and left our packet of literature in the car.

"I'll go back for it," I said as we stood on the first porch.

When I returned, the door was open and the team was already inside. *That was fast!* I thought.

"Yes, I think I would be interested in visiting your church," I heard a familiar voice begin as I entered the house.

"Great!" my trainer responded. "One of our team members is in the youth group and will be glad to tell you about their activities. He should be back any—"

"Here I am," I interrupted. Then I froze. No wonder the voice sounded familiar! Facing me in that living room was Emilio! "Hi!" I began, extending a hand.

But Emilio did not take my hand. "You're from the same church?" he asked.

I swallowed. "Yes. Emilio—"

"It's a friendly church where we study the Bible," my trainer explained, obviously puzzled by the sudden change in Emilio's attitude.

"I would not be interested in attending your church," Emilio said. "You will excuse me now, please."

"Yes, of course," my trainer agreed, frowning. "May we give you some free literature—"

"No, thank you," Emilio said, walking to the door. "Good-bye."

"Emilio," I began. But the expression on his face convinced me that it was indeed time to leave. "I'm sorry," I managed on the way out. "But I'll be back."

"Don't bother," he told me.

I felt sick as we left that house. He treated me just as if I had been the one who did those terrible things to him at the restaurant! And I couldn't blame him.

I'd be back, though. I couldn't let him believe that my behavior and lack of courage was what being a Christian was all about.

w w j d   p o w e r   s t a t e m e n t
You have the power in every relationship in your life to draw others to or away from God.

s c r i p t u r e
Stay on good terms with each other, held together by love.
HEBREWS 13:1

173

The Unmasking

By Mike Chapman

Well, he's done it again, I told myself, glancing around to see if anybody else thought the youth director's latest idea was as dumb as I did. Of course from the back row it's pretty hard to see facial expressions.

"I know some of you came tonight expecting to see the video I've been telling you about for the past month," Dave went on.

"That's exactly why I came," I agreed.

"But I guess it got lost in the mail or something, because it hasn't arrived yet," he continued. "Maybe next week."

So why don't you just dismiss us and let us take off? I felt like asking. I didn't, of course. Lonnie Adams was sitting right next to me and he was a new Christian. I wasn't going to do anything to set a bad example for him. Not on purpose anyway.

"So this is the way it'll work tonight," Dave explained. "We're putting Galatians 6:2 into practice and we'll do it by breaking into small groups of about five each. Once you get your group organized, introduce yourselves around the circle and simply start sharing whatever's on your mind. Don't worry, we'll do it in stages."

Dumb! I thought. *Dumb! Dumb! Dumb!*

"Now there's a tendency to just share the good things the Lord has been doing in your life," Dave said. "That's okay for a couple minutes, but that verse in Galatians tells us to 'bear one another's burdens' and that means opening up to the others in your group, and taking off that protective mask most of us hide behind."

This whole idea is bothering me, I wanted to tell him.

"It's not easy, but it's scriptural and it will help you grow," Dave promised. "Okay, let's break into groups of five."

There was a lot of noise and confusion as the groups were formed. It would have been a good time to sneak out without being noticed, and I probably would have if Lonnie hadn't been there.

Since Lonnie and I were sitting right next to each other we just stayed where we were. Joe Fergus turned his chair around to join us and so did Claudia Reynolds and Diane Grossinger.

"Well, I guess we have our five," Joe announced.

Real good, Joe, I thought.

"One, two, three, four, five," Claudia counted.

I gotta get out of here! I told myself.

"Does everybody know everybody?" Diane asked.

We all looked at each other. I could hardly stand the excitement.

"I don't think I know you," Claudia decided, focusing on Lonnie.

Lonnie blushed. He blushes real easy—especially around girls.

"This is Lonnie Adams," I said. "Lives on my block."

"Oh yeah, you were in my English class last semester," Joe remembered.

"Do you have a sister named Gloria?" Diane questioned.

"No," Lonnie replied. "But I have a brother named Jeff."

"You're kidding!" Claudia exclaimed. "So do I!"

"Maybe you're related," I inserted.

Fortunately the youth director interrupted us before Claudia and Lonnie started climbing their family trees.

"Okay, you should have introduced yourselves by now," Dave said from up front. "The next step is to share something about yourself with the group."

Claudia told about getting a job and how that was an answer to prayer because there was a pink dress in the window of some store downtown that she just had to have. I thought I was gonna be sick.

"I've been a Christian for over three years!" Diane exclaimed.

"I've been a Christian for a month," Lonnie said, blushing.

Then they all looked at me. "How about you, Keith?" Claudia began.

"Everything's fine," I replied. "I'm a Christian and everything's great." I shrugged. "What else can I say?"

I didn't have to say anything else. Dave's voice rose above the rumble. "You should be finished sharing something about yourself," he told us. "And you probably know something about the people in your group that you didn't know before. Right?"

He was right about that, I had to admit. Pink dress!

"We're coming to the hard part," Dave went on. "I want you to go around the circle and tell something that is hurting you right now, spiritually or otherwise. Be open and honest."

There was mostly silence in the room for a few seconds, then spurts of embarrassed laughter.

"Well, I might as well start," Joe decided, swallowing.

I studied him. He was a big muscular guy, popular and all that. What kind of problems could he have?

"There's this new transfer from Colby High," he continued. "He plays quarterback, same as me, and he's good. The coach is talking about letting him start in the game against Taft. I have to admit that some of the feelings I've had toward that guy—and the coach—aren't very Christ-honoring, if you know what I mean. So I guess I could ask you guys to pray for me about my attitude."

"Well, my problem is with my sister," Claudia began. "She gets into everything I own and my parents act like she's an angel or something."

"Just a week ago we found out that my aunt has cancer," Diane said.

It was Lonnie's turn and for once he wasn't blushing. Well, not much anyway.

"I want my parents to become Christians," he managed, "my brother, too. So far they aren't interested."

That was all and then everybody was waiting for me to bare my soul. They could keep waiting, as far as I was concerned. I had an image to maintain, after all.

"Keith, you must have some hurt to share," Claudia said.

"Yeah, I got up in the middle of the night to get a drink and stubbed my toe," I admitted.

Nobody thought that was too funny.

"Everything's fine," I insisted.

"You mean nothing's bothering you?" Joe wanted to know. "You aren't having any trouble?"

"Well, things could be better at work," I confessed, getting mad just thinking about it. "My hours are being cut because the boss' nephew needs a job. It really isn't fair." I took a breath. It felt kind of good getting my feelings out in the open. That surprised me. "It must be sort of the way you feel about this new guy on the team," I told Joe.

All five of us just started talking about stuff then—well, I guess Lonnie mostly listened—and it was amazing how much we had in common. Maintaining a consistent prayer life and keeping up with devotions was hard for everybody in the group and we all had questioned our relationship with Christ at one time or another.

"Even you, Keith?" Diane asked.

"Even me," I admitted with a grin. I hadn't planned to open up the way I did, but it was sort of contagious. And once I got started it just seemed like the most natural thing in the world.

Praying in our little group was really a good experience, too. Claudia got a little carried away, but there was still something special about praying for people who had really shared their problems in such a personal way.

After youth group was over I began to wonder if I had said too much. I had been a Christian for a long time, after all. Joe and Claudia and Diane weren't exactly new Christians, either. What was a baby Christian like Lonnie going to think, hearing a bunch of supposedly mature believers admit that their lives weren't always so great?

"Too bad the video didn't come," I began as we walked home.

"I'm glad it didn't," Lonnie replied. "I was beginning to think something was wrong with me," he went on. "You and most of the other guys at church always go around acting like everything's fine and you don't have any problems or anything."

"Lonnie—"

"But I've had a lot of problems since I've accepted Christ," he continued. "Up until tonight I thought it was just me. So I'm glad that video didn't come and we got to talk."

"I guess I am too."

w w j d   p o w e r   s t a t e m e n t

A lot of people use sarcasm as humor or as a shield to protect themselves in an uncomfortable situation. The problem is that sometimes it can be hurtful or can detract from a meaningful experience for someone else.

s c r i p t u r e

Rash language cuts and maims.
but there is healing in the words of the wise.

PROVERBS 12:18

Metamorphosis

By Kent Phillips

It was the last place I wanted to be. I mean what guy wants to spend a perfectly good Monday night listening to some kids with questionable talent pound a piano?

But when your kid sister is playing in a recital and your strong-willed mother believes that the whole family should offer "moral support," you find yourself on the back row of the women's club. Period.

"What about dad?" I asked.

"Your father had to work late," Mom reminded me.

Miss Cathcart started the recital with her beginning students, which was fine with me. The songs were really short, and it was kind of funny when the little kids made a mistake or waved to their parents.

But as the kids got bigger, the songs got longer. I glanced at the program.

"Oh no, Martha Elizabeth Dunhill is next!" I hissed.

Mom gave me a threatening look and put a finger to her lips, so I didn't say what I was thinking. Of all Miss Cathcart's students, Martha Elizabeth was the absolute worst. She had been taking for years too.

Martha Elizabeth was no kid, by the way. She was about my age, and in fact we went to the same junior high. We weren't exactly friends, but we usually said "hi" when we passed each other in the hall.

As her fingers touched the keyboard, sour notes filled the air. No kidding, it was the worst-sounding stuff in the history of the universe.

"What's the name of this song anyway?" I asked.

Mom pointed to it in the program. "The Butterfly," she whispered. "By Grieg."

"Should've stayed in the cocoon!" I hissed.

"Not another word, Timothy!" Mom ordered, her face flushed.

But the kid sitting next to me on the other side had overheard what I said and giggled. "Should've stayed in the cocoon!" he repeated gleefully, snickering.

I tried not to laugh, so I snorted, which was even worse. That made the kid next to me laugh, out loud this time, and suddenly I lost it. I couldn't stop laughing, no matter how hard I tried.

At least not until Martha Elizabeth pounded her fists on the piano keys and stomped offstage. That had never happened before. I became very quiet very fast.

I don't know if my sister played well or not. I didn't even hear her, too wrapped up in my own thoughts and what Mom was going to do to me after the recital.

But she turned it around. "What are you going to do about this, Tim?" she wanted to know while we were waiting for Stephanie.

"Do about what?" I asked innocently.

"You've been a Christian long enough to know that what you did was wrong."

"Maybe I could pray for forgiveness?" I suggested hopefully.

"That's good," Mom agreed, "but it's not enough," Mom added.

I swallowed. "Uh, maybe I could apologize to Miss Cathcart?"

"And who else?" she wanted to know.

I looked at her. "Not Martha Elizabeth!"

"Think of all the money Mr. and Mrs. Dunhill have invested in piano lessons," she went on.

"Apologize to them, too?" I was feeling sick.

"Of course maybe your father can come up with some interesting alternatives," Mom continued.

"I'll apologize," I decided quickly.

Well, might as well get it over with, I told myself the next day at school.

"Timothy!" she said when I walked up to Martha Elizabeth before school. "I was hoping I'd see you today!"

I cleared my throat. "You probably want to talk about last night, huh? Look, Martha Elizabeth—"

"Thanks for saying what you said," Martha Elizabeth interrupted.

I listened for sarcasm. There was none. "You were glad I smarted off?" I asked. "But—"

"Oh, my parents were upset by what you said and what I did, but it worked out great," Martha Elizabeth assured me. "I've been wanting to quit piano lessons for a long time and last night they finally realized that their daughter is not going to become a famous concert pianist. I'm going to study art—I may actually have some talent for it!"

I looked at her. I had known Martha Elizabeth for a long time without ever realizing how pretty she was.

"Uh, what are you doing at noon, Martha Elizabeth?" I heard myself ask.

"Eating lunch," she replied with a giggle. "Why? And call me Marti. I dropped the Martha Elizabeth a long time ago, even if Miss Cathcart still put it in her recital programs that way."

"I-uh-I thought maybe we could have lunch together," I went on, blushing, "you know, in the cafeteria."

"I owe you a lot for rescuing me from piano lessons, Timothy."

"Tim," I corrected in my deepest voice.

The bell rang then and we started off toward first period together. Mom wanted a full report on my apology to Martha Elizabeth—I mean Marti. She'd get one, all right, but it would be edited!

I had never asked a girl to eat lunch with me before, or do anything else, for that matter. Maybe it took a butterfly to get me out of my cocoon!

w w j d   p o w e r   s t a t e m e n t
Self-control is another one of the fruits of God's spirit at work in our lives. When we faithfully seek Him and spend time in His word and in prayer, the fruit of self-control will begin to show.

s c r i p t u r e
God's Spirit makes us loving, happy, peaceful, patient, kind, good, faithful, gentle, and self-controlled. There is no law against behaving in any of these ways.

GALATIANS 5:22-23 CEV

My Cousin's Secret Weapon

By Clint Baxter

My name wasn't on the list. I guess I could've lived with that, except for one thing. Brent's name was right up there at the top. He had done it to me again.

I hardly knew my cousin until his dad—my uncle —was transferred out here a year ago. At first Brent and I got along okay, but it soon became apparent that he was better at stuff than I was.

There were no jobs available, but he found one anyway. "Where?" I had wanted to know.

"Food World."

I stared at him. It was just around the corner, a lot closer to my house than his. "You're kidding!"

But he wasn't, of course. Brent always managed to make things come out his way. I figured he had a secret weapon.

He was a good student too. After the first semester I tried to make sure that Brent and I weren't in the same classes. It wasn't always possible. We both wound up taking Mrs. Hobson for English. I didn't mind. English was one subject that always came easily for me.

Unfortunately Mrs. Hobson decided that English included spoken language as well as written language.

"Each of you will prepare a five-minute speech," she announced early in the semester.

Mrs. Hobson advised us to talk about something we knew about, so I chose photography. I thought I knew a lot about it, but when I got up to give my speech, I froze. What came out of my mouth was mostly dull facts about shutter speed and types of film that nearly put the whole class to sleep.

Nobody expected too much when Brent got up to talk about his butterfly collection, but within a minute he had everyone roaring with laughter—me included. In five short minutes he had not only enlightened us with a lot of stuff we didn't know about butterflies, but he had entertained us at the same time. Miss Hobson was so entertained she gave him an A; I got a C.

Basketball was something else, though. This was going to be the year I made the team.

"I hear you're going out for basketball," Brent said one afternoon.

"Yeah, I am."

"Me, too."

"Good." I wasn't overly enthusiastic, but it didn't bother me. I was slightly taller than Brent. Besides I had seen him play in gym class a few months earlier. He was only fair.

"Want me to pick you up for that thing at church tonight?" he questioned.

I frowned. "What thing?"

"You know, that inner-city project."

"Uh no, I won't be able to go—too much homework."

Also I thought it sounded like a rotten idea. Our youth pastor decided that we should go down to this housing development one night a week, get to know some of the kids, and tutor them on a one-to-one basis.

I went the first night and it was a real mess. Those inner-city kids were rowdy and didn't seem one bit impressed that we had given up an entire evening to help them out. I had no intention of going back.

"By the way, Dave tells me that Brent is trying out for the basketball team," Dad began one night. "How about you, Ryan?"

"Yeah, I am," I assured him.

"Want to shoot a few baskets after supper?"

"Thanks, but I'm kind of tired tonight," I decided. It was nice of Dad to offer, but I played basketball at school all the time; I was definitely ready for the tryouts.

Or at least I thought I was. The coach lined us up and let us take ten free throws first. I made six out of ten, which was pretty good, but some of the other guys were making eight or nine out of ten, including my cousin. When did he get so good? What was his secret weapon anyway?

"I'll post a list of the guys who made it on the bulletin board Monday afternoon," Coach Larson told us an hour later. "Thanks a lot for coming out."

Of course my name wasn't on the list and Brent's was. And to make matters worse, that was the day when he was coming to stay with us for a few days while his parents were out of town. I couldn't even escape him at home!

"Congratulations on making the team," I forced myself to say when I entered the house and saw him sitting at the kitchen table.

"Thanks, Ryan," he replied. "You'll make it next time. Want to shoot a few baskets?"

"No thanks," I said. "Have to write my outline for that speech Mrs. Hobson assigned us."

I went up to my room, but it was a little hard to concentrate with the basketball thumping against the garage door every couple of seconds.

"Now I know what your Aunt Margaret meant," Mom said suddenly, entering the room with some clean T-shirts.

I frowned. "About what?"

"Brent's basketball workouts," Mom explained. "According to Margaret he shoots baskets for hours every day."

I nodded. *No wonder he was so good,* I thought. I really hadn't spent much time practicing at all, not by comparison.

He excused himself right after supper and went up to his room. Walking past the door later I heard him talking. I listened. If that was his speech it didn't sound very funny, and he stumbled around for words too.

An hour or two later, after watching some television, I went past the room again. *Brent was still practicing, only it seemed a lot smoother than before,* I thought, frowning. I planned to read mine over a couple times—once I thought of a topic—and let it go.

The phone rang just as I was sitting down at my desk. It was the youth pastor. "Ryan, we need more people involved in our inner-city project. How about it?"

"Well," I began.

"Brent's probably told you about the boy he's been tutoring," Mr. Reynolds went on. "Cordell prayed to receive Christ last week," the youth pastor continued. "Several kids have, in fact. It's been kind of hard, but we're starting to see results. Pray about it, Ryan."

"Yeah, I will," I promised half-heartedly. *Just because Brent led some kid to Christ didn't mean I could,* I thought, passing the guest room again.

I heard his voice, so I listened. He was still going over his speech! I couldn't believe that guy! *And he'll probably get another A,* I thought disgustedly. *If I spent that much time on mine I could get an A, too.*

So why don't you? I asked myself.

Who has the time? I answered.

You do! And you probably would've made the basketball team if you had put in enough time working out! You might've even got that job at Food World if you had hung in there instead of deciding you didn't have a chance!

I frowned. Was that the real difference between Brent and me? He was willing to put in the extra time and energy to get what he wanted and I wasn't?

I was still standing there when Mom's voice came up the stairs. "Ryan, that special you wanted to see is coming on."

I started for the staircase, then stopped. "Thanks, but I have too much homework, Mom." It would be hard to change some of my priorities, but change them I would. My cousin needed a little competition!

wwjd power statement

Self-discipline is a a fruit of God's spirit and a sign of self-care. If you care about yourself, you will take care of the concerns of your life, your responsibilities, reputation, and testimony.

scripture

So prepare your minds for service and have self-control. . . . In the past you did not understand, so you did the evil things you wanted. Be holy in all you do, just as God . . . is holy.

1 PETER 1:13-15 NCV

Shattered Dreams

By Al Burns

I couldn't even close the screen door quietly. It banged shut, announcing my arrival.

"That you, Rob?" Mom called from the kitchen.

"It's me," I replied, heading for my room. All I wanted to do was be alone.

She appeared in the doorway. "Supper won't be ready for two hours."

I felt like telling her, in no uncertain terms, that I probably wouldn't feel like eating supper later, but I didn't. She'd just ask what was wrong and I'd tell her and she'd try to cheer me up and I couldn't handle that at the moment.

"It's been a rough day," I added. "Think I'll lie down for a while."

I stretched out across the bed, hoping that sleep would come instantly, giving me some relief from my depression. *It's your own fault,* I told myself. *It was stupid to try out for the team.*

Personally I thought I had a chance this time. I gave it my best shot, just as I had when I tried out for the track team, the football team, and the basketball team. When I came in dead last during track tryouts I knew I was finished, and I was admittedly too small for football and too short for basketball. But tennis?

True, about half of my serves went into the net; but I did manage to return a few serves. Some of the other guys weren't much better.

Let me make it, Lord, and I'll give You all the credit, I had prayed as I walked toward the bulletin board outside the coach's office.

I studied that list for a couple of minutes, almost like I expected my name suddenly to appear. But it hadn't, of course. Another dream shattered.

Why, God? I asked as I lay across the bed. He had to know how much I liked sports. Suddenly there was a knock at my bedroom door. "Rob, are you asleep?" Mom's voice asked.

I wanted to be, but I wasn't. "No, Mom," I replied, sitting up. "Come on in."

She opened the door. "I hate to bother you," she said, "but I made cookies this afternoon. Would you mind taking some to that new family at the end of the block?"

I did mind, but I stood up. "I'll take them."

"I believe they have a boy around your age," she went on.

I wasn't in the mood to be social, but I could go through the motions. *Maybe nobody will be home,* I thought.

But a nice-looking lady came to the door right away. I introduced myself and told her why I was there.

"How nice!" she exclaimed, taking the cookies. "Tell your mother how much I appreciate this!"

"I will," I promised.

"You must meet my son," she continued. "Just a second, please."

The coach could've put me on the second team, I told myself as I was waiting.

"I'm sorry," our new neighbor announced suddenly. "Marc's asleep. I know he'll want to meet you, though. Please stop by again. And don't forget to thank your mother for the cookies," she called.

I nodded. Mom knew how to make good cookies, all right. In fact, she had a talent for cooking. My sister's talent was music, and Dad could fix just about anything.

And then there's me, I thought. *Mr. No Talent.*

"Hi, Rob!" one of the kids in the neighborhood yelled suddenly. "We were playing doubles till Scott had to go home. Will you fill in? We've got an extra racket."

"No thanks," I replied. *Besides, haven't you heard?* I felt like adding. *I'm no good at tennis; just ask the coach!*

I went home and relayed the new neighbor's undying gratitude to my mother for her cookies.

"You had a call while you were out," Mom went on.

I frowned. I didn't get many calls. "From whom?"

"Somebody from the church," she said. "Volleyball practice will be tomorrow night."

Not that I had any intention of going. I was giving up sports. Well, maybe it was the other way around. They had given me up and I might as well face the fact that I was no athlete.

Mom was waiting for me when I got home from school the next day. "Mrs. Talbott just called," she began.

I looked at her. "Mrs. Who?"

"Our new neighbor," she explained. "Marc is anxious to meet you."

I wasn't especially anxious to meet him. The newly formed tennis team had started workouts that afternoon.

Five minutes later I was following Mrs. Talbott down the hall to Marc's room. I wanted to ask why he didn't just come out and meet me in the living room, but I kept my mouth shut.

I found out for myself. Lying in a hospital bed was a guy about my age. He smiled when I entered the room and stuck out a hand. "Hi, I'm Marc Talbott," he said.

"Rob Winslow," I replied.

It didn't take long to discover that Marc was paralyzed from the waist down, the result of a bicycle accident a year earlier. He was very open about it and seemed to accept the situation.

"There is a slight chance that I'll walk again," he added, "but I'm leaving that in God's hands."

"Are you a Christian?" I asked. "So am I!"

"Yeah, I don't know how I would've handled this if it weren't for the strength that God has given me," Marc said. "I went through a period of bitterness and all that, but my pastor stuck with me and helped me understand that verses like Romans 8:28 are either true or they aren't."

I didn't answer.

"I must've heard that verse about being content regardless of the circumstances a million times," Marc went on. "But the more I thought about it, the more I realized that I could easily have been killed in that accident and that God kept me alive for a reason."

I didn't know what to say.

"I was planning to become a professional football player," Marc continued, "so after the accident I figured my future was shot. 'Try something else,' my pastor kept telling me."

"And did you?" I asked.

"Yeah, I tried painting, but when Mom said she liked my horse picture I knew my career as an artist was limited."

I frowned. "How come?"

"It was supposed to be a dog!" Marc exclaimed with a grin. "Then the pastor suggested I try writing my story. I did and writing came really easy for me. I've sold several short stories and now I'm working on a book. I still like football and hope to do some coaching someday," Marc said. "Just because I can't play doesn't mean I can't enjoy the game, after all." He looked at me. "Are you into sports at all, Rob?"

"A little bit," I heard myself reply. "I'm not good enough for the varsity teams at school or anything, but there's a church volleyball team I might play on."

"Hope I can get to one of the games sometime," Marc answered.

I thought about Marc as I walked home a little later. Paralyzed, and he was still trusting God and looking to the future. And I was all upset because I hadn't made the tennis team at school!

Okay, so maybe I wasn't so great at sports. So what? God obviously had something else planned for me. Wasn't that enough?

"Rob, can you play?" the same kid who had asked me the day before yelled.

I started to say "no," but glanced back at the Talbott house and nodded my head. I had two arms and two legs that still functioned. It was the least I could do.

w w j d   p o w e r   s t a t e m e n t

It's not hard to look at what others have and feel sorry for yourself for what you lack. But God gives abilities, talents, and opportunities to each of us and expects us to use them wisely.

s c r i p t u r e

Then you will say to the Lord, "You are my fortress, my place of safety; you are my God, and I trust you."

PSALM 91:2 CEV

The Weekend I'll Never Forget

By Cindy Wainwright

My father, who will be forty-three in May, acted like a little kid when the official notice arrived. "I made it!" he announced triumphantly, waving the letter and almost jumping up and down. "I'm the new regional manager!"

"That's real nice, Daddy," I added from the breakfast table where I was having a bowl of cereal.

"And listen to this," he went on, still about two feet off the ground. "Your presence is requested at the executive officers' annual meeting next weekend in San Francisco. All expenses will be paid by the company, and your wife is cordially invited to accompany you."

"San Francisco?" Mom echoed, breathlessly. "Oh Stan, we haven't been there since our honeymoon!"

"Wow, that really is nice," I agreed. "Too bad it's only for two!"

"I hadn't thought of that," Mom replied quickly, a frown working its way across her forehead. Dad just smiled absently in my direction, still excited about his new appointment.

"I was only kidding!" I told Mom "I don't want to go. I can't. I have a date with Darryl on Saturday."

It turned out that my wanting to go along wasn't the part that concerned her. "We can't go off and leave Carla home alone," she began. "Stan! Are you listening?"

"What's that?" Daddy asked, reading his letter for about the fiftieth time.

"Mother, I'm nearly seventeen!" I reminded her.

"What's wrong?" Daddy wanted to know.

"Stan, put down that letter and listen!" Mom exclaimed. "What will we do with Carla next weekend if we go to San Francisco?"

"There's no 'if' about it," Dad corrected firmly. "We're going, all right. I've waited five years for this promotion and I want you there with me, Lois."

Mom was undeniably pleased, even though there was still concern in her eyes. "But what about Carla?"

"I think you're underestimating our daughter," Daddy answered, looking at me in a special way. "She's no longer a child, you know. She's a young woman, and I believe she's more than capable of managing her own life for one weekend."

"Thank you, Daddy," I said. "I appreciate your trust."

"It has nothing to do with trust," Mom insisted. "It just isn't safe. I was reading a story in the paper about a—"

"Oh Mother!" I interrupted, hoping Daddy would come to my rescue.

But he didn't. "Your mother's right," he said. "I'd rather you didn't stay alone. Why don't you ask a girl friend to spend the weekend?"

"I'll ask Mandy," I replied.

I called Mandy and gave her the full rundown. "It's okay," she told me a moment later. "At least for Friday night. I'm not sure about Saturday, though. Sometimes I baby-sit for the Reinharts on Saturdays. I won't know until the middle of the week."

I hung up and went to tell my parents.

"She can stay both nights?" Mom asked.

For a second I almost said "yes," but somehow I couldn't. "Probably," I replied. Then I explained about the baby-sitting job.

"But suppose the Reinharts need her for Saturday night?" Mom questioned.

"Then I'll just ask someone else," I said simply.

That seemed to satisfy Mom, so we didn't discuss it after that.

We hadn't dated much, but I liked Darryl a lot more than I wanted him to know, and my stomach always felt kind of fluttery when I was near him.

"What have you heard from Mandy?" Mom asked Thursday night.

"She's planning to come over about seven tomorrow evening," I replied.

"What about Saturday?"

"Mrs. Reinhart hasn't called, so she's planning to spend Saturday night here, too," I said. "She's going out, but so am I. Neither one of us is planning to stay out late, though."

At five o'clock the next afternoon, Mom and Daddy were ready to leave for the airport.

"Have a good time."

"We will honey," Daddy promised. "Your mother and I will be able to enjoy this trip more completely than some parents because we have absolute faith and trust in you. That means a lot to us."

"It means a lot to me, too, Daddy," I managed, swallowing. "You'd better go now or you'll miss the plane."

Mandy arrived at seven and we watched television for a while. Fortunately Mandy and I had been friends for so long that I didn't have to entertain her. She even brought her books along and did some homework.

We slept late the next morning and were having a leisurely breakfast when the phone rang. It was Mom, just checking to see if everything was okay. I assured her that everything was fine.

I had no sooner hung up when the phone rang again. This time it was for Mandy.

"Mrs. Reinhart?" she repeated, frowning and looking at me. "Tonight? Well, I guess it'll be all right."

"Are you baby-sitting tonight, after all?" I asked.

"Yes," Mandy replied, making a face. "It's one of those last minute deals that I hate, but if I turn them down they're liable to get somebody else permanently."

"But I thought you had plans," I reminded her.

"It was nothing definite," she explained. "The youth group is going out and Tom Patterson asked if I was going. I told him I would be if I didn't get a baby-sitting job. He'll understand."

"I hope my parents will," I said.

"What do you mean?"

"They think you're spending the night here."

"I still can," Mandy replied. "The Reinharts hardly ever stay out past midnight. I'll have him drop me by here instead of going home—that is, if you'll be back by then!"

"Darryl knows I have to be in by eleven."

Darryl picked me up at seven-thirty and we went to a basketball game. I wasn't wild about sports, but it was apparent that Darryl was. So I showed as much enthusiasm as possible.

After the game we went out to get something to eat and then home. There was something about being with Darryl that made the time fly by. I could hardly believe it was nearly eleven.

"I remember what your dad told me about your curfew the first time I took you out," Darryl said. "And I like to stay in good with dads! Where is he tonight, by the way?"

I explained about Dad's promotion and the weekend in San Francisco. "Mom called this morning." We got out of his car and walked to the porch together.

"You mean you're home all alone?" he asked.

"No, they didn't want me to stay alone, so my friend Mandy is staying with me," I corrected. "But she is baby-sitting tonight." I fished the key out of my purse and inserted it in the lock.

"Maybe I'll come in for a minute," he suggested.

"Well, I don't know," I replied. I wanted him to, but I wasn't sure if my parents would approve.

"I really should check the place out," he went on. "You know, to make sure nobody's in there."

We went from room to room together, Darryl looking inside closets and under beds. I felt very safe with him next to me.

"Well, nobody's here," he announced.

"Thanks—"

Suddenly I was in his arms and he was kissing me—hard. At first I tried to break away, then I just relaxed and kissed him back. Again and again and again.

"Darryl, we shouldn't," I told him finally, gasping.

"Why not?" he whispered. "We're alone and nobody'll know. I really like you, Carla."

"I like you, too," I admitted, "but—"

"But nothing," he interrupted gently.

I had often wondered what I would do if a guy pressured me about sex. I had been convinced that I could handle myself in any situation. But that wasn't how I felt as Darryl held me close. My heart was pounding and I knew I was weakening.

"Your parents won't be back until tomorrow night," he reminded me, "and they were the ones who didn't want you to be alone!"

He said it as a joke, almost as if deceiving parents was something to be proud of. I remembered what my father had told me before he and Mom left for the airport. He trusted me, and I had no interest in betraying that trust.

"You'd better go now," I managed as firmly as possible.

"Carla—"

"Now."

I was standing in the open door, watching as Darryl drove off and puzzled by his casual attitude about sex—almost as if it didn't really matter and he was

just seeing if I would give in—when another car
stopped at the curb and Mandy got out.

We had been friends for years, but I was never quite
so glad to see her as I was right then.

"What's wrong?" she asked when she reached me.

"Come in and I'll tell you," I answered. "I'll never
forget this weekend!"

w w j d p o w e r s t a t e m e n t

**Remember two key principals about dealing with sexual
pressure. 1. Decide ahead of time that you will make decisions
about your sexual behavior based on God's word, not on how you
feel. 2. Make every effort to stay out of situations where your
convictions might be compromised.**

s c r i p t u r e

*So run away from sexual sin. Every other sin
people do is outside their bodies, but those
who sin sexually sin against their own bodies.*

1 CORINTHIANS 6:18 NCV

Foolproof

By Alan Cliburn

It was Tuesday afternoon and we were heading back to the warehouse, Joel and me. I couldn't believe I was actually getting paid good money just to drive around town, but I wasn't complaining either. There was more than driving involved, of course. Joel and I delivered orders for Office Warehouse, which included furniture like desks and filing cabinets.

On this particular Tuesday the truck was in the shop, so Mr. Kramer let us take one of the company cars. Fortunately there was no furniture to deliver, just packages. One of us could have handled it easily, but Mr. Kramer wanted us both to go.

"Might as well start learning how to do the paperwork, Sam," he told me before we left the warehouse.

The paperwork was a piece of cake. We just had to get somebody to sign for the merchandise at every stop. We had several deliveries in the same vicinity. Maybe that's why we finished so soon.

"Hey, turn left at the next corner," Joel said suddenly.

"We've worked hard enough for one afternoon," he went on." Let's take a little break. Pull up there in front of Harry's." Harry's was a "family recreational center," with video and computer games and stuff like that.

"Are you kidding?" I replied. "We have to get back to the store. Mr. Kramer knows we didn't have a lot of deliveries. Besides. . . ."

"Relax," Joel interrupted. "I mean, will you just trust me to work it out? I guarantee that it'll be okay."

He opened the door and got out, but I just sat there behind the steering wheel. Joel was always working the angles and so far he hadn't gotten caught. This was different, though. This time he was asking me to go along with him.

"Are you coming or not?" he demanded.

"I don't know," I answered. "It doesn't seem right."

"Don't be wound up so tight," he advised. "Or is having fun against your religion?"

For a second I nearly wished I hadn't opened my mouth to Joel about my faith, but I had. "I just believe in giving a guy his money's worth and Mr. Kramer isn't paying me to play."

"Kramer won't know anything about it," Joel hissed, leaning through the window on his side of the car. "What's the matter, can't you Christians do anything?"

That just about did it. The last thing I wanted was to give Joel a negative impression of being a Christian, but at the same time I wasn't quite dumb enough to give in. Still, I was tempted. "What'll we tell Mr. Kramer if we get back an hour late?"

Joel grinned. "We had a flat tire!"

"Yeah, but we didn't. Besides, he'll want to see a receipt if we got it repaired."

"We didn't get it repaired," Joel informed me. "We just put on the spare ourselves. We had some trouble with the jack, that's why it took so long. It's foolproof! Come on."

I knew I'd never get through to Joel if he thought Christianity was nothing but rules and regulations. I could make up the extra time at the warehouse later and he'd never know the difference. But something told me it was still wrong, regardless of how much rationalizing I did.

"I'm going back to work, Joel," I heard myself say.

"Don't be a jerk all your life," he began.

I answered him by starting the motor. I guess he knew I wasn't kidding, because he got in, slamming the door shut behind him. "I won't forget this, Turner," he snapped.

"You guys are back early," Rex Keller said as I parked the car. He ran the loading dock for Mr. Kramer.

"Yeah, we are," Joel agreed, giving me a nasty look.

"It was a light load," I added, ignoring Joel.

"We can use some help inside," Rex went on.

"Thanks to you, we'll be working in that hot warehouse all afternoon when we could be at Harry's," Joel hissed.

Joel wasn't kidding about the warehouse. It was like an oven, with little ventilation. Admittedly I had second thoughts about my decision as perspiration started running off my body a few minutes later. Joel kept his distance too, working at the other end of the building. Up until that day we had gotten along pretty well, despite our differences.

"Joel, Sam, I'd like to see you in the office," Mr. Kramer announced suddenly. It was cool in his office. I could have sat there for the rest of the day! "Was there some reason why you didn't turn in your routing sheet, Joel?" Mr. Kramer asked.

Joel gave me a superior, amused look. "Sam was in charge of the paperwork today," he replied.

"Oh no!" I groaned. "Left it in the car! Be right back." I stood up and headed for the door.

"You can get it later," Mr. Kramer assured me. "Have a seat, Sam. I really called you in here to commend you for the work you've both been doing lately. I've gotten nothing but good reports from customers for your fast, courteous service."

"Thanks a lot," I said.

"Yeah, thanks," Joel added.

"A job of this type requires men who are trustworthy," Mr. Kramer continued. "Once you leave the store you're pretty much on your own. Unfortunately not everyone can handle this kind of freedom and I was admittedly apprehensive about hiring guys your age." Joel and I just sat there.

"No more," Mr. Kramer went on. "I now have total confidence in you. I hope you'll both be with us for a long time."

"Fine with me," Joel replied.

"Me too," I agreed, "except it'll have to be part-time when school starts."

"Yes, I understand that," Mr. Kramer answered. "In fact, your honesty when you applied was one reason I hired you."

"Oh, he's real honest," Joel said, giving me a look. Naturally Mr. Kramer didn't catch the sarcasm.

"I'll let you get back to work now," Mr. Kramer decided. "By the way, did you have any trouble with the car, Sam?"

I frowned. "Trouble? No, none at all."

"Good. After you left, I remembered that the car you took doesn't have a spare tire," Mr. Kramer explained. "We'll see that it doesn't happen again."

Joel swallowed. "No spare?"

"I'm just glad you didn't have a flat," Mr. Kramer said with a smile. "That'll be all. Oh, let me have that routing sheet as soon as possible, Sam."

"Yes, sir," I agreed, quickly leaving the office. Joel was right behind me, though.

"Hey, Sam, wait up!" he whispered.

"Have to get that routing sheet," I replied, trying hard not to laugh.

"Did you know we didn't have a spare?" Joel wanted to know.

"No, of course not," I answered truthfully.

"Oh man, if I had told Kramer we had a flat and changed it ourselves. . . ."

"But you didn't," I reminded him. "I'd better get that routing sheet."

I hurried on to the parking lot, grinning all the way. Joel and his foolproof scheme! If I had given into temptation and gone along with it I would have been the fool. An unemployed one.

w w j d   p o w e r   s t a t e m e n t

To be stable is to be reliable and consistent in your behavior and actions so that you can be counted on.

s c r i p t u r e

You have been born again, and this new life did not come from something that dies, but from something that cannot die. You were born again through God's living message that continues forever.

1 PETER 1:23 NCV

Staying in Shape

By Mike Chapman

Mom was paying bills when I left the house. "And just where are you off to?" she asked.

"I have a date with a couple of dumbbells," I replied.

"Chris, that's no way to talk about your friends," she admonished.

"Mom, I'm going to work out," I answered, grinning and holding up my gym bag as proof.

"But you just got home from school," she said. "Didn't you work out there?"

"That was basketball practice," I said. "Now I'm going to lift weights," I explained. "See you later."

"If you expect to play on my team you'll get rid of the flab!" Coach Forrest had barked the first day of tryouts. He looked at us and shook his head.

"Frankly, most of you won't be able to take it, and that's fine with me. I only want the men who can."

Right then I decided I was going to be one of those "men" who made the team. When my arms were turning to jelly on the thirty-fourth push-up, I wasn't so sure, but seeing other guys collapsing all around me just convinced me to work harder.

"Is he a coach or a drill sergeant?" Jacob Winslow wheezed as we took a lap around the gym.

"This is good for us," I replied, even though my legs were telling me they were undergoing cruel and unusual punishment.

"Another lap!" the coach yelled.

There were groans, and some of the guys dropped out—but not me.

"I feel like I've been run over by a truck," Jacob complained on the way home. "How about you?"

"I'll live," I replied. "I'm gonna make the team too."

"Good luck," Jacob said. "Are you coming to Bible study tonight?"

"I'm too tired. I want to get to bed early so I'll be ready for tomorrow."

And I was ready the next day—unlike half of the guys who didn't show up for a second day of torture.

"We'll probably cut this number in half," Coach Forrest warned. "One! Two! One! Two! A little more enthusiasm, gentlemen!"

The muscles I had used the day before were screaming in pain, but I pushed myself. I was no quitter. Jacob wasn't either, I guess, because he was there too.

"You should have been in Bible study last night," he told me as we walked home. "We're starting a new project," Jacob went on. "We'll visit people who have visited the church and share Christ with them."

"Good. Guess we'll find out tomorrow—who made the team, I mean."

"Right," Jacob agreed. "Well, see you later. Think about joining us for the witnessing class."

"Yeah, sure," I said. But I didn't think about it. I was too busy thinking about making the team. My muscles may have been sore, but I kind of liked all the pressure I was putting on myself. Besides, I didn't need to attend a class to learn how to witness.

Jacob and I made the team, and I started putting more and more time into working out and getting in shape.

On one particular afternoon, the weight room at the fitness club was almost deserted. *What is this?* I wondered. There were a few of the older guys around, but hardly anybody my age.

"Excuse me," I said to one of the older guys. "Are you using these dumbbells?"

"Help yourself," he replied. He glanced at me. "You're in good shape for someone your age."

"Thanks," I said, feeling a little embarrassed. I took the weights to the nearest incline board.

"You know, Henry," I overheard that guy telling his friend, "I used to be built like that."

"So what happened?" Henry asked.

It was hard not to snicker. The first guy had a big potbelly and was obviously out of shape.

"Oh, I got the flu and then I got weak, and the weaker I got the less I felt like working out," the first man explained. "I figured I'd wait until I was feeling strong again."

You get stronger by working out, not waiting until you suddenly feel strong. I felt like telling them that. I was living proof too. I was really weak before Coach Forrest got ahold of me. But the more I worked out, the stronger I got.

I was doing some triceps extensions when Jacob finally showed up. "Can I work in?" he began.

"Okay," I answered. "Of course you'll have to reduce the weight a little."

"Very funny," he replied, starting to use the same weight I had been using. "Hey, you weren't kidding! I can barely budge it!"

I shrugged. "Told you so."

He did his set, then looked at me. "You have really gotten stronger the past couple of months."

"I've been working at it," I said simply. "Pays off."

"We've been missing you at church," he said

"I'm there every Sunday," I reminded him, starting another set.

"Yeah, but I'm talking about at Bible study and other stuff like that," Jacob continued. "You're missing out on most of the activities."

I finished my set. "There's only so much time in a day, you know. Your turn."

"I have a guy I want you to meet, Jacob told me. "He's new in my neighborhood, and he's a fan of yours," Jacob explained. "He's seen you play in a few basketball games. Why don't you come over to my place Saturday afternoon?" Jacob suggested. "We can play basketball, and you can meet Graham."

So I did. I was going to practice shooting baskets anyway, and it didn't really matter where I did it.

"Oh, I forgot to tell you," Jacob whispered when Graham went chasing a runaway ball down the driveway. "I've been inviting Graham to go to church, but he hasn't been too interested. Maybe if you invite him, he'll come."

"Yeah, okay," I agreed.

We played for a while longer; then Jacob's mom called us in for drinks.

"I have to make a phone call," Jacob said suddenly, giving me a look. "Be back in a few minutes."

So this is invite-the-guy-to-church time, I thought, not too thrilled about it. Still, it was no big deal. "What are you doing tomorrow?" I asked.

"Nothing much," Graham replied. "Why?"

"Why don't you go to church with me?" I said.

I guess I expected him to jump at the chance, since he was supposedly a fan of mine. But he didn't. "I don't think so," he answered. "I don't care anything about church. Why do you go?"

That stopped me for a second. Why did I go to church? I had never really thought about it; I just always went. "Well, to worship God," I managed. "I'm a Christian, Graham."

"So what does that mean?" he asked.

"What does it mean?" I repeated. "Well, I—I'm going to Heaven when I die and—" Suddenly my mind went totally blank, and I couldn't think of an answer.

"What if somebody doesn't believe in Heaven?" Graham asked.

There had been a time when I would've know the answer to that, but all I could do was stammer and stumble around until Jacob came back. I couldn't believe what I was hearing then. Jacob told Graham exactly how a person can receive Jesus as Savior.

"Where did you learn all that?" I questioned Jacob after Graham went home.

"In the witnessing class," Jacob explained. "I wish you'd start coming, Chris."

I wanted to tell him that I didn't have time, but I wouldn't let myself. I had as much time as anybody else; I just had to decide how to use it.

I may have been getting physically stronger with those extra workouts, but my Bible study and prayer time had really suffered. I was getting spiritually weaker all the time. My feeble attempt at witnessing to Graham had convinced me how out of shape I was—spiritually speaking, that is.

Give up the basketball team? No, it wasn't necessary to do that. But I sure made some changes in my priorities after that afternoon.

w w j d   p o w e r   s t a t e m e n t

Jesus was up against some rough competition but he stayed strong by staying in touch with his source of strength: God His Father. For us to become stronger as Christians, we too must stay close to the source.

s c r i p t u r e

Finally, let the mighty strength of the Lord make you strong.

EPHESIANS 6:10 CEV

History

By *Julie Durham*

Anxiously, I looked at the clock. Only ten more minutes to freedom. Well, actually, it would be longer than that by the time I finished my sidework.

Since Christmas, I've been waitressing in a restaurant franchise. Thank heavens this is my last week. Actually, I don't dislike waitressing. Last summer, I loved working at a family-owned restaurant. But there's a world of difference between a family restaurant and a franchise.

One difference is the pressure. Most customers don't realize I have to be at their table with water within sixty seconds after they sit down. That can be difficult, especially if I'm detained by another customer.

In a franchise, everything is timed to the second. You have to deliver the meal in so many minutes and check within three minutes to make sure everything is okay. You have to refill drinks; promptly remove empty plates; and encourage dessert at the proper time.

Besides handling at least six tables, we have to prepare desserts, drinks and some of us—me included—work the register. We often have to bus our own tables and clean any messes. Before we can go home, we have to scrub our booths and refill all salt, pepper, ketchup, and sugar dispensers.

We also have to do "sidework." Sometimes it's cleaning freezers or straightening the storage room.

My least favorite is washing the restaurant windows. We also do "prep" work, like cutting pies and scooping butter into 200 little cups. What a pain!

And then there's rolling silverware. I think that's the worst job of all. We have to spread the napkin, place the spoon and fork on top of the knife just right, roll it a certain way, and slip it into a plastic sleeve. And we have to do 200 of these before we can leave!

With all the pressure, it's easy to get upset about little things, and tempers flare. Sometimes walking through the waitress line is like walking through a combat zone. I've had some good chances to share my faith simply because the Lord has helped me keep my temper.

Finally, my shift was over, my sidework done, and I could roll my silver. Angie finished at the same time and joined me. Normally Angie's kind of talkative, but she was quiet for a change. We go to school and church together, so we're pretty good friends. I've discovered if Angie is silent, you know there's a problem.

"Did you get good tips?" I cautiously asked.

"Not really." she sighed. "They're okay, but not nearly enough. I need to either make bigger tips or work more hours."

I was surprised. She's already working eight more hours than I am—and I work too much to keep up with school.

"Why?" I asked.

"I need to start paying for some more things around the house." Angie said tersely, then bit her lips as if to seal them. That was unusual, too. Angie is never secretive.

I noticed her fingers fumbling. Several times, she had to reroll her silver because it was too crooked to pass our manager's inspection. Then she accidentally hit the pile that was accumulating by her elbow. As it fell, the silverware slipped out of the napkins and clattered across the floor.

Usually Angie finds things like that hysterically funny. But this time, she just sat and began sobbing into a napkin.

"Don't worry. I'll help you roll more." I murmured, picking up silverware.

Still crying, she gulped, "Thanks" and started rolling again.

We worked in silence for a minute. Then I decided it was time to get to the heart of Angie's tears.

"I know something's wrong. Why don't you tell me about it?"

She licked a tear off her lip. "Just a rough day, I guess." She tried to smile, but more tears edged over her long black lashes.

"I have a feeling that it's more than that," I countered. "And I think you need to talk about it. After all, what are friends for?"

She hesitated—then dropped her silverware and looked at me.

"Julie, I'm so confused lately."

"About what?" I prompted, placing a knife in the center of a napkin.

"About everything. About life. It just doesn't seem worth living anymore."

I'd heard that those were words a person sometimes used when they were thinking about suicide. But surely not Angie—she was "Miss Perfect"—a great family, a nice home, good grades, a cheerleader, and besides that, a Christian. After all, Christians were never tempted to take their own lives . . . or were they?

"What makes you feel that way," I asked, searching for the right words.

"Everything." She said hopelessly. Then the words rushed together.

"My parents are fighting like crazy—the other night I heard them talking about going to a marriage counselor. Everyone I know whose parents have gone to a marriage counselor end up getting a divorce. If they do, I'll have to help mom support the boys. Julie, if they split up I'll go crazy.

"A lot of their fights are about my brother Jon. He's been taking drugs. Dad wants to make him go to a rehab center. Mom doesn't want to. I'm worried about Jon. He's changing. And Phil's only ten, but he idolizes Jon. I'm afraid he'll follow in Jon's footsteps."

I muttered something real intelligent, like "bummer," but Angie kept talking, almost like she'd forgotten I was there. She stuffed her rolled silver into the sleeve so ferociously that it broke right through the plastic.

"And I don't know what to do about Mike. He's acting really strange . . . I think he's going to break up with me. I just couldn't stand it without Mike. . . ."

She looked at me with pain-filled eyes. "I know it's wrong for a Christian to even think about, but lately I've been wondering if it'd just be easier to end it all—to down some pills and fall asleep forever. I don't know what to do. Everything just seems so . . . hopeless."

Whew! Not exactly the conversation I'd been expecting. I knew the best thing to do was listen, but something in Angie's tone made me realize I needed to say something—that she needed some reassurance. Just talking about her problems in itself, as I'd been learning in a peer counseling class, was a request for help.

Oh, God, I cried silently, *You know I've never dealt with someone who's talking about suicide. What in the world do I do?*

For a minute, it didn't seem like God would answer my plea. But then Angie's last word rang in my mind. *Hopeless.* Maybe that was the key—to help Angie see hope.

Still praying, I spread out another napkin and mechanically plunked a knife on it.

"Angie, sometimes work really stresses me out," I started. "It's hard when the cooks take too long and burn the meal; or your customers gripe, and the manager is yelling; or you get stiffed." I stuck my rolled silver in a bag. "I used to get really upset about things like that. I'd go home with my stomach tied in knots. Then one day, I realized it was really stupid. So what if it took me ninety seconds to get to a table or if someone had to wait a minute for their coffee? An hour later, they would have forgotten all about it. And within a few hours, I realized I'd be at home with it all behind me. When things went wrong, I had to learn to just do my best. And if something went wrong that I couldn't do anything about, I had to tell myself, *In a few hours, this will be history.*

"That helps me cope better. I start to see things in perspective. I realize that the things I'm worrying about at the moment will soon all be resolved—one way or the other. Problems don't hang on endlessly. And often, the things I worry about turn out fine.

"The stuff in your life right now isn't that easy. I know you're going through some difficult problems." I paused, groping for the words. "But maybe things won't turn out as badly as you expect. Maybe a marriage counselor will help your parents do better together. And a rehab center might help Jon conquer his problem. Maybe all the things you're sure will go wrong will go right after all. This time next week, all your worries of today just might be history. Suicide won't do anything to help the problems in your family—it'll just make it worse for everybody else. For your parents, Jon, and Phil. They need you to be a strength in their lives right now."

"I hadn't thought of that," she said. Her face was streaked with mascara rivulets. She wiped it off with a napkin and blew her nose.

We were quiet for a moment, then I added. "Once, Pastor Harris said something that really stuck with me. He said we should never make any serious decisions when we're going through a valley in our lives—especially not the decision to end it all. Valleys don't last forever, Angie. If you just hold on, maybe you'll find a mountaintop on the other side of the valley. Maybe you'll find out there was cause for hope after all."

"Maybe," she contemplated, straightening her silverware stack. "But Julie, I just can't seem to get rid of the thoughts. Sometimes I lie awake at night, so tempted to sneak my mom's sleeping pills. Why can't I shake those thoughts?"

I shrugged. "Look Angie, I'm no spiritual giant, but if there's really spiritual warfare in our lives, like the Bible says, those thoughts might stem from that. Maybe suicide is a temptation, like any other temptation. Maybe Satan's trying to induce you to end it all. Maybe because if you fight it and make it through this, he knows you'll be able to make a big impact for the Lord in someone's life—maybe even in your own family."

"A temptation, huh? I never thought of that before . . . ." The tears had finally stopped. Angie's brow puckered in thought. "So if it's a temptation, then I'd need to face it like any other temptation, huh?"

"Well, I haven't thought much about it," I admitted, "but I bet you're right."

We were quiet again for a few minutes. I didn't know if I'd been any help to Angie, or if she just wrote off my words as a lecture. After a few minutes, she completely changed the subject. We began talking about school, then about the party our youth group is having next Friday night. Finally, I won't have to work and will be able to go to a youth group party again! We speculated about whether or not Matt will ask me to go with him—he's been hanging around me a lot lately.

"I've nearly become a wreck wondering if he's going to ask me to it or not!" I exclaimed. Then, by Angie's reply, I knew that some of my words had sunk in, and that maybe God had been able to use me.

She gave me a mischievous grin as she replied, "Well either way, this time next week, it will be history!"

wwjd power statement

We are not capable of solving all of our problems. There are many things that are out of our control and bigger than we are. But none of them are bigger than God. Fortunately, in a world where our pain can be so deep, our hope is not in ourselves: it is in the God we serve.

scripture

God began doing a good work in you,
and I am sure he will continue it until
it is finished when Jesus Christ comes again.

PHILIPPIANS 1:6 NCV

Overheard in the Locker Room

By Walt Carter

Chad Carter was one guy I couldn't figure out. He was really friendly and everything the first time I went to his church, so we became good buddies right away.

Or so I thought.

We went to the same high school and didn't have any classes together, but I'd still see him in the hall once in a while. That's when his behavior really bothered me.

"Hey, Chad!" I'd yell. "How're you doing?"

He'd just sort of nod and hurry on. At first I figured he was late for class, but nobody's in a hurry all the time—unless it's on purpose.

Chad avoided me in the cafeteria too. I was almost sure of it. I actually saw him duck behind a post in an attempt to keep me from seeing him, or lean over to pick up a non-existent spoon which had supposedly fallen to the floor.

Only once did we spend lunch hour together, and that was at the beginning of the fall semester. I had known him for just a week or two then. The coaches had a noon sports program set up, and anybody who wanted to play flag football could come out. Chad and I decided to try it after we finished lunch one day. It would've been fun, I guess, but I got on a team with some guys who didn't know a thing about football. Chad was on the team, too.

I'll have to admit I got really mad a few times during the game. I had been working on it but still blew up occasionally, and when I blew up I said a lot of things I shouldn't have. But I always cooled off pretty fast.

When the game was over and we went to the locker room to dress, I couldn't find Chad anywhere. It was like he had vanished. From then on, we just hardly ever spent any time together at school.

At church it was just the opposite. We got along great and talked and laughed like the buddies I thought we were.

"I'll meet you for lunch tomorrow," I'd suggest just before leaving church on Sunday.

"Uh, no," he'd answer quickly. "I can't. See you, Rick."

Of course I had a lot of friends at school—most of whom weren't Christians and didn't go to church, much less believe in Jesus—so I didn't usually think about Chad and how weird our relationship was, unless I saw him.

It could be my imagination, I thought, as he conveniently disappeared into a classroom seconds before we would've passed each other in the hall. It was possible that he really had a class in there, after all. Then I glanced at the room number and frowned. It was Miss Fitch's room; she taught sewing and nutrition!

I continued on down the hall but didn't leave the building. There was a janitor's closet next to the library. I stepped inside, leaving the door open just a crack. From there I could see almost the entire corridor, including Miss Fitch's room, but nobody could see me.

I didn't have to wait long. Chad, looking slightly embarrassed, came out of the room and continued on down the hall in the same direction he had been going previously. As far as I was concerned, that was enough evidence. Chad was definitely avoiding me! But why?

Maybe I should've just called him up and asked him, but I would've felt stupid. I decided to try an experiment instead. It might force Chad to tell me; anyway, it was worth a try.

I was waiting when Chad got to school the next day. It was early and I stationed myself at his locker. He saw me when he entered the building and paused momentarily, as if deciding what to do. Then he came toward me. The hall was nearly deserted.

"Hi, Chad!" I called out, smiling.

"Hi, Rick," he replied when he was close enough to speak without raising his voice. He opened his locker, put in some books, and took out a couple others. "I'll see you," he told me, closing the locker. "I have to go to the library and do some reading for a book report." He turned away.

"That's okay," I answered. "I'll go with you."

He seemed very aware that the halls were rapidly filling with other kids. "Anybody can use the library," he said, "but there's no talking allowed."

We started down the hall together, but not really together at all. It was as if Chad was pretending I wasn't with him. He'd answer my questions with a grunt or a nod.

"What'd you do last night?" I asked finally.

"Went to youth group at church," he said, getting the words out as fast as he could.

I was looking at Chad as he spoke—even though he wasn't looking at me—and didn't see Greg Reardon coming down the hall. Of course Greg takes up about the whole hall. He banged right into me, sending books and notes and everything else I had been carrying, crashing to the floor.

"Why don't you look where you're going, you jerk!" I yelled. I said a few other things too, which I won't repeat.

When I got my books and other stuff together, Chad was nowhere around. I didn't find him in the library, either.

As much as I tried, I didn't see Chad for the next couple of days. When I did see him on Friday, he and some other kids from church were together in the quad, talking.

"What's going on?" I asked.

"We are talking about starting an early morning prayer group," one of the girls told me. "So we're going to circulate petitions and everything," she went on, ignoring the looks Chad was giving her. "We even have these signs ready to use to advertise."

"I'll carry a sign." I picked up one that read, "Prayer Group, Tuesday mornings."

"Uh, thanks anyway," Chad said quickly, taking the sign out of my hand. "We-uh-we have all the people we need."

"Okay, then I'll take some flyers," I offered.

The other kids, except for the one girl who was new to our church, had funny expressions on their faces. Chad led me away from the group.

"I don't know exactly how to say this," he began, "but we don't want your help, Rick."

I frowned. "What are you talking about? I go to church. Why shouldn't I help?"

"You can help by leaving us alone," he went on. "Let me explain—"

I began to boil inside when he said that. Apparently I didn't live up to his expectations of what a Christian was supposed to be! That was obviously why he had avoided me like I had a disease!

"Carter, I'm sick of your—"

The principal arrived on the scene at that particular moment, so our conversation was cut short.

It wasn't until I was in fifth period that I started thinking about what Chad had told me. Who'd he think he was, anyway? It wasn't just Chad, either. All those church kids gave me weird looks when I volunteered to carry a sign or pass out flyers.

I swallowed as my anger gave way to puzzlement. Why would they treat another Christian like that? It didn't make sense.

After school I stopped by the boys' locker room to get my gym clothes. I was tying them up in a bundle when some other boys came into the locker room. They went to a locker in an aisle closer to the door, so they didn't even know I was in the room.

"Did you see those church kids trying to get attention for their prayer group?" one voice asked.

"Yeah," the second voice replied. "The principal stopped that pretty fast!"

"I thought I saw Rick Harmon with them," the first voice said.

"No, I think he was just arguing with that Chad kid," the second voice answered. "Imagine Harmon in church!" They both laughed. "He has the worst temper of anybody I know," the first voice went on, "and the worst mouth!"

"You're telling me?" the second voice questioned. "I've seen and heard him in action a couple dozen times—like the other day when Reardon accidentally bumped into him in the hall. Maybe he does go to church; he uses God's name enough!"

The first voice laughed. "Yeah! Let's go."

I sat there for a while after they left. Was that why Chad stayed away from me? Did my reputation embarrass him? And was that why he and the others didn't want me associated with the prayer group?

But I don't swear that much! I told myself. I swallowed. It wasn't true. Of course any would've been too much. And the second something went wrong, I'd express myself, usually using God's name plus a few other choice expressions. *But I always asked the Lord to forgive me afterwards,* I reminded myself.

I had never committed the problem to God, though, or asked Him to control my mouth. Maybe I even refused to admit that it was a problem. Suddenly I knew better.

A guy's locker room may seem like a strange place to pray, but I bowed my head right then and there and surrendered my temper to Him. It was a step in the right direction.

Later I told Chad about what I had done. He was glad, of course, and admitted that he probably hadn't handled the situation the way he should have, avoiding me instead of just telling me. But he was afraid to tell me. I did have a rotten temper. That's past tense. With God's help I'll keep it that way.

w w j d   p o w e r   s t a t e m e n t

There's an old adage that says "you can never not communicate." Your choice of vocabulary says much more than the words themselves. It tells others what kind of person you really are and what you truly value. If you care about what is noble and good, then your speech will reflect it.

s c r i p t u r e

Watch the way you talk. Let nothing
foul or dirty come out of your mouth.
Say only what helps, each word a gift.

EPHESIANS 4:29

My Mind Went Blank

By Alan Cliburn

It was Michelle Marsden's fault. Well, not really, but if she had been sitting up straight I probably never would have done it.

Cheated, I mean.

Okay, so I wasn't ready for the test. I admit that, but I still didn't plan to cheat. I mean, it wasn't as if I told Michelle to lean to the left while she was writing her answers or anything like that. She just did.

Even then I didn't think about copying what she wrote down. I didn't do stuff like that; I was a Christian who knew better. Sure, there had been a time when I wouldn't have given it a second thought. But when I accepted Christ a year ago, I decided to really live for Him, and that meant changing a few things in my life.

Of course this was different. The reason I wasn't ready for the test in the first place was because of church. Well, sort of anyway. I mean somebody had to volunteer to make posters to announce our next youth group activity, and God had given me a fair amount of artistic talent.

"Where's Dan?" I asked when I got to church. He was an even better artist than I was.

"Had to study for a test," Renee Kellogg replied. "He has Mrs. Quinlan for history and her tests are really monsters."

"Yeah, I know," I agreed. "I have her this semester, too. In fact Dan's in my class."

"Then what are you doing here, Aaron?" the youth director wanted to know. "Are you ready for that test?"

"Not really," I admitted. "But I can study when I get home."

The youth pastor got a phone call about then, so Renee, Mark, and I went to work on the posters. Nobody else showed up, so it took until about 9:00 P.M. to finish them all.

I didn't go straight home after we finished the posters either. Renee and Mark said they were going out for a pizza, so I decided to go along. "All that work made me hungry," I explained.

"But if you have that test tomorrow—" Renee began.

"We aren't going to stay at the pizza place all night, are we?" I asked.

"No, in fact the shorter the better," Mark replied. "I want to practice my speech for debate when I get home."

Renee and I talked him into practicing on us while we were eating. It didn't take much persuasion. I guess time just got away from us. It was 11:30 by the time I got home, and I was dead tired.

I planned to get up early and do some last minute studying before school, but that never worked for me. And especially if I had been up later than usual the night before. As it was, I got to school just as the bell rang for first hour.

"Missed you last night," I whispered to Dan as I passed his desk. "We got the posters made, though."

"Guess I'm not as good in history as you are," he replied.

"Let's get started," Mrs. Quinlan began in that take-charge voice of hers.

I was okay until I looked at the first question on the test. She was asking for battle philosophies as well as dates. Battle philosophies? My mind went blank. I glanced over the other questions, looking for an easy one. There were none. Evidently the answers were all in chapter eleven, a chapter I had never actually read.

I checked out the rest of the room. Nearly everybody was busy writing, including Dan. Paul Desmond and I were probably the only ones in the whole class who didn't know what to put down. Paul just shrugged when our eyes met briefly.

Michelle sure has nice handwriting, I thought suddenly. Easy to read, too. Before I knew what was happening, I was reading her answers, then rewriting them on my paper, except I'd change a few words around, of course. My heart was pounding so loud that I was surprised nobody sitting near me heard it, but I kept right on copying her work. Cheating. I couldn't believe that I would do anything like that, but that didn't stop me.

"Time!" Mrs. Quinlan announced as I dotted my final "i."

I sat there like a zombie as she collected the papers and reminded us of our next assignment; it was almost as if I was outside myself looking in, and I didn't like what I saw.

What did you do? I demanded of myself, at once full of guilt and shame. All those arguments which had seemed so logical when I was in the act of copying Michelle's answers fell apart as the full impact of what I had done hit me.

God, forgive me! I prayed silently as I left the building and headed for the spot where some of the church kids met for lunch. I stopped before I got there, though. I didn't feel like being around anybody right then. Besides, I felt sick to my stomach.

So what are you going to do? I wondered. What could I do? There was no way I could un-cheat, after all, and I had already asked to be forgiven.

"Hey, that was pretty clever, Hesterman," a voice began.

I glanced around to see Paul Desmond standing by a tree, hands in his pockets. "What are you talking about?" I asked, frowning.

"I'm not blind," he said. "I saw you eyeballing Michelle's paper during the test."

"Paul—"

"Listen, don't worry," he went on. "I'm keeping my mouth shut. Everything's cool."

"Everything isn't cool," I corrected. "In fact, I'm on my way to tell Mrs. Quinlan what I did right now."

"You're crazy!" he informed me, mouth open. "Why would you do anything stupid like that?"

"Because cheating was stupid," I explained. "I don't know what made me do it, but I'm telling Mrs. Quinlan."

Paul looked at me disgustedly. "I always thought you were weird, but now I'm sure of it. Does this have anything to do with your religion?"

"I'm a Christian, if that's what you mean, and Christians don't go around cheating on tests."

"Yeah, but you did," he reminded me.

"That doesn't mean I'm perfect," I answered. Right now I have to catch Mrs. Quinlan before she leaves for lunch."

"Yeah, you do that," Paul advised, stalking off toward the cafeteria.

Paul didn't seem too impressed by my honesty or the reason for it. Maybe later he'd think it over and be curious about my decision to confess.

There was no way of knowing, of course. I didn't even know what Mrs. Quinlan's reaction would be. There was no doubt in my own mind that I was doing the right thing. I guess a Christian always knows what's right, though, if he's honest with himself and with the Lord.

Of course knowing and doing are two different things.

w w j d   p o w e r   s t a t e m e n t
God's Word says that we will never be tempted beyond what we can bear. You always have access to the power of God to say "no" to temptation.

s c r i p t u r e
Take everything the Master has set out for you,
well-made weapons of the best materials.
And put them to use so you will be able to
stand up to everything the Devil throws your way.

EPHESIANS 6:11

From Tragedy to Triumph

By Cindy Wainwright

The suitcase was lying in the middle of the living room rug when I dashed into the house. Suddenly I forgot all about telling Mom that her brilliant, talented daughter had passed algebra.

It was a black suitcase, old and battered, and the identification tag read "Mrs. Gayle Perkins." Then it gave Aunt Gayle's address in Fairmount.

I put my books down quietly and listened for voices. There were none.

"Mom?" I called out apprehensively. "I-I'm home."

Then a door opened and closed in the hall and Aunt Gayle appeared, a finger to her lips. "Shhh," she whispered, "your mom's resting."

I swallowed. "But Aunt Gayle," I began softly, unable to stop myself, "what's wrong? Mom was okay when I went to school this morning. She was fine."

"It's too early to tell," Aunt Gayle said. "She collapsed right after lunch. Luckily your father was here. He called me."

"Is there anything I can do?" I wanted to know.

"Pray, honey," she answered simply.

Mom was feeling better that night and wanted to get up, but Aunt Gayle and Dad insisted she stay in bed. I had a feeling they knew more than they were telling me. I was fifteen; I had a right to know what was going on. After all, she was my mother. I confronted Dad while Aunt Gayle was doing the dishes.

He looked at me with tired, swollen eyes and suddenly I didn't want to know whatever he knew. He led me into the den and closed the door.

"Only very basic tests have been made so far," he told me. "At the hospital tomorrow—"

"The hospital!" I interrupted. "Daddy—what's wrong?"

"Dr. Reimers believes your mother may have cancer, Bethany."

I was momentarily paralyzed.

"We didn't want to tell you until it was definite," Dad went on. "She'll spend several days in the hospital while tests are conducted."

"But Mom's always been so healthy," I began, swallowing.

"Not all cancer is terminal, honey," Dad reminded me.

"I know," I answered, forcing a smile. "Maybe with surgery she'll be fine."

"That's the spirit," he said. "Now you'd better run help your Aunt Gayle with the dishes.

I nodded as I hurried out of the den. But I didn't go right to the kitchen. I couldn't. Tears filled my eyes and wanted to spill down my cheeks. I had been able to hold them back while I was with Dad, but now I cried silently, so Mom wouldn't hear. I went into the bathroom and washed my face with cold water.

Right there in the bathroom, my face still wet, I asked God to help my mom. At first it was formal, like I always prayed. I had asked Jesus to come into my heart when I was eight, but being a Christian had always been so casual and natural that I took it—and Him—for granted.

In the weeks that followed I grew up a lot. Mom did have cancer, and it was serious; but she wasn't "at death's door," or anything like that. She was able to be up and around, and Aunt Gayle went back home.

My own prayer life became a real source of strength and communication. I could feel the love of God in my life. It brought our whole family closer together.

Several months later, the black suitcase again greeted my return from school. Aunt Gayle was in the kitchen, preparing supper.

"Where's Mom?" I asked cautiously.

"In the hospital, honey," Aunt Gayle replied. "She broke her legs today."

I thought I was ready for anything but the news caught me off guard. I stared at my aunt. "Both of them?"

"I don't understand it, either," she said. "Your father is there now. I'm sure he'll explain everything when he comes home."

Dad looked exhausted when he came in an hour later.

"What is it?" I wanted to know. "How did she break her legs?"

"The cancer has spread to her bones," he said. "She'll be bedridden the rest of her life. We need to pray."

I didn't feel like praying; I felt like crying. But I bowed my head and closed my eyes and listened as

Dad started talking to God. It was a simple prayer. He asked God to be with Mom, of course, and for us to be able to accept whatever happened as His will.

It didn't make sense to me. How could it be God's will for Mom to have cancer? I talked to Dad about it later.

He put an arm around me and shook his head. "I don't pretend to know why things happen the way they do, honey. But I do know that Romans 8:28 says 'And we know that all things work together for good to them that love God, to them who are the called according to His purpose' (KJV). Mom is trusting in the Lord completely. That's all we can do."

I learned to be cheerful around Mom—even when she broke her legs a second time—and most of the time I really felt it. We had a relationship that few of my friends had with their parents.

Mom came to my high school graduation in a wheelchair. She was smiling and radiant, a real testimony to some of my non-Christian classmates who knew of her illness.

I moved right into the college group at church. It wasn't long before I heard about their outreach program, where they'd put on a musical program and then individually talk to members of the audience about Christ. I was all for it until I found out that we would be gone for nearly five days. That stopped me. Mom was growing weaker. I couldn't be away from her for that long.

But when Mom heard about the trip, she wanted to know why I wasn't going. Eventually she got it out of me, and then insisted that I go. I did, and it was one of the most rewarding experiences of my life. Three months passed, and our group went on another evangelical outreach trip. There was no question that I would go.

If this were fiction instead of fact, I suppose Mom would have suddenly begun to improve. But it didn't work out that way at all. As the end of summer approached, she grew much weaker. There were many nights when we thought she was gone.

At the same time, the college group was planning its final trip before the fall semester began. I think everyone at church was surprised when I signed up— Mom had been on the prayer list for weeks. But I knew Mom wanted me to go.

Almost from the beginning it was obvious that this would be the most effective outreach project our group had attempted. It was well planned, we were well trained, and the community was backing us one hundred per cent.

I had said good-bye to Mom Friday before we left, of course, but I didn't realize that it would be for the final time. Halfway through that weekend I received a call from Dad. Mom had died.

Of course it was a blow, I'd be lying if I said otherwise, but I felt peace and serenity inside, too— peace and serenity that only a Christian can have at such a tragic moment. I remained with the church group for the entire weekend, instead of rushing home. I knew I could do nothing at home, but there was much to be done for Christ in the little resort town where we were staying. I had the opportunity to witness to many more kids before the weekend was over.

But the most wonderful thing happened Sunday night. The woman who had opened her home to five of the girls from our church—me included—came to our final musical program. When Stella, the guitar player, spoke to her afterward, that woman asked Jesus to come into her life and save her soul.

"The girl whose mother died has something I want," she told Stella, referring to me.

I had stopped questioning why Mom had to have cancer a long time ago and learned to trust that God is always in control.

w w j d   p o w e r   s t a t e m e n t

When tragedies happen, it's okay to cry. Remember that when Jesus lost friends He loved, He expressed His grief and pain. Sometimes there are no words to take the pain away. But, like Jesus, we are to place our faith solely in God and bring our wounded hearts to Him.

s c r i p t u r e

You're blessed when you feel you've lost what
is most dear to you. Only then can you be
embraced by the One most dear to you.

MATTHEW 5:4

Lessons from a Firefly

By Julie Berens

The sound of laughter drifted through the open window where Jenalyn O'Connor lay on her bed staring at the ceiling. She knew it was her little brother, Bobby, and his friend, D.J., out on a firefly expedition.

"I wish my biggest problem was catching lightning bugs," Jenalyn said to the stuffed tiger at the foot of her bed. "Why does life have to get so hard when you turn fifteen?"

The tiger just stared back at her. *Typical,* Jenalyn thought. *No one has any answers for me—except Mom. She's got my life all mapped out.*

As much as Jenalyn loved her mom, she didn't love her mom's plans for her future.

"I've heard of boys carrying on in their father's footsteps," Jenalyn had told her best friend April just a few days ago, "but not of girls following in their mother's. Just because my mom always wanted to be a nurse doesn't mean I want to be one. She talks about nursing like it's her ministry or something."

"With all the people she helps, I'm sure it is," April had replied. "Anyway, Jena, your mom's not a mind reader. If you don't want to be a nurse, tell her. She'll understand."

Jenalyn wasn't so sure. With a mom and two sisters who were nurses, Jenalyn felt like she'd be a traitor if she said she was more interested in helping out at summer kindergarten camp than working at the hospital. Besides, being a candystriper, becoming an R.N., and working at Providence Hospital was a family tradition. It was planned. It was expected. But it was not what Jenalyn wanted to do with her life. Working at the kindergarten camp for the summer and becoming a teacher was.

In fact, Jenalyn had been helping out at a kindergarten class for a couple of months now as part of a special program at school. Since her last class was study hall, Jenalyn was dismissed early to work with the younger kids.

It was there she'd met Tanika and discovered that by drawing silly pictures she could get the little girl to talk and laugh when no one else could. And then there were Garrett and Simon. They loved the game she invented where she would draw a part of an animal and then add other parts until one of the boys would guess what the animal was. Mrs. Shaw, the kindergarten teacher, had remarked how good she was with the kids.

A knock on the door interrupted her thoughts. Even before the door opened, Jenalyn knew it was her mom leaving for work.

"Everything's set for you to start at the hospital," Mrs. O'Connor said as she came to sit on the corner of Jenalyn's bed. "I even picked up your uniform for you."

Jenalyn couldn't think of anything to say, so she just nodded.

"We're going to have such fun together, Jenalyn," her mom continued. "I'll show you around, and we can have lunch together. It'll be just like when your sisters were candystripers. I know you'll love nursing and helping other people as much as we all do."

"Sure, Mom," Jenalyn said without enthusiasm.

"Anything you need to talk to me about, honey?" Mrs. O'Connor asked, pushing back Jenalyn's bangs. Jenalyn opened her mouth to tell her mom about the kindergarten camp, but when she saw the look in her mom's eyes, she stopped. She didn't want to put out the light of the dream she saw there. "No, Mom," she said, "everything's great."

When her mom left, Jenalyn got off the bed and went to the window. She pulled back her curtain and stared at the stars. "Lord, I don't know what to do," she whispered. "I don't want to disappoint my mom, but I don't even like the thought of being a nurse. Hospitals depress me." She sighed. "I really like helping out at kindergarten—especially with Tanika."

She stared at the small white lights in the sky. "But then there's all that stuff about honoring your parents. My mom has always dreamed her girls would be nurses. Trisha and Betsy are. Am I supposed to, too?" She paused, waiting for an answer. "If I am, could You have one of those stars blink twice for 'yes' and three times for 'no'?" Jenalyn continued to stare at the sky, but nothing happened. "I didn't think so."

"Hey, Jena, come on down and count our lightning bugs," Bobby shouted. He and D.J. held up their jars for inspection. The fireflies fluttered about, blinking on and off.

"Not now, Bobby. I'm busy," she called back.

"Bobby, it's late. Time to get ready for bed," Jenalyn heard her mom call from the back deck.

Bobby and D.J. said their good-byes and headed inside. Next, Jenalyn heard the pounding of Bobby's feet on the stairs and then her brother burst into her room.

"You need more light in here," Bobby said as he came to the window with his jar of fireflies. "Good thing I brought these for you." He handed Jenalyn the jar. Its yellow glow brightened the room just a little. "Mom said I need a bath, so will you watch these? She said no glass in the bathroom." He was gone before she could reply.

Jenalyn looked in the jar. Fifteen fireflies. Not bad for a night's work. "Okay, bugs, blink twice for 'yes' and three times for 'no,'" she said with a smile. Her smile disappeared as the light in the jar grew dimmer.

Even with the holes poked in the lid, Jenalyn didn't think the fireflies would survive the night. They weren't meant to be bottled up so Bobby could scare away shadows in his room with "nature's nightlights" as he called them. They were supposed to be flying around outside.

Suddenly the fireflies lit again, and Jenalyn was startled to see the reflection of her face in the glass. It looked like she was caught in the jar with the bugs. As the light in the jar dimmed again, a small light inside of Jenalyn began to burn brighter.

"Being cooped up in this jar isn't why God created you," Jenalyn said. "Just like being cooped up in a hospital doing a job I'd hate isn't why God created me." She wanted to unscrew the jar lid and let the bugs fly out of her open window right now, but she knew that wouldn't be fair to Bobby. She also knew that taking the job as a candy striper at the hospital wouldn't be fair to herself or her mom. She had to follow the light of her own dream, not someone else's.

Cradling the jar of fireflies under her arm, she headed downstairs to talk to her mom. She'd talk to Bobby about letting them go, but right now she wanted to show the lightning bugs to her mom and explain about feeling trapped in a dream that wasn't her own. She'd tell her mom about Tanika and Garrett and Simon too—about how it felt to help other people and the joy it brought her. As she walked, she said a prayer that her mom would understand—about the fireflies, about breaking tradition, about following a new light, about the joy of a dream set free.

<u>w w j d   p o w e r   s t a t e m e n t</u>

Truth is more than just confessing when you have done something wrong. It means being true to the person that God made you to be.

<u>s c r i p t u r e</u>

But when the Spirit of truth comes, he will lead you into all truth. . . . he will speak only what he hears, and he will tell you what is to come.

JOHN 16:13 NCV

Louder Than Words

By Cindy Wainwright

I heard the news about Keren while I was washing out beakers for Mr. Coleman in the science lab after school.

"Come on, Maya, let's go," Gracie Martin said, sticking her head inside the door. "Pew! What's that awful smell?"

"We did an experiment with sulfur today," I replied. "It always smells like this."

"How come you have to clean up?" Gracie wanted to know. Then she nodded knowingly. "Don't tell me— you volunteered. Right?"

"You said not to tell you," I reminded her. "But somebody had to do it, and Mr. Coleman went to a faculty meeting."

"Maya, have you ever wondered what would happen if you didn't do all the things you do?" Gracie asked.

I blushed slightly. "I don't do so much."

"I think people take advantage of you," Gracie went on, "and what do you get out of it anyway?"

"Christians are supposed to help others," I began. "Don't you remember how Jesus washed His disciples' feet?"

"Oh, that reminds me!" Gracie exclaimed. "Keren Duncan's a Christian!"

I stared at Gracie in disbelief. "Keren? But how? When?"

245

"I don't know any of the details," Gracie admitted. "Look, I can't take this smell another second or I'll pass out. I'll wait for you outside."

"Don't bother, I'm not going straight home," I replied. "I have to stop by Mrs. Hamilton's house and do her laundry. Her arthritis is acting up again."

"Maya!"

"See you at church tonight," I said.

"Okay," Gracie agreed, a disgusted look on her face.

Keren Duncan a Christian! I thought as I rinsed out the last few beakers. It was hard to believe. She was one of the most popular girls in school and always seemed to be so self-satisfied.

I didn't know her very well, even though we lived in the same neighborhood and had several classes together. Her friends were members of the student council and that type; mine were less well known around school, people like Gracie who kept out of the spotlight.

"You should invite Keren to come to youth group," someone had suggested to me once. "She may be pretty, but that doesn't change her spiritual condition."

I knew that was true and would've been glad to invite Keren to our youth group—or even share my personal testimony with her—but I couldn't. I was so shy that I barely said anything at all unless I knew the other person really well.

So someone else had to invite Keren. I think Carla Winters finally did, because Keren came several times with her. Carla was so outgoing that she probably kept witnessing to Keren until it sunk in, I decided.

The air was cool and crisp as I hurried toward Mrs. Hamilton's little house. It was just a block from the school and she was always glad to see me. I felt the same way about her.

I hadn't been helping with her laundry and other chores very long. I didn't even realize she was there and needed help until the youth pastor told about this senior citizen in our church who could use some assistance.

"She was a teacher in our Sunday school until her arthritis prevented her from regular attendance," he added. "Any volunteers?"

No one else raised a hand, so I did, keeping it up just long enough for the youth pastor to see it.

I arrived at home from Mrs. Hamilton's just as Mom was fixing dinner. "Maya, would you mind taking a pot of soup over to Mr. Bigelow? He hasn't been well, and his wife is in the hospital."

Keren and her father were getting out of the car when I passed their house on my way to Mr. Bigelow's tiny cottage on the corner.

"Hi, Maya!" Keren sang out.

"Hi," I replied.

"Could I talk to you for a second?" she asked.

"I'll stop on my way back," I promised. "I have to get this soup to Mr. Bigelow while it's hot."

I rang the bell when I reached the cottage, but he didn't answer. "Mr. Bigelow!" I called.

When there was no response, I tried the door. It was unlocked. *Maybe he really is sick,* I thought, suddenly concerned. I opened the door and walked inside. "Mr. Bigelow?"

I heard a muffled groan and then saw him, lying on the living room rug. "Help me!" he whispered hoarsely.

The phone was out of order, so I raced out the front door. Keren and her father were still unloading groceries from their car.

"It's Mr. Bigelow!" I called. "Come quick!"

In a matter of minutes an ambulance had been called and was on its way.

"Thank goodness you were home," I told Keren and her father as the ambulance attendants were loading Mr. Bigelow onto the stretcher. "I don't know what I would've done if you hadn't been."

"But we don't deserve any credit," Keren insisted. "If you hadn't brought that soup over here he could've been there for days without anyone finding him."

"Maybe," I agreed. "Right now I'd better fix something to eat."

Keren frowned. "You mean here? But if Mr. and Mrs. Bigelow are both in the hospital, who—"

I answered her question by pointing at a furry face peeking out from under the couch.

"A kitten!" Keren exclaimed.

"There are four of them," I said. "Not counting the mother cat. And they're probably all hungry."

"Can I help you feed them?" Keren asked.

"Okay," I agreed. "Come on."

We found an ample supply of cat food, and all four kittens—plus their mother—appeared in the doorway at the sound of the can opener.

"I'll put everything away when they're finished," I told Keren. "You can go if you want."

"Not yet," Keren replied. "I have something I want to tell you. Remember I wanted to talk to you later?"

"I almost forgot," I admitted. "With all the excitement, I mean."

Keren smiled. "I wanted you to know that I'm a Christian now."

I nearly told her I already knew, but changed my mind. "That's wonderful, Keren! I'm sure you'll never regret it."

"I'm sure I won't, either," she said.

"I know Carla must be thrilled," I went on.

"Carla?" Keren repeated. "I don't think she knows. She was absent today, and I haven't had a chance to call her."

"But I just assumed that she was the one who led you to the Lord," I explained, frowning slightly.

"Well, she certainly did have a lot to do with it," Keren agreed. "She took me to church and youth group and told me what being a Christian was all about. Your pastor made the steps necessary to accept Jesus very clear."

I nodded. "Then your decision was based on what a lot of people said, not just one."

Keren smiled. "No, it was mostly because of one person, Maya. And it had nothing to do with what she said, because she didn't say anything!"

I shook my head. "I don't know who you mean."

"I mean you!" Keren exclaimed, laughing,

I stared at her, mouth open. "Me? But I—"

"I used to go to Sunday school when I was little," Keren went on. "That was before we moved here. The thing I remembered most about Jesus from the stories we heard was that He helped people and wanted to do things for others. But most of the so-called Christians I knew only cared about themselves."

She obviously wanted to talk, so I remained silent. Besides, I was still in a state of shock.

"When I saw you at youth group that first night, you volunteered to help some old lady with her housework. I thought that was beautiful. I've been watching you a lot since then, Maya, even though you weren't aware of it. You're always doing things for people and never get, or even expect, credit for it!"

"Doing things for other people can be its own reward," I said simply, a little embarrassed.

"Anyway, I wanted what you have, and that's why I asked Jesus to come into my heart last night," Keren told me. "So thank you very much, Maya."

I wanted to speak, but couldn't right then. With that big lump in my throat I could barely smile. Still I knew that Keren got the message.

w w j d   p o w e r   s t a t e m e n t

People are watching you. You are a walking, talking, living, breathing testimony for Jesus every day as you go to school or work or hang out at home.

s c r i p t u r e

A good person gives life to others;
the wise person teaches others how to live.

PROVERBS 11:30 NCV

Worrywart

By Teresa Cleary

Erin Fulton stood in line at the grocery store and glanced at her watch. She sighed. She'd never get to her older sister's house by 3:30. She'd told Betsy she would pick up diapers for four-month-old Nathan, but she hadn't expected it to take so long.

"Hurry up, hurry up, hurry up!" she said under her breath to the lady in front of her who was digging in her purse for a nickel. Erin checked her watch again and moaned. It was already 3:45. Fifteen minutes less to talk to Betsy and there was so much to tell her.

Finally the lady found her nickel and moved through the line. Erin quickly paid for the diapers and hurried out to her bike. She pedaled as fast as she could while holding the diapers in one hand and steering with the other.

Erin parked her bike against the side of Betsy's garage and raced to the back door. Through the window she saw Betsy bouncing Nathan, while a bottle heated on the stove.

"Come on in, Erin!" Betsy called over Nathan's cries. "I have my hands full!"

"Sorry I'm late," Erin said, setting the diapers down on the table. "Hope you weren't worried."

"No," Betsy said with a smile. "I figured you got stuck at school or the lines at the store were horrible, as usual. Besides, you're the worrywart in the family, not me."

Erin had to admit her sister was right. She was notorious for worrying about everything.

251

Before Betsy had gotten married and the family still took vacations together, Erin was always the one who asked Dad if they had enough gas or if he was obeying the speed limit so that they didn't get pulled over. In fact, whenever there was a problem in the family, someone was sure to quip, "Let Erin worry about it."

Erin sat down at the table. "Well, if you'd heard Dad and Mom talking last night, you'd be worried too."

Betsy took the bottle from the stove, tested the milk, and gave it to Nathan. His crying stopped.

"Wish my problems could be solved that fast," Erin sighed.

Betsy sat down next to her sister. "Okay, what's up? What are you worried about now?"

"Dad was talking about work last night and he told Mom they're laying people off in June. One hundred engineers will lose their jobs and he might be one of them."

Erin stood up and paced the kitchen. "If Dad loses his job, we'll probably have to move. That means I'll have to say good-bye to my friends, good-bye to you, Tom, and Nathan, and good-bye to any chance of being captain of the drill team next year."

"You forgot good-bye to the youth group," Betsy said without a smile, but with a twinkle in her eyes.

"It's not funny, Betsy," Erin wailed. "My world is falling apart, and you're joking about it."

"Sorry Erin, but I think you're overreacting." Betsy put Nathan over her shoulder to burp him. "I know there are problems at the factory, but Dad has more seniority than most guys there. Layoffs won't happen until June. That's three months away, and you've already got yourself tied up in knots."

"I can't help it," Erin moaned. "I'm a born worrier. You know that. Whether it's Monday's project, Thursday's tryout, or Friday's test, I start worrying about it ahead of time. That way I'm prepared."

"You gotta stop it, Erin, or you'll end up with an ulcer or warts or something," Betsy told her.

"Warts?"

"Yeah," Betsy laughed. "Worry warts!"

"Real funny," Erin said, her temper flaring, "but tell me you never worry. When you look at all the crime and drugs in the world and then you look at Nathan, tell me you don't worry about him."

Betsy shook her head. "Am I concerned? Yes. Worried? No. Those problems may be bigger than I can handle, but they're not bigger than God."

Betsy put Nathan in his swing and walked over to where her Bible lay on the counter.

"Don't quote me Matthew 6," Erin said. "Dad and Mom do it so much I know the verses by heart."

She recited in a squeaky voice, "Therefore I tell you, do not worry about your life, what you will eat or drink; or about your body, what you will wear. Is not life more important than food, and the body more important than clothes? Look at the birds of the air; they do not sow or reap or store away in barns, and yet your heavenly Father feeds them. Are you not much more valuable than they? Who of you by worrying can add a single hour to his life? . . . Therefore do not worry about tomorrow, for tomorrow will worry about itself (Matthew 6:25-27, 34 NIV.)

"Brilliant, Erin," Betsy said, giving her sister a hug. "You've memorized the verses; now what are you going to do about them?"

"What am I supposed to do?" Erin said, moving away from her sister and flinging her hands into the air.

"I think something like that would be very effective," Betsy replied.

"Like what?" Erin thought her sister must have gone nuts. Betsy threw her hands in the air as dramatically as Erin had. "Give your worries away," she said.

"Yeah, like someone else wants my problems," Erin retorted. She shook her head. She'd come to Betsy for help, and instead she was more frustrated than before.

"Look, I gotta go," she said. "Mom's probably putting dinner on the table, and I don't want her to wor—"

Betsy smiled slightly. "I'll call and tell her you're on your way. Thanks for getting the diapers. Your money is on the counter."

Erin kissed Nathan and stomped out the back door. She hoped the ride home would clear her head, but even the wind rushing by her ears seemed to whisper, "Worry!"

Later that night, Erin sat on her bed with her Bible open. *What am I supposed to do, Lord?* she thought. She smiled as she remembered Betsy's response. "Give your worries away," her sister had told her.

Even though Erin had dismissed that advice, she hadn't forgotten it. In her mind she began to replay all her worries—real and imagined. After she'd thought of everything she could, she clenched her hands into fists like she was actually grabbing all those worries.

Lord, I usually try to handle all my problems on my own, Erin admitted. *I realize now, I can't handle any of them without Your help, so I give them to You.* Erin opened her fists and raised them to heaven.

At first she felt a sense of peace; then almost as quickly as she had sensed her worries disappear, she felt them creeping back into the corners of her mind.

I guess I'm not very good at this yet, Lord, she admitted.

But then another thought pushed back the worries. *Do not worry about tomorrow. . . .*

"All I can do is my best," Erin said aloud to herself. "That's all the Lord wants."

She almost laughed. "And it's not like I have to do this alone. God will be there to help," she said, "because He loves me—Erin Fulton—worry warts and all."

w w j d   p o w e r   s t a t e m e n t

Worry is evidence of a lack of trust. Take all of the things you are worried about today and place them in the hands of the God Who loves you completely. He can be trusted.

s c r i p t u r e

Do not worry about anything, but pray and ask God for everything you need. And when you pray, always give thanks. And God's peace which is so great we cannot understand it, will keep your hearts and minds in Christ Jesus.

PHILIPPIANS 4:6-7 NCV

Additional copies of this book and
other titles in the *WWJD* series
are available from your local bookstore.

WWJD for Kidz

WWJD Pocket Bible

Answers to WWJD

Answers to WWJD Journal

Honor Books
Tulsa, Oklahoma